Invasive Electrophysiology for Beginners

Springer Nature More Media App

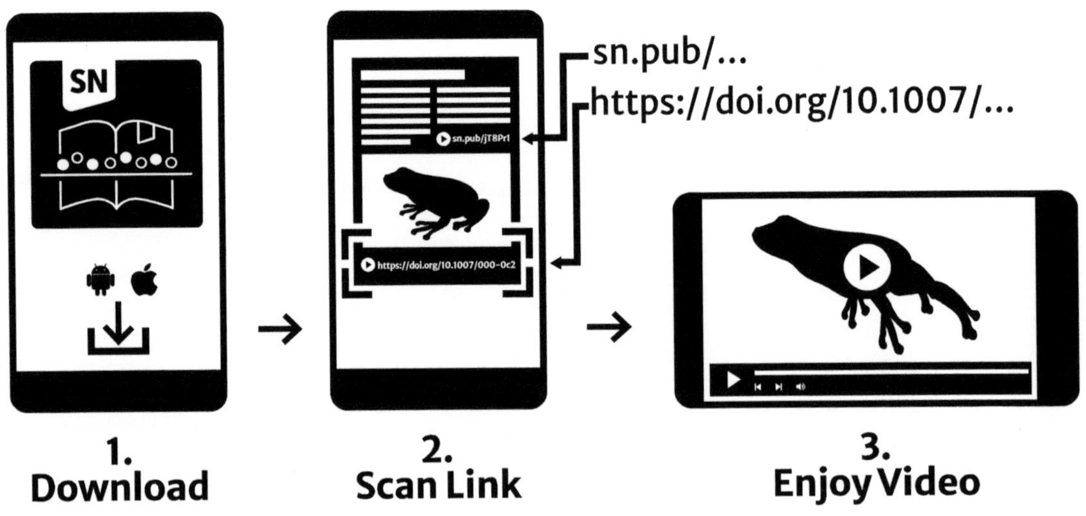

Support: customerservice@springernature.com

Leon Iden · Martin Borlich ·
Philipp Sommer

Editors

Invasive Electrophysiology for Beginners

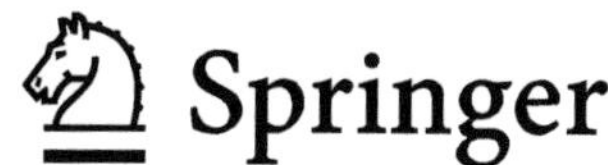

Editors
Leon Iden
Herz- und Gefäßzentrum
Segeberger Kliniken GmbH
Bad Segeberg, Germany

Martin Borlich
Herz- und Gefäßzentrum
Segeberger Kliniken GmbH
Bad Segeberg, Germany

Philipp Sommer
Klinik für Elektrophysiologie/
Rhythmologie, Herz- und
Diabeteszentrum NRW
Bad Oeynhausen, Germany

This work contains media enhancements, which are displayed with a "play" icon. Material in the print book can be viewed on a mobile device by downloading the Springer Nature "More Media" app available in the major app stores. The media enhancements in the online version of the work can be accessed directly by authorized users.

ISBN 978-3-662-70157-7   ISBN 978-3-662-70158-4   (eBook)
https://doi.org/10.1007/978-3-662-70158-4

Foreword

The friendly invitation to write a foreword for a textbook on cardiac arrhythmias elicited two feelings in me: on the one hand, the feeling of aging, because usually only "older semesters" receive such an invitation, and on the other hand—and connected with it—the realization that over the years, I have somewhat lost the proximity to direct application. Essentially, both are correct, albeit somewhat painful. However, I am very happy to fulfill the editors' request to give the book a hopefully appropriate classification and correct perspective with a foreword.

Interventional electrophysiology has undergone an outstanding development over the last (at least) 40 years and, like hardly any other field in medicine, has promoted the most important patient values, a better and/or longer life, in an incredible way. The interventional and thus in many cases also curative treatment of people with highly symptomatic and sometimes even life-threatening cardiac arrhythmias is indeed a great achievement of medicine. The "seniors" among the rhythmologists still have a vivid, rather dreadful, memory of the bleak era of antiarrhythmic drug treatment. With the clinical development and establishment of ablation therapy, the foundation for modern interventional rhythmology was laid. In a breathtaking developmental ride, electrophysiologists managed, step by step and with great consistency in the 1980s and 1990s, to overcome a new hurdle in the interventional treatment of cardiac arrhythmias every 2–3 years. From AV node ablation to the successful ablation of accessory pathways, modulation of the AV node, ablation initially of typical and atypical atrial flutter, and also ventricular arrhythmia, this was, even from today's perspective, an almost incredible success story. With the successful treatment of atrial fibrillation, a treatment option for an arrhythmia that is prevalent to an endemic extent was also successfully developed and established.

The present specialist book on interventional therapy for cardiac arrhythmias excellently summarizes the achievements in a current "Perspective 2022." In addition to the important basics of ablation therapy, the different forms of cardiac arrhythmias are presented and addressed in a practical, understandable, and comprehensible manner. The focus of the individual chapters is on the safe and effective treatment through catheter ablation. In doing so, the current state of knowledge on the pathophysiology of arrhythmias is excellently linked with modern interventional therapy options. At this point, special thanks are due to all those who have driven the successful development of interventional electrophysiology through knowledge and conviction, but also through courage and determination. Many of the decisive advances on the way to establishing ablation treatment as standard therapy have been achieved by European electrophysiologists, with significant contributions from German electrophysiology as well—the contributions of this book also bear witness to this. I very much hope that the reading will also serve as an incentive to take on further challenges in the interventional management of cardiac arrhythmias and to develop (even) better solution strategies.

I wish this excellent textbook wide dissemination and recognition and all readers much joy in reading it. Special thanks go to the editors – also for the kind invitation to this foreword.

Gerhard Hindricks

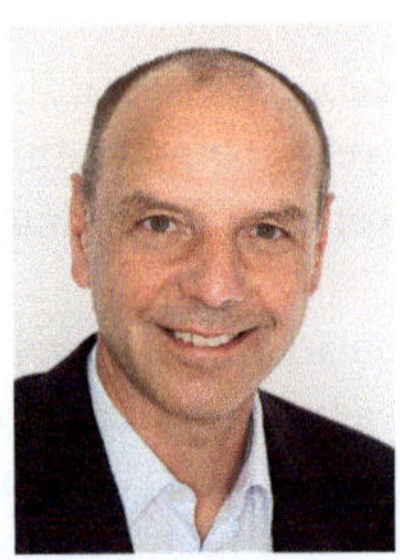

Preface

Dear friends of invasive electrophysiology!

For over 20 years, ablation has been performed regularly and increasingly frequently in many centers. Often with great intensity, but also often in smaller centers with lower case volumes. Getting an idea of what invasive electrophysiology actually means, how it works, and what the treatment goals are is not so easy – we had to realize that there is hardly any suitable literature in the German-speaking world that can provide a good overview for beginners in this field.

Thus, the idea for our book project "Invasive Electrophysiology for Beginners" was born – many great colleagues were immediately ready to contribute articles on the respective topics, and so we can proudly present a practical guide that will be as helpful as a companion in everyday life as it will be as a work for evening reading.

For one thing is important: that electrophysiology is conducted at an excellent level and that we can provide our patients with an optimal treatment strategy based on current knowledge.

And now have fun reading, learning, and puzzling.

Leon Iden　　　　Martin Borlich　　　　Philipp Sommer

PS: We deliberately refrain from differentiating between female and male forms in this book—electrophysiologists of all genders should always feel addressed.

Contents

Abbreviations

Abl	Ablation catheter (short form)
ACT	activated clotting time; activated coagulation time
AH	Interval between atrial signal and His
ALARA	"As low as reasonably achievable"; radiation protection principle
AP	Accessory pathway
AP	anterior-posterior; X-ray image, in which the beam path in relation to the body goes from front (anterior) to back (posterior)
ARVC	"Arrhythmogenic right ventricular cardiomyopathy"; arrhythmogenic right ventricular cardiomyopathy; Synonym: ARVD
AVNRT	AV node reentry tachycardia
AVRT	Atrioventricular reentrant tachycardia
CCW	"counterclockwise"; indication of the propagation direction of typical atrial flutter
CF	"contact force"; contact pressure
CHA2DS2-VASc-Score	Scoring system for calculating the thromboembolic risk in AF
CL	"cycle length", cycle length
CPVT	"Catecholaminergic polymorphic ventricular tachycardia"; catecholaminergic polymorphic ventricular tachycardia
CRT	Cardiac resynchronization therapy
CS	"coronary sinus"; coronary venous sinus
CT	Computed tomography
CT	Crista terminalis
CTI	Cavotricuspid isthmus
CW	"clockwise"; indication of the propagation direction of typical atrial flutter
DAD	"Delayed afterdepolarization"; late afterdepolarization
DGK	German Cardiac Society
DOAC	"Direct oral anticoagulants"; direct oral anticoagulants; Synonym: DOAC, NOAC
EAD	"Early afterdepolarization," early afterdepolarization

EAT	Ectopic atrial tachycardia
ECMO	"Extracorporeal membrane oxygenation"; extracorporeal membrane oxygenation
EF	"Ejection fraction"; left ventricular ejection fraction
EGM	"Electrogram"; Elektrogramm
EKG	Electrocardiogram
EP	Electrophysiology
EPS	Electrophysiological study
FAM	"Fast anatomical mapping"; method for 3D creation of maps in the CARTO system
FAT	Focal atrial tachycardia
FBI	"Fast—broad—irregular" (– tachycardia)
FP	"Fast pathway"; faster conduction pathway
FTI	"Force time integral"; force-time integral
HCM	Hypertrophic cardiomyopathy
HFS	High-frequency current
HPSD	"High power short duration"
HRA	High right atrium
HV	Interval between His and ventricular signal
IABP	Intra-aortic balloon pump
ICD	"Implantable Cardioverter" Defibrillator; implantable cardioverter defibrillator
ICE	"Intracardiac echocardiography"; intracardiac echocardiography
IEGM	"Intracardiac electrogram"; intracardially derived ECG
IVC	Inferior vena cava, V. cava inferior
LAA	"Left atrial appendage"; left atrial appendage
LAMRT	Left atrial macroreentrant tachycardia
LAO	"Left-anterior-oblique" projection direction
LAT	"Local activation time," lokale Aktivierungszeit
LGE	"Late gadolinium enhancement"; methodology in cardiac MRI
LIPV	"Left inferior pulmonary vein"; left inferior pulmonary vein
Long RP	Long interval between R-wave and p-wave
LR-AT	"Localized reentrant atrial tachycardia"; Localized atrial reentry tachycardia
LSI	Lesion Index; Lesionsindex
LSPV	"Left superior pulmonary vein"; left superior pulmonary vein
LV	Left ventricle
LVEDD	Left ventricular end-diastolic diameter
LVOT	"Left ventricular outflow tract"; left ventricular outflow tract
MAZE	Designation of a surgical ablation
MR-AT	"Macroreentrant atrial tachycardia"; atrial macro-reentry tachycardia
MRT	Magnetic resonance imaging

NCC	"Non-coronary cusp"; non-coronary pocket of the aortic sinus
NCX1	Na^+/Ca^{2+} exchanger
NIKM	Non-ischemic cardiomyopathy
PA	posterior-anterior; X-ray image, in which the beam path in relation to the body proceeds from back (posterior) to front (anterior)
PES	Programmed electrical stimulation
PFO	Persistent foramen ovale
PJRT	"Permanent junctional reciprocating tachycardia"; Permanent junctional reentry tachycardia
PPI	Post-pacing interval; post-stimulation interval
PV	Pulmonary vein
PVI	Pulmonary vein isolation
RAA	"Right atrial appendage", right atrial appendage
RAO	"Right-anterior-oblique" projection direction
RF	Radiofrequency
RIPV	"Right inferior pulmonary vein"; right inferior pulmonary vein
RSPV	"Right superior pulmonary vein"; right superior pulmonary vein
RV	Right ventricle
RVOT	"Right ventricular outflow tract"; right ventricular outflow tract
Short RP	Short interval between R-wave and p-wave
SMA	Superior mitral valve annulus
SOP	Standard Operating Procedure; standard procedure
SP	"Slow pathway," slow conduction pathway
SVC	Superior vena cava, V. cava superior
SVT	Supraventricular tachycardia
TA	Tricuspid valve annulus
TCL	"Tachycardia cycle length", cycle length of the tachycardia
TEE	Transesophageal echocardiography
TIA	Transient ischemic attack
TK	Tricuspid valve
TSP	Transseptal puncture
TTE	Transthoracic echocardiography
TTI	"Time to isolation"; time until isolation (of the pulmonary vein)
VBP	"Ventricular Premature Beat"; ventricular extrasystole; Synonym: VES, PVC
VES	Ventricular extrasystole
VHF	Atrial fibrillation
VKA	Vitamin K antagonist
VOP	"Ventricular Overdrive Pacing"; Ventrikuläre Übersteuerungsstimulation (method for differentiating SVT)
VT	Ventricular tachycardia
WOI	"Window of interest"
WPW	Wolff-Parkinson-White (syndrome)

About the Editors

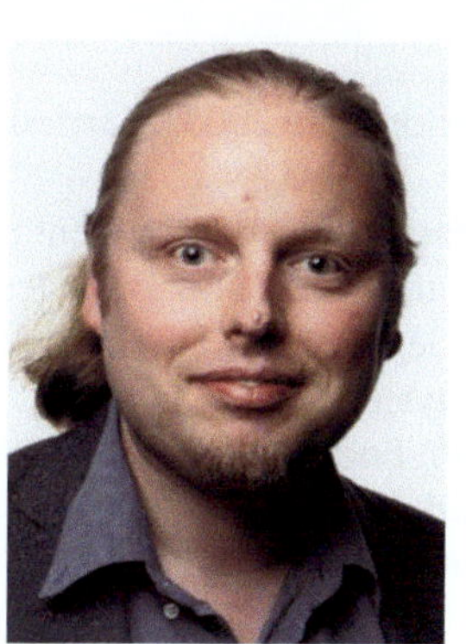

Leon Iden

- Year of birth: 1985. Doctor since 2011. Married, 2 children
- EP since 2012. Training in Segeberg and as a Fellow at the German Heart Center Munich. Since 2016, head of electrophysiology at the Heart and Vascular Center Bad Segeberg.
- What I love about EP: The perfect synthesis of craftsmanship, intellectual work, and teamwork.
- What I don't like about EP: AF redos with isolated veins.
- Besides EP, my favorite activity: Photography.
- What I would like to be able to do: Play a (rhythm) instrument.
- Favorite arrhythmia: Atypical atrial flutter.
- The book is great because it includes the things I would have liked to know from the beginning. Segeberger Kliniken GmbH, Bad Segeberg, Germany, e-mail: leon.iden@segebergerkliniken.de

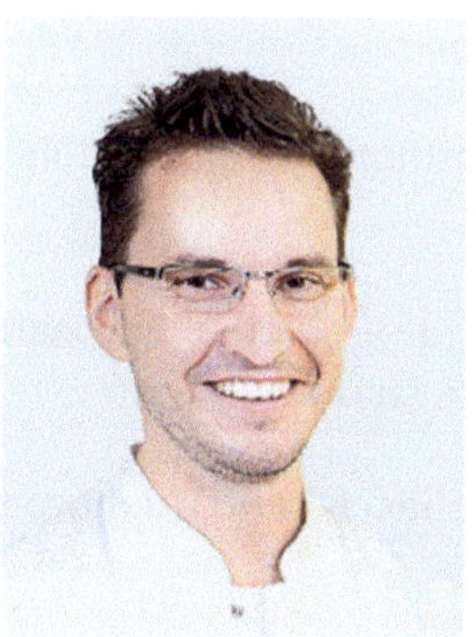

Martin Borlich

- Year of birth: 1986. Doctor since 2013. Married, 2 children
- EP since 2014. Specialist training at the Heart Center of the Segeberger Clinics until 2020, active as a Fellow at the Heart Center Leipzig in 2017.
- Currently Senior Consultant of the Invasive Electrophysiology Section, Heart Center Bad Segeberg
- What I love about EP: The moment when the tachycardia ends under ablation.

- What I don't like about EP: When a VT ablation is planned and high amiodarone levels prevent inducibility.
- Besides EP, my favorite activity: Karate training for my children
- What I would like to be able to do: Fly light aircraft like Cessna or Piper
- Favorite arrhythmia: AVRT
- The book is great because it conveys the basic knowledge of EP in a structured and clear manner. Segeberger Kliniken GmbH, Bad Segeberg, Germany,
  e-mail: martin.borlich@segebergerkliniken.de

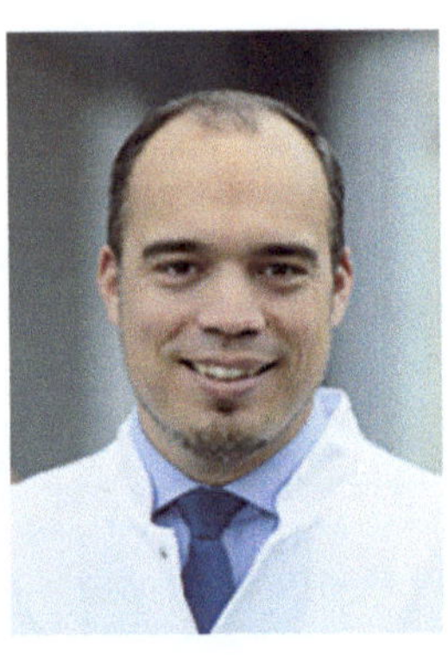

Philipp Sommer
- Year of birth: 1975. Doctor since 2003. Married, 2 children
- EP since 2003. 15 years at the Heart Center Leipzig, since 2018 at the Heart and Diabetes Center NRW in Bad Oeynhausen Director of the Clinic for Electrophysiology.
- What I love about EP: Focused, technology-heavy, and curative work.
- What I don't like about EP: When the technology fails.
- Besides EP, my favorite activities are: Running, golfing.
- What I would like to be able to do: Run more than 10 km. Less than 10 strokes per hole.
- Favorite arrhythmia: Atypical atrial flutter
- The book is great because it is practical and easy to understand. Herz- und Diabeteszentrum NRW, Bad Oeynhausen, Germany,
  e-mail: psommer@hdz-nrw.de

Contributors

Till Althoff Arrhythmia Section, Cardiovascular Institute, Hospital Clínic, University of Barcelona, Barcelona, Spanien

Christian von Bary Klinik für Innere Medizin I – Kardiologie und Pneumologie, Rotkreuzklinikum München, München, Germany

Hendrik Bonnemeier Klinik für Kardiologie, Helios Klinik Cuxhaven, Cuxhaven, Germany

Martin Borlich Herz- und Gefäßzentrum, Segeberger Kliniken GmbH, Bad Segeberg, Germany

Felix Bourier Klinik für Herz- und Kreislauferkrankungen, Deutsches Herzzentrum München, München, Germany

Sonia Busch Medizinische Klinik II, Klinikum Coburg GmbH, Coburg, Germany

Julian K. R. Chun Cardioangiologisches Centrum Bethanien – CCB, Frankfurt a. M., Germany

David Duncker Hannover Herzrhythmus Centrum, Klinik für Kardiologie und Angiologie, Medizinische Hochschule Hannover, Hannover, Germany

Lars Eckardt Klinik für Kardiologie II: Rhythmologie, Universitätsklinikum Münster, Münster, Germany

Heidi Estner Medizinische Klinik und Poliklinik I, LMU Klinikum der Universität München, München, Germany

Melanie Gunawardene Abteilung für Kardiologie und Internistische Intensivmedizin, Asklepios Klinik St. Georg, Hamburg, Germany

Christian-Hendrik Heeger Klinik für Rhythmologie, Universitäres Herzzentrum Lübeck, UKSH Campus Lübeck, Lübeck, Germany

Leon Iden Herz- und Gefäßzentrum, Segeberger Kliniken GmbH, Bad Segeberg, Germany

Marc Kottmaier Zentrum für Herzrhythmusstörungen Augsburg, Neusäß, Germany

Charalampos Kriatselis Klinik für Innere Medizin – Kardiologie, Angiologie, Nephrologie und konservative Intensivmedizin, Vivantes Klinikum Neukölln, Berlin, Germany

Jakob Lüker Abteilung für Elektrophysiologie, Herzzentrum der Uniklinik Köln, Köln, Germany

Andreas Metzner Universitäres Herz- und Gefäßzentrum Hamburg-Eppendorf, Hamburg, Germany

Tilko Reents Klinik für Herz- und Kreislauferkrankungen, Deutsches Herzzentrum München, München, Germany

Laura Rottner Universitäres Herz- und Gefäßzentrum Hamburg-Eppendorf, Hamburg, Germany

Vanessa Sciacca Klinik für Elektrophysiologie/Rhythmologie, Herz- und Diabeteszentrum NRW, Ruhr-Universität Bochum, Bad Oeynhausen, Germany

Dong-In Shin Klinik für Kardiologie, Herzzentrum Niederrhein, Helios Klinikum Krefeld, Krefeld, Germany

Christian Sohns Klinik für Elektrophysiologie/Rhythmologie, Herz- und Diabeteszentrum NRW, Ruhr-Universität Bochum, Bad Oeynhausen, Germany

Philipp Sommer Klinik für Elektrophysiologie und Rhythmologie, Herz- und Diabeteszentrum NRW, Bad Oeynhausen, Germany

Daniel Steven Abteilung für Elektrophysiologie, Herzzentrum der Uniklinik Köln, Köln, Germany

Dierk Thomas Klinik für Kardiologie, Angiologie, Pneumologie, Zentrum für Innere Medizin, Universitätsklinikum Heidelberg, Heidelberg, Germany

Roland R. Tilz Klinik für Rhythmologie, Universitäres Herzzentrum Lübeck, UKSH Campus Lübeck, Lübeck, Germany

Stephan Willems Abteilung für Kardiologie und Internistische Intensivmedizin, Asklepios Klinik St. Georg, Hamburg, Germany

Electrophysiological Mechanisms of Cardiac Arrhythmias

Martin Borlich

1.1 Introduction

Cardiac arrhythmias arise from disturbances in the formation or conduction of impulses, which can also occur in combination. Bradycardic arrhythmias arise from either sinus node dysfunction or impaired conduction in the cardiac conduction system. The fundamental mechanisms for the development of tachycardic arrhythmias are considered to be increased automaticity, triggered activity, and reentry.

Automaticity refers to the ability of cardiomyocytes to spontaneously depolarize and generate impulses without prior stimulation (pacemaker function). Increased automaticity includes the physiologically increased automaticity of cells with primary pacemaker function (e.g., sinus tachycardia during fever) and the abnormally increased automaticity in disturbances and deviations of the regular excitation process (e.g., supraventricular extrasystoles). Triggered activity is the initiation of impulses in cells caused by depolarizing oscillations of the membrane potential, referred to as afterdepolarizations. They occur as a result of preceding action potentials and can be divided into early (EAD—"early afterdepolarization") and late (DAD—"delayed afterdepolarization") afterdepolarizations. These can manifest, for example, as early-onset ventricular extrasystoles and trigger life-threatening ventricular arrhythmias.

In reentry, an anatomical or functional substrate allows sustained circulating excitation. A spreading depolarization wave does not extinguish after the initial tissue activation but reactivates the site of the original excitation. This mechanism is the most common cause of arrhythmias. AV nodal reentrant tachycardia (AVNRT) or atrial flutter, for example, are based on reentry mechanisms.

The diagnosis of the underlying mechanism of a cardiac arrhythmia is significant for the selection of appropriate pharmacological or interventional therapy. Invasive electrophysiological studies provide clues about the mechanism through the spontaneous behavior of the arrhythmia and the response to standardized electrophysiological stimulation maneuvers. A definitive proof of the underlying mechanism is not always successful, as these can occur simultaneously and transition fluidly into one another.

▶ The fundamental mechanisms for the development of tachycardic arrhythmias include **increased automaticity**, **triggered activity**, and **reentry**.

M. Borlich (✉)
Segeberger Kliniken GmbH, Bad Segeberg, Germany
e-mail: martin.borlich@segebergerkliniken.de

1.2 Disturbances of Automaticity

1.2.1 Automaticity and Hierarchy of Pacemaker Function

The cells of the excitation formation and conduction system are hierarchically organized. Their defining characteristic is the ability to depolarize spontaneously, gradually, and diastolically, generating new action potentials upon reaching a threshold. The normal automaticity of the sinoatrials node determines the heart rate under physiological conditions (see Fig. 1.1).

Spontaneous diastolic depolarization, essential for pacemaker function, arises from a net increase in intracellular positive charges during diastole. (Anumonwo and Pandit 2015).

Cells of the sinoatrial node lack specific potassium channels (K^+ inward rectifier I_{K1}), which are involved in stabilizing the resting membrane potential in other cardiomyocytes. Outward potassium currents are carried by delayed rectifier potassium channels (I_K), which are responsible for repolarization. These voltage-dependent potassium channels are inactivated after the maximum diastolic potential, thus enabling early diastolic depolarization. The decline of the outward K^+ current is followed by the activation of inward ion currents. With the hyperpolarization of the cell membrane, specific inward channels, known as "funny channels" (I_f), are opened. They allow an influx of Na^+ and, to a lesser extent, K^+ ions into the cell interior and are primarily responsible for the slow depolarization in this phase 4 of the action potential (DiFrancesco 2010). Additionally, Ca^{2+} channels (I_{CaT}) open and allow an inward current of Ca^{2+} ions. This triggers local calcium releases from the endoplasmic reticulum and accelerates the final part of the diastole. Rising intracellular calcium concentration activates the Na^+/Ca^{2+} exchanger (NCX1), which transports three Na^+ ions into the cell for one Ca^{2+} ion and generates a net influx of positively charged ions into the cell. Upon reaching the threshold potential of approximately -40 mV, a new action potential is generated. This rapid depolarization and thus the beginning of the new action potential in the sinoatrial node is carried by the opening of L-type calcium channels and not by a sodium influx as in the working myocardium. With this depolarization, inward channels (I_f, I_{CaT}, I_{CaL}) close again, and repolarization begins anew (Issa et al. 2018). The interplay of time- and voltage-dependent ion channels, which underlies the pacemaker activity, is referred to as the "membrane clock" and interacts strongly with intracellular Ca^{2+} signaling ("calcium clock") for the joint regulation of the automaticity of pacemaker cells (Carmeliet 2019).

The cells of the sinoatrial node reach the action potential threshold under physiological conditions earlier than subordinate cells in the hierarchy of the specific conduction system. Their slower diastolic depolarization is interrupted by the conducted action potential. This determines the heart rate by the sinoatrial node. Since spontaneous diastolic depolarization is a normal property of these cell groups, it is considered "normal" or physiological automaticity.

The pacing rate of the pacemaker cells of the sinoatrial node is influenced by the maximum diastolic potential, the threshold potential for triggering an action potential, and the rate of diastolic depolarization. The activity of the sympathetic and parasympathetic nervous systems controls this pacing rate. Parasympathetic influences on the sinoatrial node and the AV node slow the rate of impulse generation by increasing K^+ conductance (hyperpolarization). This prolongs the time to reach the threshold potential. The sympathetic nervous system increases the discharge rate of the sinoatrial and AV nodes through β1-adrenergic stimulation by increasing the net influx of ions, resulting in an acceleration of diastolic depolarization. Similarly, medications or electrolyte shifts can influence the heart rate.

1.2.2 Increased Automaticity

Cells that do not belong to the specific excitation formation and conduction system do not spontaneously depolarize under physiological

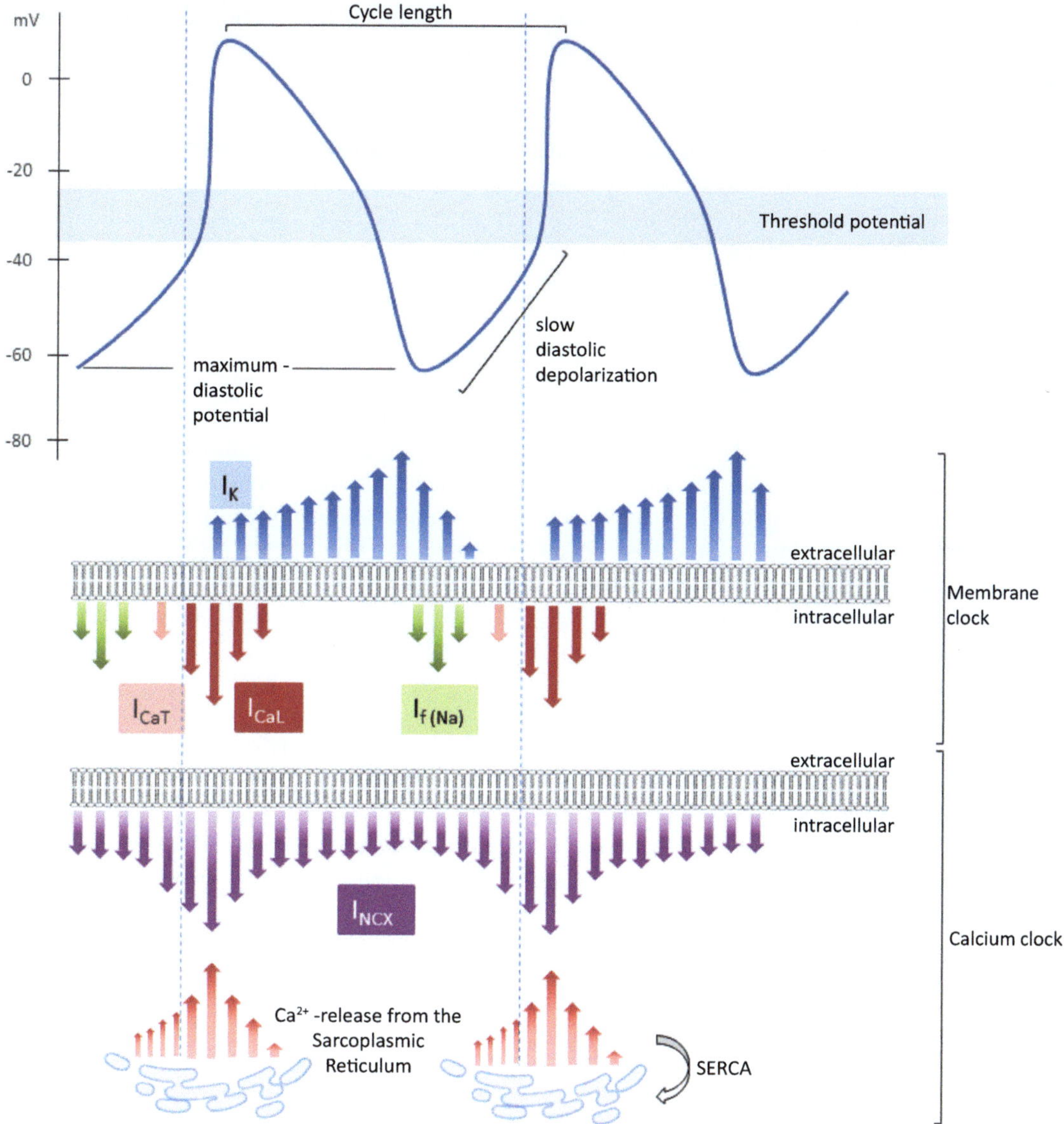

Fig. 1.1 Principle of automaticity in sinus node cells. The course of the membrane potential in sinus node cells (*top*) and the involved ion currents (*middle*) and components of the "calcium clock" are shown. The diastolic depolarization is characteristic of pacemaker cells. The opening of voltage-dependent If channels ("funny channel") and ICaT channels results in slow depolarization through a net influx of positively charged ions. The increase in intracellular Ca^{2+} concentration during diastolic depolarization leads to a local release of Ca^{2+} from the sarcoplasmic reticulum (Ca^{2+}-induced Ca^{2+} release). The sodium-calcium exchanger (NCX1) is also activated, generating a net influx of positively charged ions. Upon reaching the threshold potential, rapid depolarization begins through the opening of L-type calcium channels (ICaL) (no Na^+ influx as in working myocardium). Repolarization occurs through increased conductivity of potassium channels (Ik). The Ca^{2+} pump SERCA transports calcium ions back into the sarcoplasmic reticulum, thereby lowering the intracellular Ca^{2+} concentration (adapted from Murphy C, Lazzara R. Current concepts of anatomy and electrophysiology of the sinus node. J Interv Card Electrophysiol. 2016 Jun;46(1):9-18).

conditions. However, in, for example, ischemic regions of the heart, more positive resting membrane potentials can occur, which can trigger spontaneous depolarization (depolarization-induced automaticity). The difference between physiological and abnormal (mostly increased) automaticity is thus that the excitation process of the cells exhibiting increased activity deviates from their normal course. Not only can a lower resting membrane potential lead to abnormal automaticity, but also altered potassium conductivity or abnormal release of Ca^{2+} from the sarcoplasmic reticulum. This results in a change in the excitation process of the cells, resulting in bradycardia or tachycardia (see Fig. 1.2).

Increased automaticity is not very susceptible to suppression by overstimulation. It can be well treated with medication such as beta-blockers or antiarrhythmics, or specifically terminated by ablation (Zipes et al. 2017). Cardiac arrhythmias based on increased automaticity include, for example, inappropriate sinus tachycardia, focal atrial tachycardia, (supra-)ventricular extrasystoles, or certain (often idiopathic) ventricular tachycardias. Increased automaticity as a cause of arrhythmias is not as common as triggered activity or the reentry mechanism.

▶ Clinical arrhythmias based on the mechanism of increased automaticity include focal atrial tachycardia, inappropriate sinus tachycardia, (supra-)ventricular extrasystoles, and certain forms (often idiopathic) of ventricular tachycardia.

1.3 Triggered Activity

Triggered activity refers to the initiation of impulses in heart muscle cells that occurs as a result of afterdepolarizations following previous action potentials. They occur either early during the repolarization phase of the preceding action potential (early afterdepolarizations = EAD) or late after the completion of repolarization (delayed afterdepolarizations = DAD). If these depolarizing oscillations of the membrane potential are large enough to reach the threshold potential for triggering a new action potential, this is considered triggered (see Fig. 1.3). Single extrasystoles or sustained tachycardias can be the result.

1.3.1 Early Afterdepolarizations (EAD)

Early afterdepolarizations (EAD) are oscillations in the membrane potential that occur

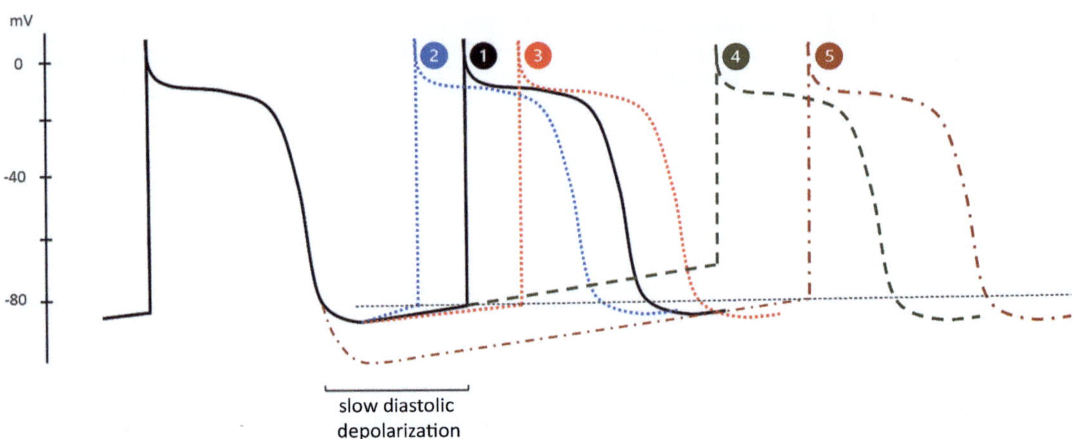

Fig. 1.2 Influence of regular automaticity using the example of a His-Purkinje cell. Two action potentials under physiological conditions are shown (*1*). His-Purkinje cells exhibit spontaneous diastolic depolarization. The cell's impulse rate is increased by accelerating diastolic depolarization (*2*) and is slowed by delaying diastolic depolarization (*3*), increasing the threshold potential (*4*), and starting diastolic depolarization from a more negative resting membrane potential (*5*)

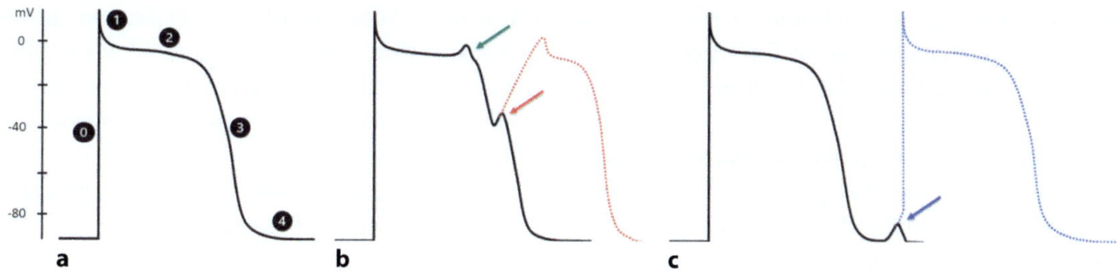

Fig. 1.3 Action potential of the working myocardial cell and types of afterdepolarizations. **a** The action potential can be divided into five phases. Phase 0 describes the rapid depolarization (fast upstroke). Repolarization begins after an initial peak (Phase 1), reaches a plateau (Phase 2), transitions into final repolarization (Phase 3), before the resting membrane potential is re-established (Phase 4). **b** Early afterdepolarizations (EAD). Shown are Phase 2 EAD (*green arrow*) and Phase 3 EAD (*red arrow*). Exemplarily, the triggering of another action potential after an early afterdepolarization in Phase 3 is shown (*red, dashed*). **c** Late afterdepolarization (DAD). Shown is a late afterdepolarization in Phase 4 after complete repolarization. This DAD triggers another action potential (*blue, dashed*)

during repolarization and shift the membrane potential in a depolarizing direction. Any prolongation of the action potential favors EAD. The normal repolarization of myocytes relies on a critical balance between depolarizing inward currents and repolarizing outward currents during the action potential plateau. During Phases 2 and 3 of the action potential, the net membrane current is normally directed outward. Factors that temporarily shift the net current inward during this phase can generate EAD or trigger EAD-related arrhythmias. The cause can be a reduced repolarizing K^+ conductance or an increase in the net inward current (Na^+ or Ca^{2+}). EAD can occur in Phase 2 (plateau phase of the membrane potential) or Phase 3 of repolarization. The upward impulses of the action potential triggered by Phase 2 EAD are mediated exclusively by Ca^{2+} currents (Na^+ channels are inactivated). EAD occurring in Phase 3 arise from more negative membrane potentials. Here, the depolarizing currents can be caused by Na^+ and Ca^{2+} currents (Wit 2018). Regardless of whether the EAD are subthreshold or trigger new action potentials, the temporal and spatial heterogeneity of repolarization can create a substrate prone to arrhythmias. Conditions that prolong the repolarization phase and favor EAD include structural heart diseases with delayed repolarization, electrolyte disturbances (e.g., hypokalemia and hypomagnesemia), bradycardias, congenital

long QT syndromes, or therapy with class IA and III antiarrhythmics (Issa et al. 2018). EAD-mediated triggered activity is a common mechanism for the initiation of polymorphic VT and Torsades de Pointes tachycardias (Weiss et al. 2010). Bradycardias and prolonged QT intervals favor the development of EAD-mediated sustained arrhythmias.

1.3.2 Late Afterdepolarizations (DAD)

Late afterdepolarizations occur in phase 4 of the action potential, i.e., after the completion of repolarization. They can trigger another action potential or occur subthreshold. The cause is Ca^{2+} overloads in the cell plasma, which occur, for example, in myocardial ischemia, digitalis overdose, or increased catecholamine concentrations. Under physiological conditions, Ca^{2+} influx into the cell plasma occurs during the plateau phase (phase 2) of the action potential and activates the release of Ca^{2+} from the sarcoplasmic reticulum, the cell's Ca^{2+} store. Subsequently, Ca^{2+} is actively transported back into the SR via the intracellular transporter SERCA. Ca^{2+} is transported out of the cell via the Na^+/Ca^{2+} exchanger. This periodic change in intracellular Ca^{2+} concentration forms the basis for the orderly contraction of heart muscle cells.

Under pathological conditions, Ca^{2+} overload leads to secondary release of Ca^{2+} from the sarcoplasmic reticulum. The Na^+/Ca^{2+} exchanger (NCX1) again transports Ca^{2+} out of the cell, but the membrane potential becomes more positive due to the transport of Na^+ ions into the cell. If the amplitude of the late afterdepolarization is sufficient to trigger another action potential or triggers a series of action potentials, extrasystoles or sustained tachycardias can occur. Rapid spontaneous or stimulated heart rates favor the development of arrhythmias. Likewise, areas with cells in which subthreshold DADs occur can create a substrate that favors cardiac arrhythmias (Amoni et al. 2021; Wit 2018).

Clinical examples of DAD-induced arrhythmias include focal atrial tachycardias, junctional ectopic tachycardias (JET), and polymorphic catecholaminergic VT (CPVT).

For pharmacological therapy, Ca^{2+} channel blockers, beta-blockers, or class Ib antiarrhythmics such as lidocaine can be used.

If possible, overstimulation can be performed. Arrhythmias based on triggered activity can be effectively terminated with this stimulation maneuver. This is due to the increased activity of the Na^+/K^+-ATPase, which is caused by the increase in intracellular Na^+ concentration as a result of the numerous previous action potentials during overstimulation.

1.4 Reentry

Under physiological conditions, an electrical impulse is generated in the sinoatrial node, followed by a wave of excitation spreading over the myocardium and the specific conduction system, leading to depolarization of the ventricles and thus to an orderly heart action. The excitation wave extinguishes at the end of the cycle because the refractory period of the cells is long compared to the duration of the excitation spread. In reentry tachycardias, there is a circulating excitation. For initiation, a unidirectional conduction block is required, where a part of the circuit does not conduct or is unexcitable (e.g.,

refractory). Subsequently, the excitation moves in a single direction, circling around a non-electrically excitable area, returning to its starting point, and beginning again on the same path.

▶ A unidirectional conduction block is essential for the initiation of reentry.

The tachycardia ends when a part of the conduction pathway is interrupted or temporarily blocked. The reentrant circuit can take on a variety of sizes and shapes and include different types of myocardial cells (e.g., atrial and ventricular cells) (Tse 2016).

Two types of reentry are distinguished (see Fig. 1.4):

1. **Anatomical Reentry**: In this type of reentry, the excitation travels along anatomically predetermined pathways. Centrally, there is an electrically non-excitable area. The size of the excitation circuit is stable, and the frequency of the tachycardia depends on the path length and conduction velocity. Part of the circuit is fully or partially repolarized "excitable gap", thus becoming electrically excitable again and maintaining the tachycardia. The cycle length depends on the wavelength (conduction velocity × effective refractory period) and the excitable gap. Examples of tachycardias with anatomical reentry as the underlying mechanism are atrial flutter, AV reentry tachycardia (AVRT), AV node reentry tachycardia (AVNRT), and scar-associated ventricular tachycardias.

2. **Functional Reentry**: Here, a circulating excitation arises in areas without clearly defined anatomical boundaries. The path of excitation in functional reentry is determined by the different electrophysiological properties (refractoriness, excitability, and conduction velocity) of the tissue through which the electrical excitation circulates. In contrast to anatomical reentry, functional reentry lacks fixed anatomical boundaries, making it variable, unstable, and dynamic in size and location. A partially non-excitable myocardial area or scar tissue constitutes the substrate

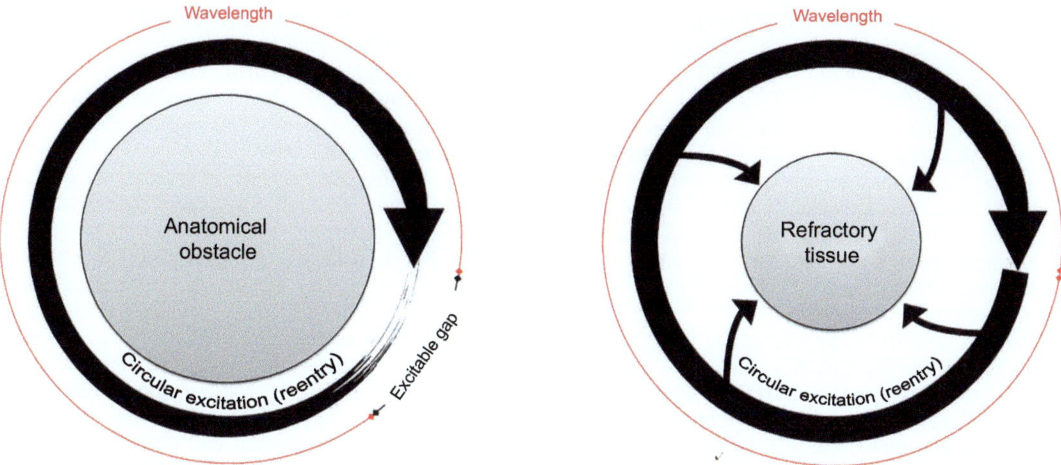

Fig. 1.4 Anatomical reentry (**a**) and functional reentry (**b**). In anatomical reentry, the excitation (*black*) circles around an anatomical, non-conductive obstacle. A part of the circuit is fully or partially excitable ("excitable gap"). In functional reentry, the excitation circles around a core of refractory tissue that is no longer excitable after the initiation of reentry through continuous stimulation. The stimulation of the circulating wavefront is just sufficient to excite the tissue ahead of it, which is in its relative refractory period (partially excitable gap). Here, the "leading circle" concept of functional reentry is illustrated.

for a conduction block. This is referred to as the "leading-circle reentry" concept. The central area of the functional block develops during the initiation of the reentry. Subsequently, it is kept refractory by continuous electrical stimulation during the reentry. There is no fully excitable gap on the circuit as in anatomical reentry. For the sake of completeness, the concept of the "spiral wave" as another biophysical theory of functional reentry should be mentioned (Comtois et al. 2005). Arrhythmias with functional reentry as the underlying mechanism include atrial fibrillation or forms of atypical atrial flutter (multiple reentry circuits) (Leonelli et al. 2017).

Reentry mechanisms are the most common cause of cardiac arrhythmias. Understanding the underlying mechanisms of tachycardia and their visualization through modern 3D mapping systems enables targeted treatment for long-term rhythm control. Pharmacological therapies aim to alter the ratio of wavelength (distance the excitation front travels in its own refractory period) to the path length of the circuit so that the circulating excitation cannot be maintained.

The wavelength changes by influencing the propagation speed or the effective refractory period (Rolf and Möckel 2016). Interventional therapy often targets the critical isthmus of the circuit, i.e., the site of slow conduction. In multiple functional reentries that can maintain atrial fibrillation, for example, the therapy targets the initiatingtriggers, e.g., by isolating the pulmonary veins.

▶ Reentry is a very frequently observed mechanism of arrhythmias in the EP lab. The mechanism can be characterized by certain stimulation maneuvers such as entrainment and usually well visualized and specifically treated using modern 3D mapping systems.

References

Amoni M, Claus P, Dries E, Nagaraju C, De Buck S, Vandenberk B, Willems R (2021) Discrete sites of frequent premature ventricular complexes cluster within the infarct border zone and coincide with high frequency of delayed afterdepolarizations under adrenergic stimulation. Heart Rhythm 18(11):1976–1987. https://doi.org/10.1016/j.hrthm.2021.07.067

Anumonwo JM, Pandit SV (2015) Ionic mechanisms of arrhythmogenesis. Trends Cardiovasc Med 25(6):487–496. https://doi.org/10.1016/j.tcm.2015.01.005

Carmeliet E (2019) Pacemaking in cardiac tissue. From IK2 to a coupled-clock system. Physiol Rep 7(1):e13862. https://doi.org/10.14814/phy2.13862

Comtois P, Kneller J, Nattel S (2005) Of circles and spirals: bridging the gap between the leading circle and spiral wave concepts of cardiac reentry. Europace 7(Suppl 2):10–20. https://doi.org/10.1016/j.eupc.2005.05.011

DiFrancesco D (2010) The role of the funny current in pacemaker activity. Circ Res 106(3):434–446. https://doi.org/10.1161/CIRCRESAHA.109.208041

Issa Z, Miller JM, Zipes DP (2018) Clinical arrhythmology and electrophysiology E-book: a companion to Braunwald's heart disease. Elsevier, pp 51–79

Leonelli F, Bagliani G, Boriani G, Padeletti L (2017) Arrhythmias originating in the atria. Card Electrophysiol Clin 9(3):383–409. https://doi.org/10.1016/j.ccep.2017.05.002

Rolf S, Möckel M (2016) 273e Grundlagen der Elektrophysiologie. In: Suttorp N, Möckel M, Siegmund B, Dietel M (Hrsg) Harrisons Innere Medizin, 19. Aufl. ABW

Tse G (2016) Mechanisms of cardiac arrhythmias. J Arrhythm 32(2):75–81. https://doi.org/10.1016/j.joa.2015.11.003

Weiss JN, Garfinkel A, Karagueuzian HS, Chen PS, Qu Z (2010) Early afterdepolarizations and cardiac arrhythmias. Heart Rhythm 7(12):1891–1899. https://doi.org/10.1016/j.hrthm.2010.09.017

Wit AL (2018) Afterdepolarizations and triggered activity as a mechanism for clinical arrhythmias. Pacing Clin Electrophysiol. https://doi.org/10.1111/pace.13419

Zipes DP, Jalife J, Stevenson WG (2017) Cardiac electrophysiology: from cell to bedside E-book. Elsevier, pp 453–463

Energy Sources for Ablation and Their Mechanisms

Christian-Hendrik Heeger and Roland R. Tilz

2.1 Introduction

The goal of cardiac ablation is the cauterization of the tissue underlying the arrhythmia. Ultimately, the precise application of the respective energy leads to an acute cell death in the target region and ideally to permanent scar formation. Both thermal systems using heat energy (radiofrequency current, laser) or cold energy (cryotherapy) as well as, more recently, non-thermal systems such as irreversible electroporation (so-called pulsed-field ablation) are used. Each energy source has specific properties as well as advantages and disadvantages. A good knowledge of the available methods is essential for learning ablation strategies, improving outcomes, and avoiding complications (Table 2.1).

Supplementary Information The online version contains supplementary material available at https://doi.org/10.1007/978-3-662-65797-3_2. The videos can be accessed individually by clicking the DOI link in the accompanying figure caption or by scanning this link with the SN More Media App.

C.-H. Heeger (✉) · R. R. Tilz
Klinik für Rhythmologie, Universitäres Herzzentrum Lübeck, UKSH Campus Lübeck, Lübeck, Germany
e-mail: christian.heeger@uksh.de

R. R. Tilz
e-mail: roland.tilz@uksh.de

▶ As energy sources for ablation, both thermal systems using heat energy (radiofrequency current, laser) or cold energy (cryotherapy) as well as, more recently, non-thermal systems such as irreversible electroporation (so-called pulsed-field ablation) are used.

2.2 Radiofrequency Current

Of all the methods mentioned, the historically oldest procedure is radiofrequency ablation. This form of energy can be used to treat any cardiac arrhythmia. In this process, thermal tissue damage is generated using high-frequency alternating current (300–750 kHz) (Fig. 2.1).

In the most commonly used unipolar ablation, the catheter tip acts as one electrode and a large surface electrode on the patient's skin as the second electrode. In the rarely used bipolar ablation, a second catheter tip is used instead of the skin electrode.

Lesion formation is complex and depends on various factors such as power, catheter stability, contact force of the catheter on the tissue, size of the ablation electrode, and cooling rate (blood flow and catheter irrigation). The target tissue temperature for this type of ablation is at least 50°C, as permanent cell damage occurs at this temperature. At higher temperatures, the risk of carbonization of the ablation electrode increases, which can lead to an ischemic stroke during ablation in the left atrium. Tissue temperatures >

L. Iden et al. (eds.), *Invasive Electrophysiology for Beginners*, https://doi.org/10.1007/978-3-662-70158-4_2

Table 2.1 Overview of the energy sources used in invasive electrophysiology

Energy Source	Radiofrequency Current	Laser Energy	Cold Energy	Electroporation
Lesion Principle	Thermal	Thermal	Thermal	Non-thermal
Myocardium Specific	No	No	No	Yes
Advantage	Universally applicable (all arrhythmias treatable) Single-shot PVI Very good data	Single-shot PVI Endoscopic ablation	Single-shot PVI Stability Partially reversible lesions (AVNRT) Very good data	Single-shot PVI Myocardium specific, non-thermal, no direct contact needed
Disadvantages	Collateral damage	Collateral damage, only usable for ablation in atrial fibrillation	Collateral damage, only usable for ablation in atrial fibrillation and as single-tip catheter for SVT	So far, little data
Ablation Systems	Single-tip catheter Radiofrequency balloon (Heliostar, Biosense Webster)	Laser balloon (X3, Cardiofocus)	Cryoballoon (AFA-Pro, MDT/POLARx, Boston Scientific) Single-tip (FREEZOR, MDT)	Farapulse (Boston Scientific)

PVI Pulmonary vein isolation

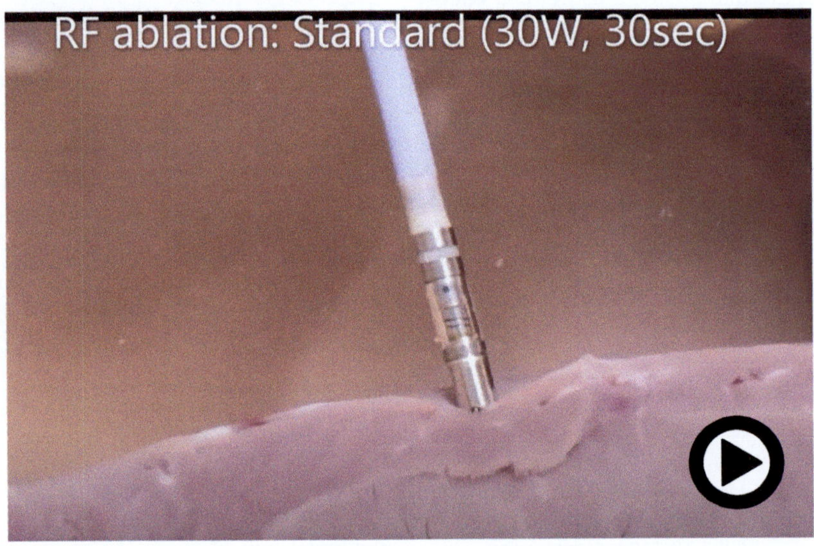

Fig. 2.1 RF ablation (30 W) for 30 s with associated lesion formation on the myocardium in a water bath. A *Qdot* ablation catheter from Biosense Webster was used (https://doi.org/10.1007/000-d2e)

80°C lead to a higher risk of a "steam-pop" phenomenon, where gas explosion in the tissue can cause perforations (Fig. 2.2).

Excessively high tissue temperatures can be avoided by reducing the power delivered, the application time, and the contact force. Today, irrigated and thus actively cooled ablation catheters are mainly used in the left atrium and for ventricular ablations. The advantages of cooled ablation are

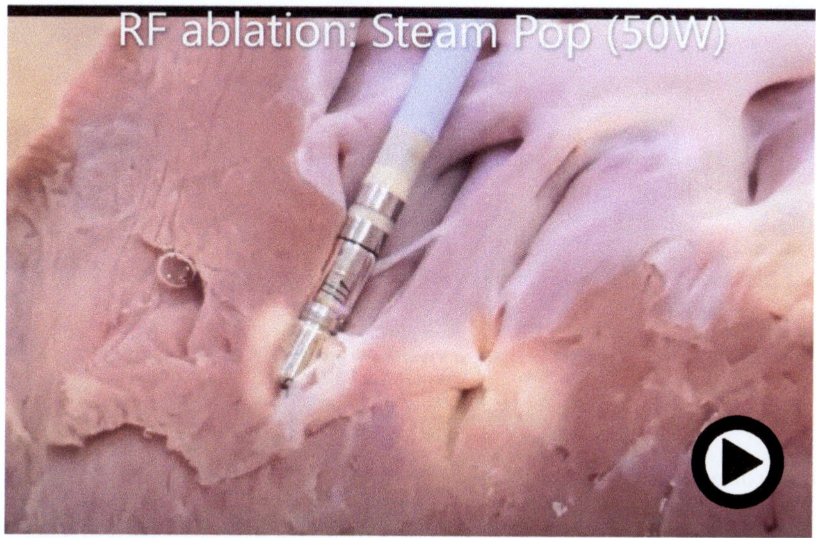

Fig. 2.2 RF ablation (50 W) with intramyocardial gas formation and explosion ("steam pop") due to a tissue temperature > 100°C. Severe complications can result. A *Qdot* ablation catheter from Biosense Webster was used; myocardium in a water bath (https://doi.org/10.1007/000-d2d)

1. the avoidance of high electrode-tissue surface temperatures and thus the reduction of the risk of carbonization ("charring"),
2. the ability to deliver more energy because the energy delivery is not limited by high catheter temperatures.

The delivery of higher energy allows the formation of larger lesions. It is important to emphasize that when power, time, and contact force are specified and not limited by high temperature, cooled lesions result in smaller lesions compared to non-cooled lesions. Additionally, cooled lesions lead to a different lesion shape (drop shape) compared to conventional ablations. Modern ablation catheters have contact force sensors at the catheter tip to precisely determine the contact of the catheter with the tissue, thereby improving lesion formation and increasing safety (Fig. 2.3; Kautzner et al. 2015; Kumar et al. 2012).

In power-controlled ablation with radiofrequency current, an application is typically performed with 30–40 W over a duration of approximately 20–60 seconds. From a physical perspective, energy transfer and lesion formation in radiofrequency current ablation occur in two ways. Initially, due to the high current density in the tissue beneath the catheter tip, there is direct heating of the tissue caused by tissue resistance (so-called resistive heating). Subsequently, the thermal energy is conducted through the tissue, damaging the adjacent tissue portions (so-called conductive heating). Resistive heating is brief and thus leads to relatively uniform heating of the tissue up to irreversible cell death. In contrast, conduction occurs with a time delay and spreads more slowly and indiscriminately through the tissue. Conduction often results in reversible cell damage and edema formation in the outer areas of the lesion, leading to a consequently inhomogeneous lesion. An ideal lesion should affect the entire myocardial wall without damaging the surrounding tissue, which is particularly relevant in the area of the posterior atrial wall due to its anatomical proximity to the esophagus. Cooled radiofrequency ablation initially leads to a rather small, non-transmural zone with high heat development due to tissue resistance (resistance phase), which subsequently spreads passively to deeper tissue layers through heat conduction (conduction phase). The lesion thus formed is drop-shaped, has a relatively broad zone of reversible tissue damage, and extends relatively deep into the tissue.

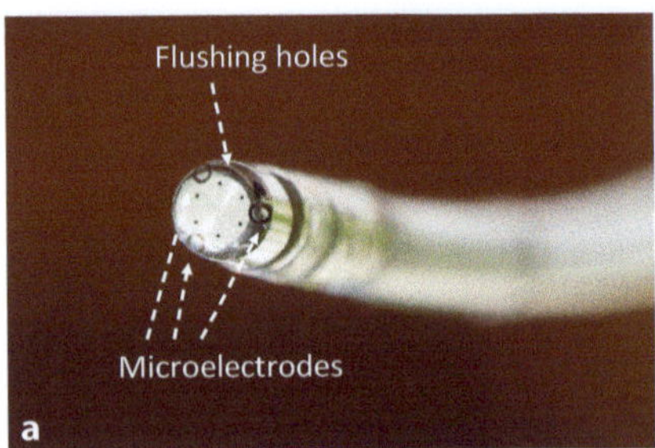

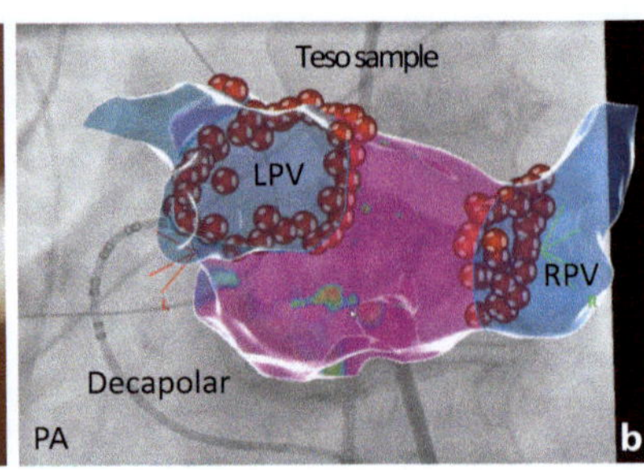

Fig. 2.3 **a** Modern cooled radiofrequency ablation catheter with contact force sensors, microelectrodes, and irrigation holes in the catheter tip. **b** 3D map of a left atrium with circumferential ablation points around the ipsilateral pulmonary veins. *RPV* right pulmonary veins, *LPV* left pulmonary veins, *PA* posterior-anterior

▶ In power-controlled ablation, the power is set fixed, and the tissue temperature is subject to relatively large fluctuations. In temperature-controlled ablation, the temperature is preset, and the power is titrated to achieve this temperature.

2.2.1 Radiofrequency Ablation Using "High Power Short Duration"

With the "High Power Short Duration" (HPSD) ablation, a novel ablation strategy with radiofrequency current has recently become available, offering several potentially significant advantages over conventional RF ablation. In this type of ablation, a very high power (at least 50 W) is applied in a short time (Fig. 2.4).

The lesions thus generated are wider and flatter than the previous lesions achieved with moderate power over a moderate time (e.g., 30 W/30 s). This characteristic makes the HPSD ablation type ideal for the treatment of atrial arrhythmias (e.g., pulmonary vein isolation). Initially, conventional ablation catheters (e.g., Smarttouch, Biosense Webster; FlexAbility/TactiCath, Abbott) were set to a maximum application of 50 W for a few seconds in power-controlled mode without special thermocouples, achieving good results in terms of effectiveness and safety. In recent years, novel ablation catheters such as the DiamondTemp (Medtronic) and the QDOT Micro (Biosense Webster) have become established in clinical practice. These catheters allow precise and rapid temperature measurement with special thermocouples placed in the catheter tip, enabling temperature-controlled ablation (Barkagan et al. 2018). The power is titrated depending on the preset target temperature, improving the safety of the ablation by avoiding excessively high temperatures and "steam pops." With these ablation catheters, it is possible to perform the so-called "very High-Power Short-Duration" (vHP-SD) ablation, which allows power from > 50 up to 90 W (Tilz et al. 2021a; Heeger et al. 2021a).

In contrast to ablation in standard mode with moderate power for a moderate time, vHPSD ablation achieves immediate high heat development during the resistance phase with a relatively large, complete transmurality. The subsequent passive conduction zone, in turn, is relatively small. The resulting lesion is significantly flatter with a narrow zone of reversible tissue damage compared to standard ablation. The flatter vHP-SD lesions are ideally suited for thin tissue, as they avoid high penetration depth and potential damage to surrounding tissue while simultaneously achieving rapid and safe transmurality. The safety and effectiveness of this novel ablation strategy have already been evaluated in clinical studies. Compared to conventional ablation, significantly shorter ablation and procedure times were observed with a high safety profile and effectiveness (Reddy et al. 2019; Tilz et al. 2021a; Heeger et al. 2021a).

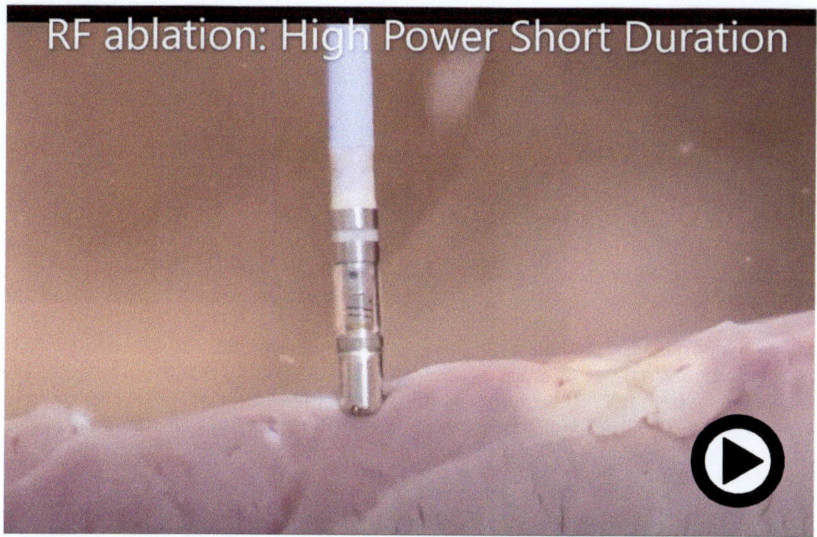

Fig. 2.4 RF ablation with "High Power Short Duration" (HPSD). Short RFA pulses with high power ensure rapid lesion formation. A Qdot ablation catheter from Biosense Webster was used; myocardium in a water bath (https://doi.org/10.1007/000-d2f)

> Ablation using "High-Power Short-Duration" represents the most modern ablation type for radiofrequency current ablation. Modern catheters with precise and tissue-proximal thermocouples are used. A lot of energy is applied in a short time, which is intended to improve both effectiveness and safety.

An important advantage of radiofrequency ablation is its versatility and adaptability. The energy can be adjusted to the requirements and can also be switched from a cooled to an uncooled mode at any time. Unlike balloon catheters (laser balloon, cryoballoon), whose application area is limited to pulmonary vein isolation for the ablation of atrial fibrillation, radiofrequency current-based single-tip catheters can also precisely and safely treat significantly more complex arrhythmias such as atrial tachycardias, AV node reentry tachycardias, and accessory pathways. Currently, this form of energy is the only one used for ventricular ablations (e.g., for the ablation of ventricular tachycardia, ventricular extrasystoles). Since 2021, in addition to single-tip catheters, there has also been an approved radiofrequency-based balloon catheter used for pulmonary vein isolation as a single-shot system. Disadvantages of radiofrequency current ablation include potential thermal damage to surrounding tissue, such as thermal damage to the esophagus, which in extreme cases can lead to the formation of an atrioesophageal fistula with high lethality.

2.3 Laser Energy

High-energy laser light can be used for the ablation of cardiac tissue. Currently, laser energy is used in laser balloon ablation for the isolation of pulmonary veins. In this process, the pulmonary veins are visualized using an endoscope integrated into the balloon, and laser energy with a wavelength of 980 nm is directly applied to the cardiac tissue under visual guidance (Fig. 2.5) (Lemery et al. 2002).

The ablation of the target tissue is achieved through the absorption and heat conversion of the light energy in the cardiac tissue. The laser balloon is filled with deuterium oxide (D_2O) and contrast medium. The D_2O allows the laser energy to pass through without absorption, thereby preventing the balloon from heating up. At the same time, it allows a clear view of the cardiac tissue via a 2F endoscope. The current version of the laser balloon is the so-called

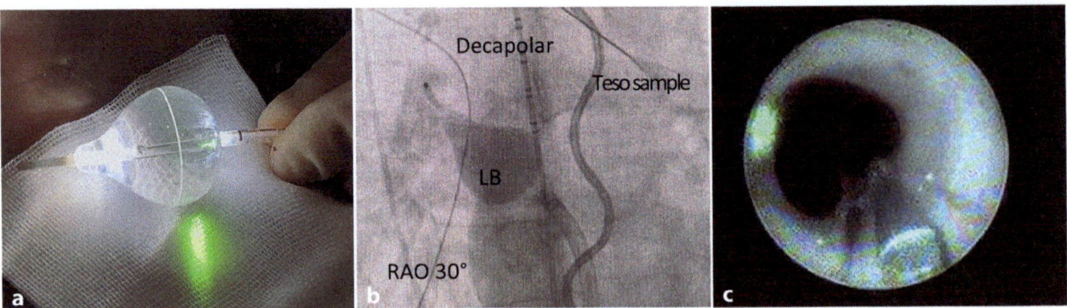

Fig. 2.5 X3 laser balloon ablation system with endoscopic view of the cardiac tissue Cardiofocus. **a** Laser balloon ablation system (X3, Cardiofocus). **b** Fluoroscopic view in RAO 30°. Teso probe: esophageal temperature probe, *LB* laser balloon. **c** Endoscopic view into the right upper pulmonary vein. *Green area*: target area for laser ablation

X3 from the company Cardiofocus. With this system, laser energy can be precisely and automatically used to perform pulmonary vein isolation (Heeger et al. 2020). Advantages of laser balloon ablation include ablation under endoscopic control, the variable balloon (with diameters ranging from 7–42 mm), and its use as a single-shot system for pulmonary vein isolation. However, this also limits the system to this application area. Ablations beyond the sole pulmonary vein isolation are not possible.

2.4 Cryoenergy

Unlike thermal ablation using radiofrequency current or laser, cryoablation involves freezing the target tissue. In this process, liquid nitrous oxide (N_2O) is used, which changes from a liquid to a gaseous state within the catheter system, leading to significant cooling of the catheter. The temperature drop occurs continuously. Temperatures of approximately $-20\,°C$ result in extracellular ice formation in the target tissue, which leads to osmotic shifts within the cell, whereas temperatures from $-40\,°C$ cause intracellular ice formation and irreversible damage to cell organelles. The rewarming of the tissue after the end of the cold application also leads to further tissue damage. By freezing the catheter to the tissue during ablation, a stable position is ensured, and dislocation of the system is prevented. For cryoablation, both single-tip catheters (Freezor, Medtronic) and two balloon catheter systems for performing pulmonary vein isolation (Arctic Front Advance, Medtronic/POLARx, Boston Scientific) are available (Fig. 2.6; Kuck et al. 2016).

Single-tip cryoablation catheters can be used for the ablation of AV nodal reentrant tachycardias (AVNRT) and para-Hisian accessory pathways. The advantage of cryoablation here lies in the fact that lesion formation is reversible if the application is terminated in time, e.g., in the case of total AV block during the ablation of the slow pathway for the treatment of AVNRT, thus avoiding permanent damage. However, this also means that recurrence rates after cryoablations in the context of AVNRT and accessory pathways are higher compared to radiofrequency ablation. Therefore, single-tip cryoablations are rarely used today.

The most important application area of cryoablation currently is cryoballoon-based pulmonary vein isolation (Kuck et al. 2016). A major advantage over point-by-point radiofrequency ablation is the fact that the cryoballoon can be used as a single-shot device for the isolation of the pulmonary veins. Often, a single (usually) 180-second application per pulmonary vein is sufficient to achieve a continuous lesion and permanent isolation of the pulmonary veins (Heeger et al. 2015). The procedure times for pulmonary vein isolation have been reduced to < 60 minutes using this method. Typical

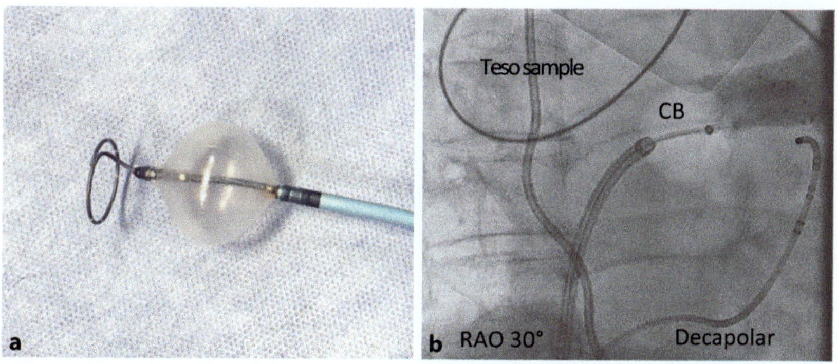

Fig. 2.6 Cryoballoon ablation system. **a** Cryoballoon ablation system. **b** Fluoroscopic view in RAO 30°. Teso probe: esophageal temperature probe, *CB* cryoballoon

complications of radiofrequency ablation such as pericardial tamponade, esophageal lesions, or pulmonary vein stenosis rarely occur. However, the risk of phrenic nerve injury is somewhat increased (Kuck et al. 2016; Heeger et al. 2021b).

2.5 Electroporation

Unlike thermal methods, electroporation uses an electric field. In this process, the cell membranes of cardiac tissue are destabilized by very short and high-energy pulses of up to 2 kilovolts. The electric field used for ablation leads to the formation of irreversible nanopores in the cell membrane, causing the collapse of the membrane potential and inducing apoptosis or necrosis with subsequent scar formation. Depending on the energy used, the changes are initially reversible, but with higher energy, they become irreversible.

A significant feature of electroporation compared to thermal methods is its relative tissue selectivity. Different tissues (myocardium and adjacent tissues such as the esophagus, nerve tissue, fat tissue, blood vessels) have different threshold values of electric field strengths for irreversible electroporation. Since myocardial cells react significantly more sensitively to electrical impulses and have lower threshold values of field strengths for irreversible electroporation than the surrounding tissues, this property is of great importance for catheter ablation. This specific property has already been extensively investigated and demonstrated in animal models (Kaminska et al. 2012). According to this, the cell membranes of myocardial structures are destabilized by field strengths of 400 V/cm, while for cell membranes of non-myocardial tissues, up to 9 times higher field strength is required for irreversible electroporation. Initial studies in humans show similar observations (Fig. 2.7; Reddy et al. 2021).

The advantages of this property are of immense importance for catheter ablation, as adjacent structures such as the esophagus and the phrenic nerve can be injured, especially during catheter ablation of atrial fibrillation. As a relatively new method, there is still not much data available regarding electroporation. Therefore, its effectiveness and safety still need to be proven in clinical practice, but the currently available data is very promising.

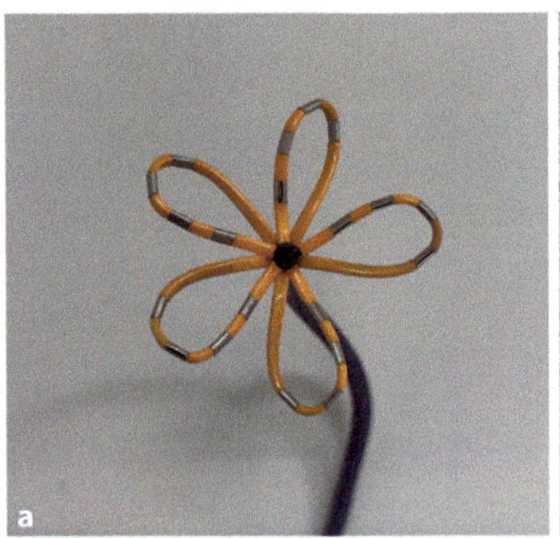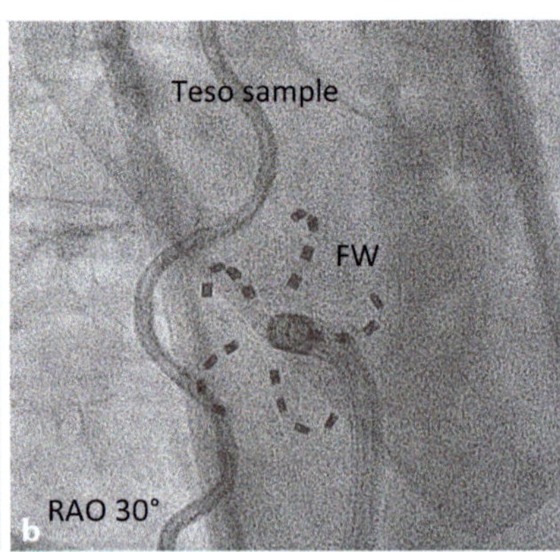

Fig. 2.7 Electroporation (Pulsed-Field Ablation) Ablation System (FARAPULSE). **a** Farapulse Ablation System. **b** Fluoroscopic view in RAO 30°. Teso probe: esophageal temperature probe, *FW* FARAPULSE Ablation System

References

Barkagan M, Contreras-Valdes FM, Leshem E, Buxton AE, Nakagawa H, Anter E (2018) High-power and short-duration ablation for pulmonary vein isolation: Safety, efficacy, and long-term durability. J Cardiovasc Electr 29:1287–1296

Heeger CH, Wissner E, Mathew S, Deiss S, Lemes C, Rillig A, Wohlmuth P, Reissmann B, Tilz RR, Ouyang F, Kuck KH, Metzner A (2015) Once isolated, always isolated? Incidence and characteristics of pulmonary vein reconduction after second-generation cryoballoon-based pulmonary vein isolation. Circ Arrhythm Electrophysiol 8:1088–1094

Heeger C-H, Tiemeyer CM, Phan H-L, Meyer-Saraei R, Fink T, Sciacca V, Liosis S, Brüggemann B, Große N, Fahimi B, Reincke S, Kuck K-H, Ouyang F, Vogler J, Eitel C, Tilz RR (2020) Rapid pulmonary vein isolation utilizing the third-generation laserballoon – The PhoeniX registry. Ijc Hear Vasc 29:100576

Heeger C-H, Popescu SS, Vogler J, Eitel C, Kuck K-H, Tilz RR (2021a) Single very high-power short-duration application for successful ablation of frequent premature ventricular contractions. Europace 24:649–649

Heeger C-H, Sohns C, Pott A, Metzner A, Inaba O, Straube F, Kuniss M, Aryana A, Miyazaki S, Cay S, Ehrlich JR, El-Battrawy I, Martinek M, Saguner AM, Tscholl V, Yalin K, Lyan E, Su W, Papiashvili G, Botros MSN, Gasperetti A, Proietti R, Wissner E, Scherr D, Kamioka M, Makimoto H, Urushida T, Aksu T, Chun JKR, Aytemir K, Jędrzejczyk-Patej E, Kuck K-H, Dahme T, Steven D, Sommer P, Tilz RR (2021b) Phrenic nerve injury during cryoballoon-based pulmonary vein isolation: results of the worldwide YETI registry. Circ Arrhythmia Electrophysiol CIRCEP121010516

Kaminska I, Kotulska M, Stecka A, Saczko J, Drag-Zalesinska M, Wysocka T, Choromanska A, Skolucka N, Nowicki R, Marczak J, Kulbacka J (2012) Electroporation-induced changes in normal immature rat myoblasts (H9C2). Gen Physiol Biophys 31:19–25

Kautzner J, Neuzil P, Lambert H, Peichl P, Petru J, Cihak R, Skoda J, Wichterle D, Wissner E, Yulzari A, Kuck K-H (2015) EFFICAS II: optimization of catheter contact force improves outcome of pulmonary vein isolation for paroxysmal atrial fibrillation. Europace 17:1229–1235

Kuck KH, Brugada J, Furnkranz A, Metzner A, Ouyang F, Chun KR, Elvan A, Arentz T, Bestehorn K, Pocock SJ, Albenque JP, Tondo C, Fire, Investigators ICE (2016) Cryoballoon or radiofrequency ablation for paroxysmal atrial fibrillation. N Engl J Med 374:2235–2245

Kumar S, Morton JB, Lee J, Halloran K, Spence SJ, Gorelik A, Hepworth G, Kistler PM, Kalman JM (2012) Prospective characterization of catheter–tissue contact force at different anatomic sites during antral pulmonary vein isolation. Circ Arrhythmia Electrophysiol 5:1124–1129

Lemery R, Veinot JP, Tang ASL, Green M, Farr N et al (2002) Fiberoptic balloon catheter ablation of pulmonary vein ostia in pigs using photonic energy delivery with diode laser. Pacing Clin Electrophysiol 25:32–36

Reddy VY, Grimaldi M, Potter TD, Vijgen JM, Bulava A, Duytschaever MF, Martinek M, Natale A, Knecht S, Neuzil P, Pürerfellner H (2019) Pulmonary vein isolation with very high power, short duration, temperature-controlled lesions the QDOT-FAST trial. JACC Clin Electrophysiol 5:778–786

Reddy VY, Dukkipati SR, Neuzil P, Anic A, Petru J, Funasako M, Cochet H, Minami K, Breskovic T, Sikiric I, Sediva L, Chovanec M, Koruth J, Jais P (2021) Pulsed field ablation of paroxysmal atrial fibrillation. JACC Clin Electrophysiol 7:614–627

Tilz RR, Sano M, Vogler J, Fink T, Saraei R, Sciacca V, Kirstein B, Phan H-L, Hatahet S, Lopez LD, Traub

A, Eitel C, Schlüter M, Kuck K-H, Heeger C-H (2021a) Very high-power short-duration temperature-controlled ablation versus conventional power-controlled ablation for pulmonary vein isolation: The fast and furious – AF study. Ijc Hear Vasc 35:100847

Tilz RR, Meyer-Saraei R, Eitel C, Fink T, Sciacca V, Lopez LD, Kirstein B, Schlüter M, Vogler J, Kuck K-H, Heeger C-H (2021b) Novel Cryoballoon Ablation System for Single Shot Pulmonary Vein Isolation – The Prospective ICE-AGE-X Study. Circ J 85:12961304

Setup in the EP Lab

Dong-In Shin

The technical, structural, and personnel requirements of a cardiac catheterization laboratory for performing catheter ablations essentially correspond to the same criteria that apply to the performance of coronary angiographies and coronary interventions (Hamm et al. 2001) and should follow the guidelines for setting up and operating cardiac catheterization laboratories of the German Society of Cardiology (Schächinger et al. 2015). Therefore, the following will focus on the specifications of an EP laboratory.

3.1 EP-specific Equipment Points

In addition to the analogies to interventional catheterization laboratories, every electrophysiological laboratory has certain equipment features, which are briefly described here.

3.1.1 EP Workstation (Recording System)

The EP workstation displays, arranges, processes, measures, and stores surface ECGs and intracardiac signals. Standard configurations include two monitors: one continuously displaying the (unprocessed) real-time image and the other used for fixed images, measurements, annotations, and data storage. Both screens must be visible in both the control room and the examination room. Typically, the EP workstation can also display data for hemodynamic monitoring (blood pressure measurement, oxygen saturation). The stimulation channel for intracardiac stimulations is selected via the interface of the EP workstation. There are connections to the stimulator, the 3D mapping system, the RF generator, and the hospital IT-system.

3.1.2 Stimulator

Via the stimulator, stimulation sequences or protocols are set, started, interrupted, or stopped. Typically, the setting for stimulation is done as cycle length (i.e., the interval between two stimuli is set) and not as frequency. In addition to fixed stimulations, various stimulation sequences can be set and partially saved as presets. The stimulator is usually operated in the control room; with some models, it is possible to attach a control unit to the examination table. The stimulator has connections to the workstation, the 3D mapping system, and the catheter connection cable slots. With some 3D mapping systems, it is possible to connect the stimulation

D.-I. Shin (✉)
Klinik für Kardiologie, Herzzentrum Niederrhein,
Helios Klinikum Krefeld, Krefeld, Germany
e-mail: Dong-in.shin@helios-gesundheit.de

© The Author(s), under exclusive license to Springer-Verlag GmbH, DE, part of Springer Nature 2025
L. Iden et al. (eds.), *Invasive Electrophysiology for Beginners*, https://doi.org/10.1007/978-3-662-70158-4_3

path directly to the mapping system and select the stimulation site in the mapping system.

3.1.3 3D Mapping System

A 3D mapping system (or multiple systems) is a fundamental component of an EP laboratory. Due to the abundance of displayed information, two monitors are usually used for display—both in the intervention room and the control room. There are connections to the RF generator and the stimulator. Some 3D mapping systems also offer the possibility of connecting to the hospital information system or RIS, e.g., for integrating cross-sectional imaging. Furthermore, communication with the fluoroscopy unit for integrating image data from the examination is possible (see also Chap. 6 and 20). The operation of the mapping system is done from the control room. Often, procedural support by clinical specialists is offered by the manufacturers. It is advisable to largely master the operation and functionality independently to work autonomously and troubleshoot in case of technical difficulties.

3.1.4 RF Generator

The generator for providing radiofrequency energy is another essential component of the laboratory. Often, the actual generator is located in the intervention room, while a remote control for setting and controlling is installed in the control room. The generator is usually connected to a pump for controlling the irrigated ablation. Various presets (irrigated/non-irrigated ablation, preset power levels) can be saved for different scenarios for easier retrieval. There are connections to both the 3D mapping system and the EP workstation.

3.1.5 Consoles

In addition to the described—typically permanently installed—components, there are various other components of an EP laboratory arranged on mobile consoles. An important example of this is the consoles for cryoablation, which, in addition to the connection options for the corresponding (balloon) catheters, also include a screen for visualizing the ablation and control elements for operation. It is possible to arrange the 3D mapping system on a mobile console as well. This solution can be used in laboratories utilized by various disciplines, but it is not optimal in terms of setup time and susceptibility to errors or the rate of technical defects.

3.2 Requirements for the Room

In principle, the EPU laboratory, consisting of the intervention room and control room (Fig. 3.1), should be located in close proximity to cardiac catheterization laboratories used for coronary interventions. The advantages lie in enabling the shared use of necessary structural units, such as monitoring stations, and at the same time ensuring close proximity to other interventional specialties (cardiology, angiology, radiology, vascular surgery).

If the EPU laboratory is also to be used for the implantation of cardiac devices, the construction planning must take into account the installation of a Class Ib room air system, which, according to existing data and recommendations, is sufficient for the implantation of rhythm devices with small incisions and preparation above the fascia. Embedding in a multidisciplinary intervention center with direct access to an intensive care unit as well as various imaging procedures (especially CT) appears to be a sensible location. Given the complexity of electrophysiological procedures and the high level of concentration required by the examination team, positioning the laboratory near a high-performance coffee machine is advised.

The room size of the EP laboratory should not be less than 40 m^2, as in addition to the necessary equipment of a cardiac catheterization laboratory, additional space units are required for housing an ablation generator, one or more three-dimensional mapping systems, pumps

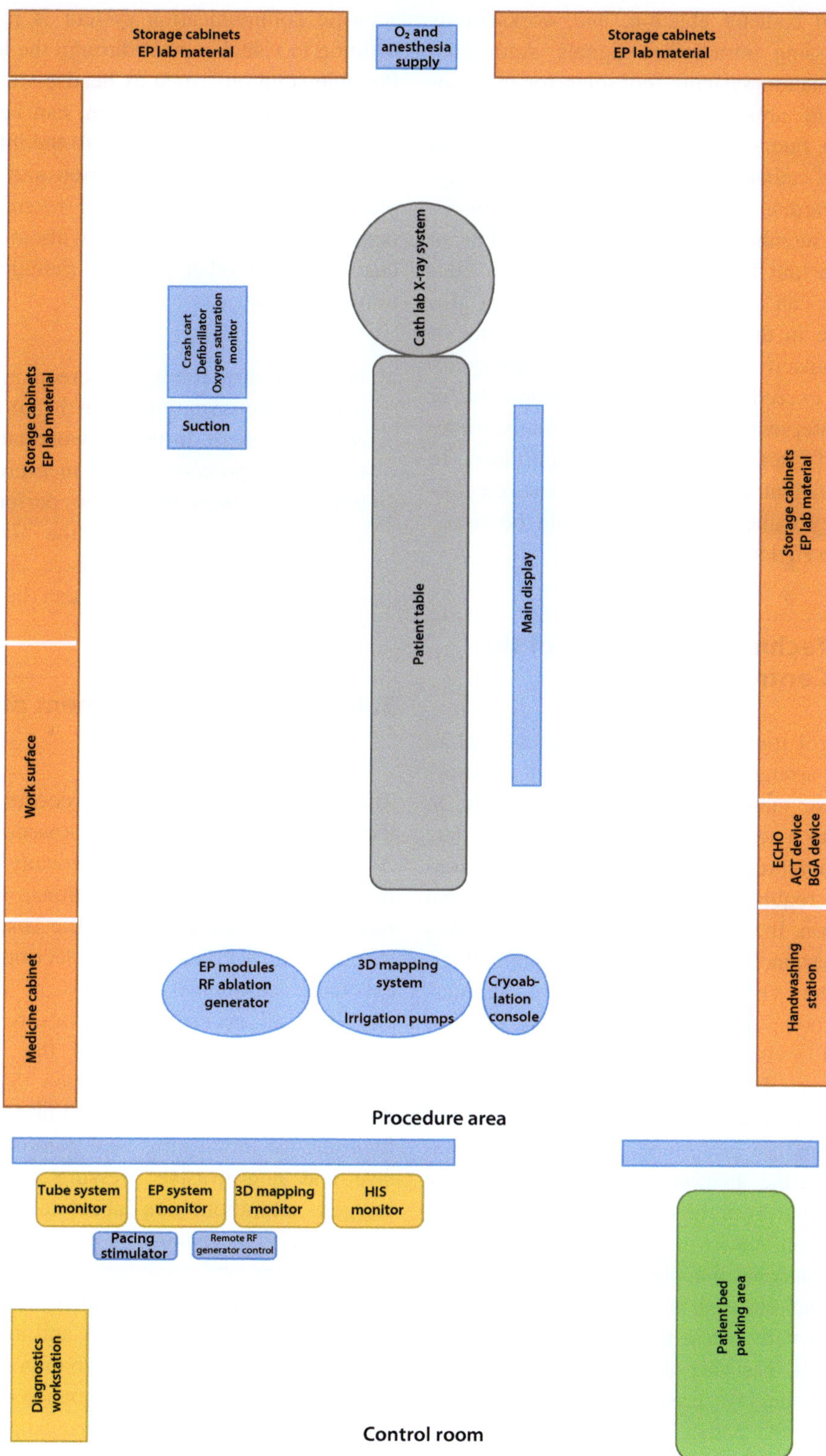

Fig. 3.1 Possible setup of an EP laboratory with the naming and location of the essential functional units for performing an electrophysiological examination

for cooled catheter ablation, and workstations for processing intracardiac signals. Additional mobile ablation systems (consoles for cryo- or pulsed-field ablation, laser ablation systems) must also find sufficient space. Particularly in the case of catheter ablation of ventricular tachycardias, cardiac support systems (IABP, extracorporeal membrane oxygenation) as well as an anesthesia unit for mechanical ventilation after intubation can regularly be used and must also find space in the EP laboratory. The extent of storage capacity for EP materials, which quantitatively exceeds the storage requirements for purely interventional cardiology many times over, is of often underestimated importance. To ensure efficient workflow and hygiene, electrophysiology catheter materials should be stored within the EP laboratory.

3.3 Technical Equipment of the Control Room

The control room must be of sufficient size to allow the arrangement of all necessary monitors for cardiac mapping and catheter ablation. In addition to a screen for transmitting X-ray data from the intervention room, two additional monitors are required for the electrophysiological workstation. In addition to a monitor that makes the intracardiac signals of the electrophysiological catheters visible in real-time from the intervention room, another post-processing monitor is needed to visualize subsequent measurements and analyses. In close proximity is the stimulator, through which manual and programmed stimulations are performed, and a remote control unit for the ablation generator to modify the energy output from the control room. The monitor series continues with separate screens for the three-dimensional mapping systems and should finally conclude with a workstation for report generation with access to the hospital information system, ensuring the retrieval of relevant findings (imaging procedures, ECG recordings, electronic patient records, lab data, etc.). To enable continuous communication between the examination room and the control room, an acoustic communication system is required in addition to visual contact through the lead glass. Portable solutions, such as headsets or a manually operated intercom system, can be used for this purpose. A partition door to the intervention room serves radiation protection and the complete shielding of the control room, allowing personnel in this area to work without the use of lead aprons or other personal radiation protection measures.

▶ In the control room, all screen information from the intervention room is mirrored and converges there. In the EP workstation, additional post-processing and measurements of intracardiac signals can be performed and saved. The stimulator and the 3D mapping system are operated from here, and settings on the ablation generator can be remotely adjusted.

3.4 Technical Equipment of the Procedure Room

The core component of the procedure room is the high-resolution X-ray fluoroscopy system. A monoplane system is technically sufficient for performing catheter ablations, whereas a mobile C-arm does not meet the basic requirements for an EP lab. Further electrophysiological basic equipment includes an emergency cart with all necessary materials required for pericardiocentesis, as well as the option for temporary pacemaker stimulation. Since many catheter ablations are performed under sedation, facilities for monitoring vital parameters (invasive and non-invasive pressure measurement, oxygen saturation) are absolutely necessary. Additionally, there must be a permanent option for suctioning oral secretions and administering oxygen. Furthermore, materials for airway management such as Guedel tubes and materials for (emergency) endotracheal intubation are needed. Finally, the immediate performance of an echocardiography, as well as the immediate determination of a blood gas analysis and the "activated clotting time" (ACT), must be technically ensured. The necessary 3D mapping systems should be permanently installed in the procedure room to ensure the highest possible preservation, especially of the cable material. For the central monitor unit of the cardiography system, if possible, a single large screen should be chosen, whose visual layout with different information units (display of intracardiac signals, 3D mapping display, vital parameters, X-ray data, additional imaging data) can be individually designed depending on the specific catheter ablation and the examiner. Comprehensive radiation protection in the procedure room, in addition to the possibility of a low-frequency fluoroscopy function using different collimation strengths by the cardioangiography system, also includes the provision of a lead protection screen with flexible lamellae, a lead under-table shield, a foot switch shield, as well as the use of lead aprons or lead mats directly on the patient's body. Personal radiation protection should consist of the use of an appropriate all-around apron, a thyroid shield, and suitable radiation protection glasses with side protection.

▶ The design of the procedure room is based on the aspects of complication management, radiation protection, and hygienic requirements.

According to DIN 1946-4 from 2008, the performance of cardiac catheter examinations requires rooms with an air cleanliness class Ib (AWMF 2013). This essentially means that almost germ-free supply air is introduced through the ceiling and usually discharged near the floor. A positive air balance is required, which includes proof of air overflow from inside to outside. Additionally, the DIN regulation also prescribes a minimum height for the supplied air from outside. Regarding the complex hygiene recommendations and the different hygiene regulations of the federal states, it seems absolutely necessary to have a hygiene report prepared in consultation with the construction planners and hospital hygiene before converting or building a new EP lab or planning a change in use of an existing cardiac catheter lab.

3.5   Personnel Equipment

For performing catheter ablations for atrial fibrillation, there are specific recommendations from the German Society of Cardiology, which were formulated in a position paper in 2017. It seems logical and sensible to follow these recommendations for catheter ablations of other arrhythmias, especially for complex cardiac arrhythmias (ventricular arrhythmias, ectopic arrhythmias), as well. According to these recommendations, the continuous presence of two members of the medical and nursing staff is required during a catheter ablation. Among the medical staff, at least one person must have the specialist qualification in cardiology and simultaneously provide proof of the additional qualification in rhythmology "Invasive Electrophysiology." On the side of the assistant staff, the continuous presence of two employees is required, who have sufficient experience in performing electrophysiological examinations and catheter ablations and have also undergone special training in handling analgesia sedation. Since many interventional electrophysiological procedures are performed under sedation (midazolam, propofol), the performing doctors must have sufficient experience in initiating, monitoring, and ending sedation in patients. This particularly includes intensive and emergency medical experience against the background of an existing specialist standard.

3.6   Structural Equipment for Complication Management

In the event of a complication during catheter ablation, in addition to the electrophysiologically trained assistant staff and doctors, other staff members from different specialties must be acutely deployable. This mainly involves the ability to involve specialized personnel from the fields of intensive care medicine, radiology, angiology, neurology, and cardiac surgery in the treatment of the complication. Generally, previously implemented, documented (SOP), and accessible process flows are necessary, which can be followed in the event of a surgical or neurological complication during catheter ablation. The technical and personnel requirements that guarantee the continuous provision of interdisciplinary complication management over 24 hours are essential features of the required structural equipment of an EP lab.

The assurance of all necessary quality criteria for performing catheter ablation in complex cardiac arrhythmias, especially in atrial fibrillation, can be certified through a positive certification process as an atrial fibrillation center by the German Society of Cardiology (Kuck et al. 2017). In a dedicated and extensive criteria catalog, prescribed minimum standards in the areas of technical equipment, personnel training, procedure frequency, complication management, structural conditions of the hospital, and pre- and post-care of treated patients must be demonstrated.

References

AWMF (2013) Anforderungen an Raumlufttechnische Anlagen (RLTA) in medizinischen Einrichtungen. Hyg Med 38(3):367–369

Hamm CW, Bösenberg H, Brennecke R, Daschner F, Dziekan G, Erbel R, für die Kommission Klinische, K. (2001) Leitlinien zur Einrichtung und zum Betreiben von Herzkatheterräumen (1.Neufassung)Herausgegeben vom Vorstand der Deutschen Gesellschaft für Kardiologie – Herz- und Kreislaufforschung Bearbeitet im Auftrag der Kommission für Klinische Kardiologie. Z Kardiol 90(5):367–376. https://doi.org/10.1007/s003920170168

Kuck KH, Böcker D, Chun J, Deneke T, Hindricks G, Hoffmann E, Willems S (2017) Qualitätskriterien zur Durchführung der Katheterablation von Vorhofflimmern. Kardiologe 11(3):161–182. https://doi.org/10.1007/s12181-017-0146-0

Schächinger V, Nef H, Achenbach S, Butter C, Deisenhofer I, Eckardt L, Kelm M (2015) Leitlinie zum Einrichten und Betreiben von Herzkatheterlaboren und Hybridoperationssälen/Hybridlaboren. Kardiologe 9(1):89–123. https://doi.org/10.1007/s12181-014-0631-7

Puncture Techniques in the Catheter Lab

4

David Duncker and Dong-In Shin

4.1 Introduction

For access routes in catheter ablations and other interventions in invasive electrophysiology, various puncture techniques are required. Usually, the venous and arterial femoral vessels are punctured. A large part of electrophysiological procedures consists of left atrial ablations, so transseptal puncture is also one of the basic skills in electrophysiological training. A good knowledge of puncture techniques can help avoid complications.

Supplementary Information The online version contains supplementary material available at https://doi.org/10.1007/978-3-662-65797-3_4. The videos can be accessed individually by clicking the DOI link in the accompanying figure caption or by scanning this link with the SN More Media App.

D. Duncker (✉)
Hannover Herzrhythmus Centrum, Klinik für Kardiologie und Angiologie, Medizinische Hochschule Hannover, Hannover, Germany
e-mail: Duncker.david@mh-hannover.de

D.-I. Shin
Klinik für Kardiologie, Herzzentrum Niederrhein, Helios Klinikum Krefeld, Krefeld, Germany
e-mail: Dong-in.shin@helios-gesundheit.de

4.2 Puncture of the Femoral Vessels

4.2.1 Materials

The puncture of the femoral vessels is performed using the Seldinger technique, which is not described in detail here (Seldinger 2008). A puncture needle (usually 18G) and a wire are required, over which the desired sheath can be introduced. Depending on the planned procedure, single or multiple venous or arterial sheaths of various sizes are needed. A right femoral approach is often preferred due to better steerability. Up to three venous sheaths are usually possible ipsilaterally without problems; for more than three or larger sheaths, it is advisable to puncture the femoral veins bilaterally. The femoral arteries are usually punctured only singularly. An incision of the skin with a scalpel can facilitate a smoother introduction of the sheaths, which is especially advisable for sheaths with a larger diameter.

▶ If performing the puncture with ultrasound support, an ultrasound device with a vascular probe, a sterile cover for the probe, and (sterile) ultrasound gel are additionally required.

A list of materials to be prepared before the puncture is shown in Table 4.1.

"

Table 4.1 Materials for Puncture of the Femoral Vessels

Local Anesthetic	e.g., Mepivacaine 2%
Syringe and Infiltration Needle	
Puncture Needle	Usually 18G
Seldinger Wire	Usually 0.035–0.038″
Sheath	Depending on catheter selection (usually 7F)
For Ultrasound-Guided Puncture	
Ultrasound Device	
Vascular Probe	
Sterile Cover for the Probe	
Sterile and Non-Sterile Ultrasound Gel	

4.2.2 Procedure

The patient should be positioned with a slightly abducted, extended leg in slight external rotation. Adequate local anesthesia of the target areas is administered beforehand. The following describes the venous puncture first and then the arterial puncture of the femoral vessels. Basically, a conventional puncture technique based on anatomical landmarks can be distinguished from an additional ultrasound-guided puncture technique. A depiction of the anatomical relationships in the femoral triangle is shown in Fig. 4.1.

4.2.3 Puncture of the Femoral Vein

The puncture of the femoral vein should be performed 1–2 cm below the inguinal ligament and before the great saphenous vein branches off, before it runs behind the femoral artery. Usually, a puncture needle with a half-filled syringe is used for the venous puncture under slight aspiration. The course of the inguinal ligament can be visualized by palpating the anterior superior iliac spine and the pubic tubercle. Especially in obese patients, the so-called "inguinal fold" is not equivalent to the course of the inguinal ligament. Subsequently, the course of the femoral artery can be palpated by locating the proximal course of the artery with one finger and the distal course with another finger through the femoral triangle. The puncture of the vein can be performed 1–2 cm medial to the artery. The puncture needle can now be advanced at a 30–45° angle parallel to the palpated course of the artery under slight aspiration. As an additional orientation for the alignment of the puncture needle, the fluoroscopic representation of the femoral head can be used, as the target region should be located distal to this bony guide structure.

Aspiration of blood indicates the passage of the vessel wall. If blood is aspirated without resistance, the needle position can be fixed with one hand, the syringe unscrewed, and then a Seldinger wire can be advanced into the vessel.

▶ A pulsatile flow from the puncture needle or already during aspiration is an indication of an arterial mispuncture.

In the event of accidental puncture of the femoral artery, manual compression for 1–3 minutes is recommended before further puncture attempts to prevent the formation of an arteriovenous fistula or a pseudoaneurysm.

In cases of low venous filling pressure, the vein may be compressed by the puncture needle, so aspiration may only be successful when the puncture needle is gently withdrawn. If the puncture attempt was not successful, no further angle changes should be made after advancing the needle to avoid uncontrolled vessel and tissue lacerations in depth; rather, a new puncture attempt should be made after slightly modifying the puncture direction and entry angle.

4.2.4 Puncture of the Femoral Artery

The arterial puncture is usually performed only with the puncture needle. The puncture of the femoral artery should be performed caudal to the inguinal ligament, as the artery runs cranially from this point as the external iliac artery and quickly becomes retroperitoneal, thus preventing

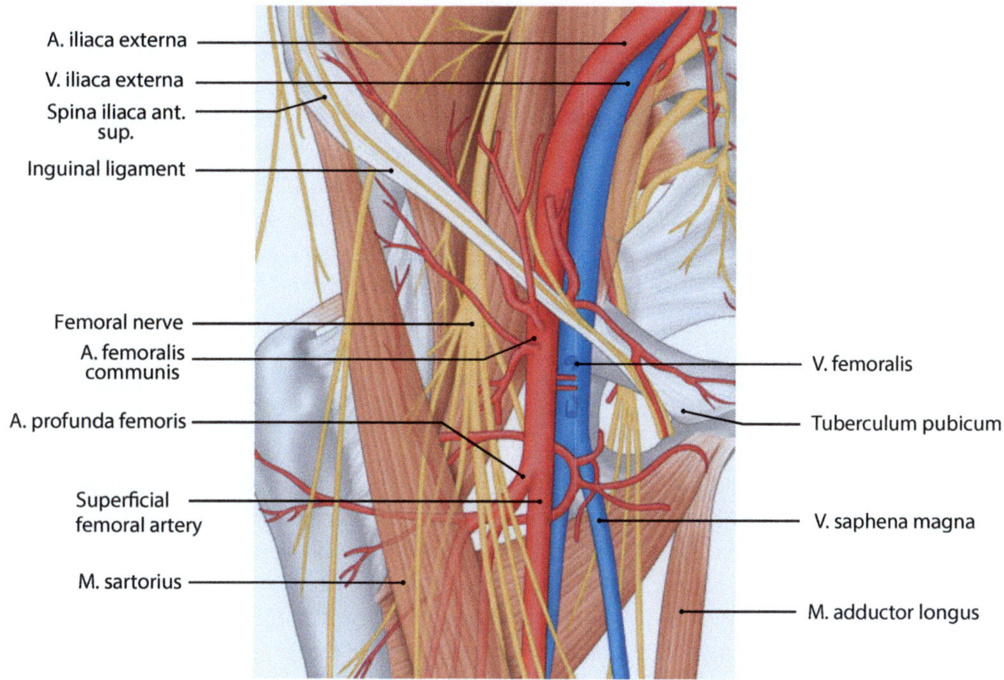

Fig. 4.1 Anatomical landmarks for the puncture of the femoral vessels. The femoral triangle is bordered cranially by the inguinal ligament, medially by the adductor longus muscle, and laterally by the sartorius muscle. Here lie the femoral vein, artery, and nerve (from medial to lateral). By palpating the anterior superior iliac spine and the pubic tubercle, the course of the inguinal ligament can be visualized, and the femoral vessels can be punctured below it. In the further course of both vessels, it can be seen here that, on the one hand, the division into the profunda femoris artery and the superficial femoral artery occurs, and on the other hand, the vein later runs behind the artery. Therefore, punctures that are too caudal should be avoided (From Duncker et al. 2021; modified after Tillman and Debus 2012)

manual compression in the event of bleeding. Additionally, the puncture should be performed caudally before the bifurcation into the profunda femoris artery and the superficial femoral artery. The puncture height should be radiologically at or slightly below the center of the femoral head; a corresponding control of the puncture height can be performed fluoroscopically. This is usually significantly more cranial than the venous puncture site. Initially, as described above, the anatomical landmarks and the course of the artery should be palpated. The puncture needle is then advanced at a 30–45° angle, and after passing through the vessel wall, pulsatile blood flow from the needle becomes visible. The puncture needle is fixed, and a Seldinger wire is introduced into the vessel.

For femoral-arterial punctures in the context of coronary angiography, a puncture using a micropuncture needle can also be performed to reduce vascular complications (Ben-Dor et al. 2020). For this purpose, instead of the usual 18G puncture needle and a 0.035″-wire, the artery is punctured with a 21G puncture needle and a micropuncture wire with a 0.018″-wire, and a 4 Fr sheath is introduced, through which angiography is then performed. The height is controlled angiographically and can be corrected if necessary. If the height is correct, the sheath is switched to a correspondingly larger sheath over the 0.035″ wire.

4.2.5 Ultrasound-Guided Puncture

The ultrasound-guided puncture provides precise information about the size and spatial relationships of the vessels, such as depth, caliber, or positional anomalies and passage obstructions. The ultrasound-guided puncture for electrophysiological examinations can reduce the rate of vascular complications to nearly zero (Brass et al. 2015; Sobolev et al. 2017; Ströker et al. 2019; Wang et al. 2019). In a recent meta-analysis, real-time ultrasound-guided puncture of the femoral vein during electrophysiological procedures reduces vascular complications, arterial mispunctures, post-procedural groin pain, and puncture time (Kupó et al. 2020).

Imaging should be used as additional information to anatomical landmarks. A distinction is made between indirect and direct ultrasound-guided puncture. In the indirect method, an ultrasound examination of the target vessels is performed before the invasive procedure, and the vessels are marked on the skin. The vessel is then punctured based on these markings. In the direct method, the puncture is performed under ultrasound using a sterile cover over the ultrasound probe. The ultrasound-guided puncture allows for an accurate depiction of the course of the vessels, the exact puncture height (considering individual differences, especially in arterial bifurcation or the positional relationship of the artery to the vein), and verification of the correct position of the needle and later the wire.

The depiction of the vessels can be done either in the transverse (short axis) or longitudinal plane (long axis). The transverse plane is usually quicker to learn and makes the depiction of smaller vessels easier. However, the longitudinal depiction allows for a more accurate visualization of the needle and the actual puncture site.

To depict the vessels, the artery is first palpated, and then the ultrasound probe is placed over the artery at the level of the inguinal ligament. The vessels can be depicted using 2D imaging and color Doppler. The vein lies medial to the artery and is usually somewhat deeper in comparison (Fig. 4.2). By compressing with the ultrasound probe, the vein can usually be easily compressed, whereas the muscle-stronger arterial wall usually shows a stable diameter. In

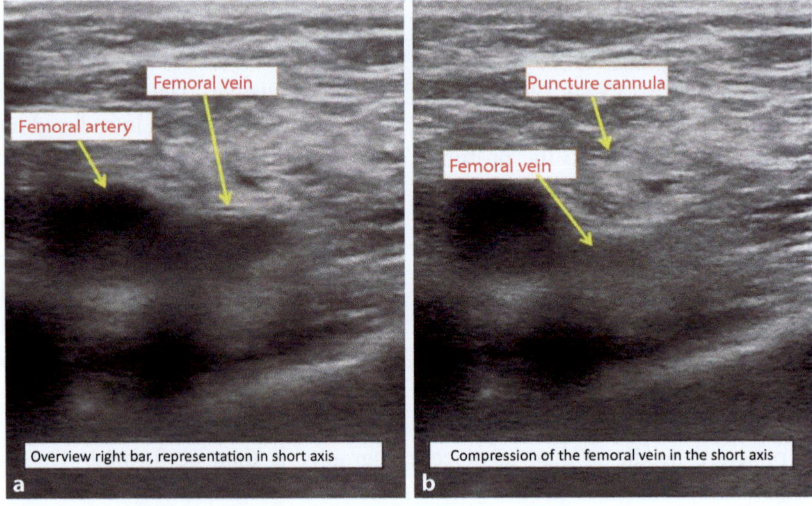

Fig. 4.2 An exemplary example of an ultrasound-guided puncture of the right femoral vein. Depiction of the femoral vein and the common femoral artery in the short axis (**a**) and compression of the femoral vein during the advancement of the puncture needle (**b**). (From: Duncker et al. 2021)

color Doppler, the artery shows a pulsatile flow, while the vein shows a constant flow.

After identifying the target vessels and the appropriate puncture height, the ultrasound probe can be held in one hand while the puncture needle is advanced with the other hand. The course of the puncture needle can be tracked in the ultrasound image. The passage of the vessel wall can be depicted, thus avoiding injury to the posterior vessel wall, which can be particularly important in patients with dehydration, high venous pressures, or under anticoagulation.

Troubleshooting in Femoral Vessel Puncture
- Very low venous filling pressure: If possible, administer fluids, puncture under Valsalva maneuver.
- In ultrasound (US), artery clearly lying above the vein: increased external rotation of the leg; puncture from further medial under US; compression under ultrasound, which can cause the vein to be compressed medially and punctured there in a controlled manner.
- Significantly hardened tissue after multiple ablations: pre-dilation with smaller sheaths, ascending dilation, and if necessary, incision/expansion of the already made tissue incision with a scalpel.

After successfully placing one or more Seldinger wires into the desired vessels, the corresponding sheaths can then be introduced. Each sheath should then be carefully aspirated and flushed free of air. If vascular anomalies or vascular injuries are suspected, a contrast agent injection can be performed.

4.3   Transseptal Puncture

4.3.1   Materials

The basic equipment for transseptal puncture (TSP) consists of a puncture needle and a long sheath with an associated dilator. The long sheath is usually a fixed, i.e., non-steerable sheath that has a typical pre-bend. In principle, a long steerable sheath can also be used for TSP, which requires a correspondingly longer TSP needle. This can be helpful, for example, in dilated atria or re-ablations as an alternative. The degree of pre-bend of the fixed sheaths is generally between 45 to 55° with a typical sheath length of 63 cm. To ensure smooth advancement of the ablation catheter, an inner diameter of 8 to 8.5F should be chosen. The sheath system usually includes a guide wire with a diameter between 0.032 to 0.035 inches. The most common TSP needles have a distal curvature angle between 30 to 55° and must be selected in a length compatible with the sheath system (usually 71 cm). The so-called "needle-wire system" is a 120 cm long nitinol guide wire with a diameter of 0.014 inches (SafeSept wire, Pressure Products, San Pedro, CA, USA), whose distal end consists of a sharp and J-shaped bent tip. Within the sheath-needle system, this tip initially shows a straight alignment to pierce the interatrial septum straight through, before it deforms into a J-shape after passing through the septum and can thus be advanced atraumatically into the left atrium. A selection of typical sheaths and needles for TSP are shown in Fig. 4.3.

4.3.2   Procedure

Preparation
First, under fluoroscopic control (AP view), the long sheath with dilator is placed over a guide wire in the superior vena cava. The alignment of the sheath tip is achieved by rotating the sheath clockwise so that the flush port of the sheath is directed towards the patient and, in reference to a clock face, comes to rest at about 5 o'clock. After removing the guide wire, the TSP needle is introduced through the sheath without the needle tip protruding beyond the distal end of the dilator, thus still being completely within the sheath system. It is important that the advancement of the needle in the sheath is done with the needle stylet left in place, so that

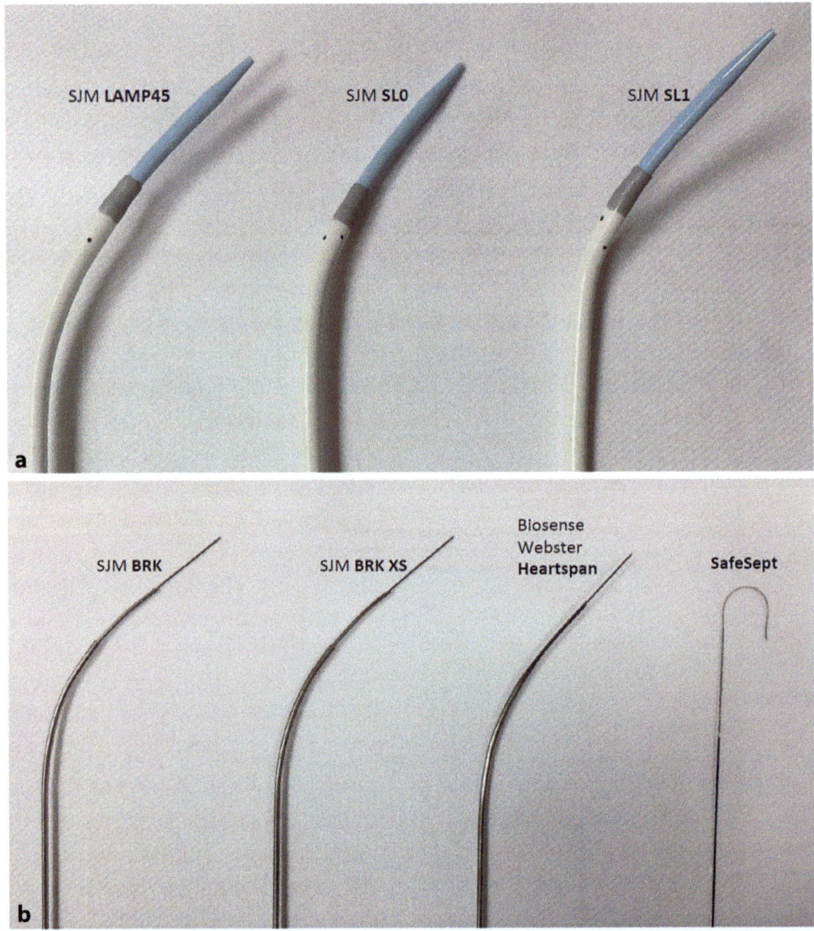

Fig. 4.3 Selection of typical sheaths and needles for transseptal puncture. **a** Three different fixed sheaths with dilator with different curvatures and widths. **b** Three different TSP needles with different curvatures; SafeSept wire with sharpened and pre-bent tip for direct puncture. (From Duncker et al. 2021)

no plastic material can enter the lumen of the needle tip. After placing the needle, the stylet can be removed, followed by aspiration of air and subsequent flushing of the needle through a stopcock system. The subsequent transseptal puncture can be performed under invasive pressure measurement at the needle tip or under control by applied contrast medium.

Alignment of the Sheath-Needle System and Puncture of the Fossa ovalis

First, the alignment of the puncture system is performed in an RAO 30° view. The tip of the puncture system should point in a line towards the septum and have a similar alignment to the diagnostic catheter in the coronary sinus (Fig. 4.4a). In the LAO 40–60° view, a perpendicular direction to the septum is simultaneously presented (Fig. 4.4b). The slow retraction of the puncture system in an LAO view now takes place. Helpful here is the LAO angulation in which the diagnostic RV/His catheter runs directly towards the examiner, as this LAO plane usually indicates the tangential course of the septum (Fig. 4.4b). During the retraction, two typical jumps towards the interatrial septum are usually observed. The first jump indicates the passage of the aortic bulb, the second jump indicates the movement of the puncture system during the transition from the muscular part of the septum to the fossa ovalis. After the second jump, the entire system is slightly retracted and then placed on the septum with a forward movement, resulting in a tent-like tightening ("tenting") of the septum towards the left atrium (Fig. 4.4c). As a visual aid, the septum can be marked and made visible in most cases by administering a small amount of contrast medium (Fig. 4.4c).

At this point, a check of the anteroposterior alignment of the system in an RAO projection (30°) can be performed, and the CS-synchronous movement of the puncture needle can be confirmed. Under fluoroscopic and/or echocardiographic control (TOE or intracardiac ultrasound),

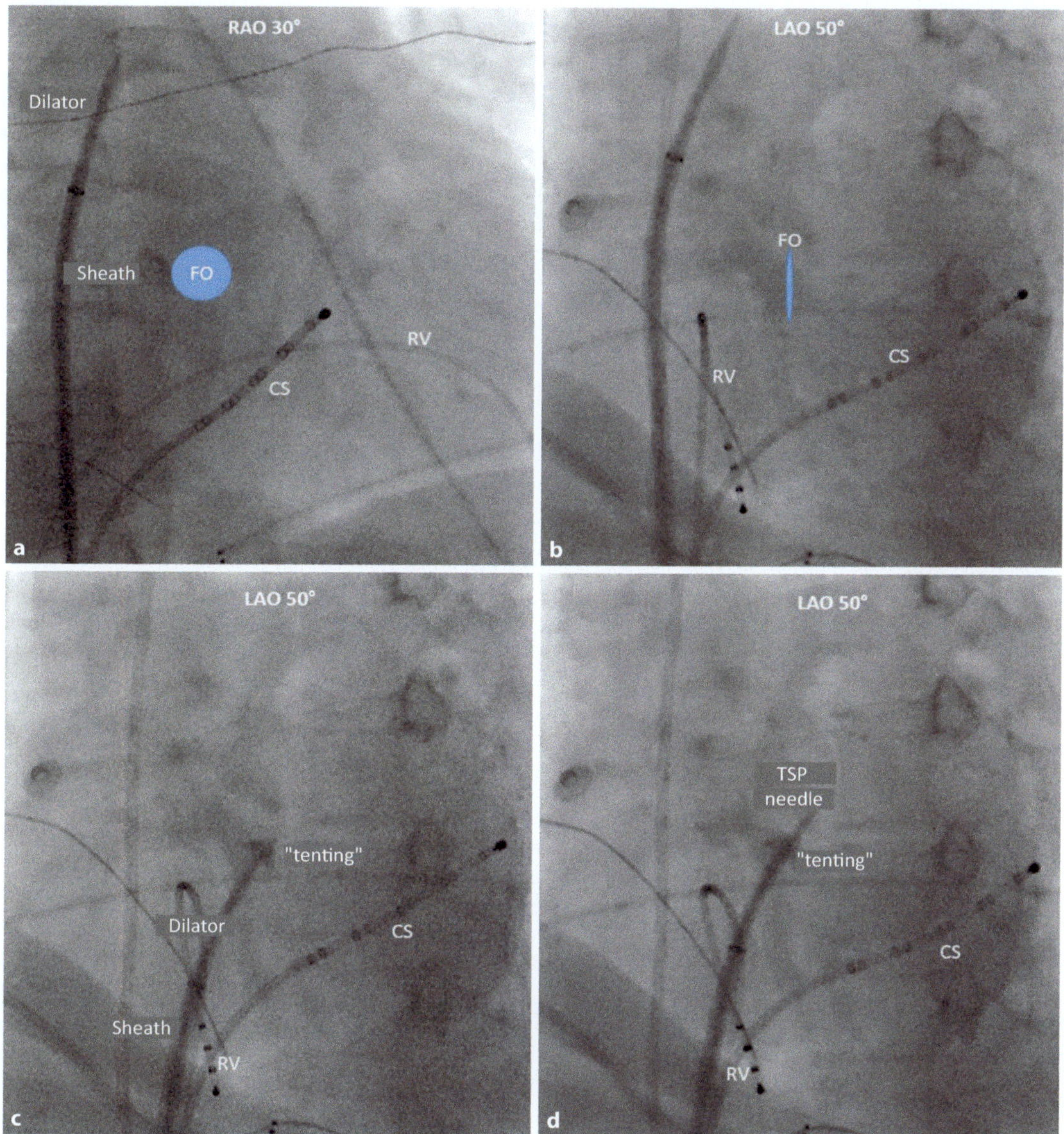

Fig. 4.4 Alignment of the sheath-needle system and puncture of the fossa ovalis (FO). **a** Alignment of the puncture system in RAO view towards the FO by clockwise rotation. **b** Alignment of the puncture system in LAO view towards the septum. **c** Retraction and "tenting" of the septum with the dilator tip and contrast medium marking. **d** Advancement of the TSP needle and puncture of the septum. (From: Duncker et al. 2021)

the advancement and passage of the TSP needle through the septum is performed (Fig. 4.5, Video 4.1). The correct needle position can be secured by confirming a left atrial pressure curve and/or administering contrast medium into the left atrium. The dilator and finally the long sheath are then advanced into the left atrium over the needle tip. Alternatively, after removing the needle, a wire-guided advancement of the sheath including the dilator into the left atrium is performed, followed by the joint removal of the wire and dilator. After the secure placement of the sheath tip in the left atrium, blood aspiration is performed after removing the dilator and the TSP needle to avoid a possible air entry into the left atrium, followed by continuous flushing of the sheath. At the latest, a weight-adjusted intravenous administration of heparin with a target ACT (activated clotting time) of > 300 s must be administered.

4.3.3 Problems During the Puncture

ST Segment Elevations/Pressure Drop after Puncture
If ST segment elevations (primarily in the inferior limb leads II, III, and aVF) are observed

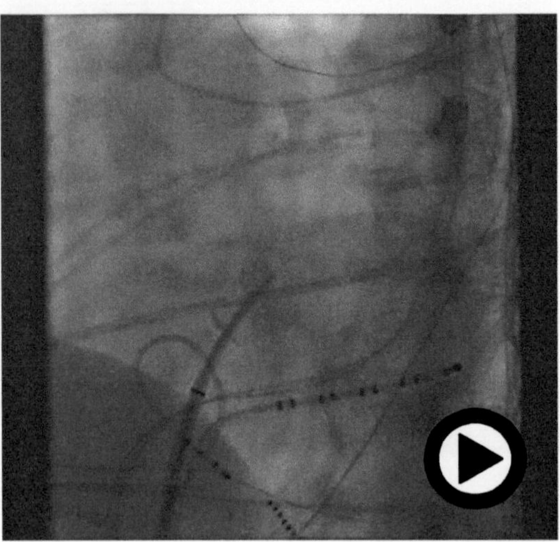

Fig. 4.5 Performing a transseptal puncture in the LAO projection (https://doi.org/10.1007/000-d2g)

immediately after puncture and insertion of the sheath system into the left atrium, air embolism is the most likely cause. This peracute ECG change can be accompanied by hypotension, ventricular tachycardia, or AV block.

▶ Although in most cases the consequences of an air embolism resolve spontaneously, it must be possible to administer volume, antiarrhythmics, or catecholamines as clinically required.

Immediately, the placement of a sheath in the femoral artery should be considered to obtain arterial blood pressure measurement and to enable coronary angiography. In any case, aspiration through the used transseptal sheath should be performed to prevent further air passage. Differential diagnostically, the described changes can also be caused by a vasospastic and neuronally mediated reflex (Bezold-Jarisch-like reflex), which leads to a transient coronary spasm through activation of vagal regulation during TSP. Usually, the ST segment elevations are immediately reversed after the administration of atropine.

Absence of Inward Movement of the Puncture Needle during Withdrawal
If no typical inward jumps are visible during the withdrawal movement of the puncture system, the correct alignment of the sheath-needle system must be checked. With correct alignment, a dilation of the right atrium is often found, so that the needle tip remains too far from the septum and does not fall into the fossa ovalis during withdrawal. This can only be overcome by manually pre-bending the TSP needle. Care must be taken to bend the needle proximally to the existing bend apex to increase the reach. It is important to avoid kinking the needle, as this can make it difficult to register a pressure curve and administer contrast medium (Fig. 4.6).

Floppy Septum
With a hypermobile or aneurysmal ("floppy") septum, problems occasionally arise for the required passage of the needle tip through the septum, as it can stretch dangerously far towards

the free wall of the left atrium, thus posing the risk of perforation when the needle passes through the septum and atrial wall. After achieving sufficient "tenting," the system's own introducer stylet of the TSP needle can be used to pierce the septum. Due to the small diameter of the stylet, passage through the septum is usually achieved with very little force. The advancement of the needle into the left atrium over the stylet is then easier and can be followed by the placement of the dilator or sheath (Fig. 4.7).

Fibrotic Septum

Especially in patients with structural heart diseases, after cardiac surgeries, or previous transseptal procedures, the interatrial septum can appear fibrotic, making a TSP significantly more difficult. In addition to the aforementioned use of the needle stylet, the Safe-Sept wire can also be used here. After "tenting" the septum using the sheath-needle system, the Safe-Sept wire is advanced through the lumen of the TSP needle to the septum. The sharp and very thin tip of the wire then pierces the interatrial septum with a straight alignment until it reaches the left atrium. Due to the lack of guidance of the TSP needle, the sharp wire tip now takes on a curved J-shape and can be advanced far into the left atrium or the left upper pulmonary veins. The lying wire now serves as a guide wire for the following TSP needle and the sheath system (Fig. 4.8).

Finally, the possible use of the NRG©-RF TSP needle (Baylis, Montreal, Quebec, Canada), whose tip is capable of applying RF energy, allows the septum to be passed without the use of extraordinary force. Alternatively, the use of the conventional puncture needle and the ablation generator is also described, whereby the application of energy is only possible after deactivating the impedance limits of the generator.

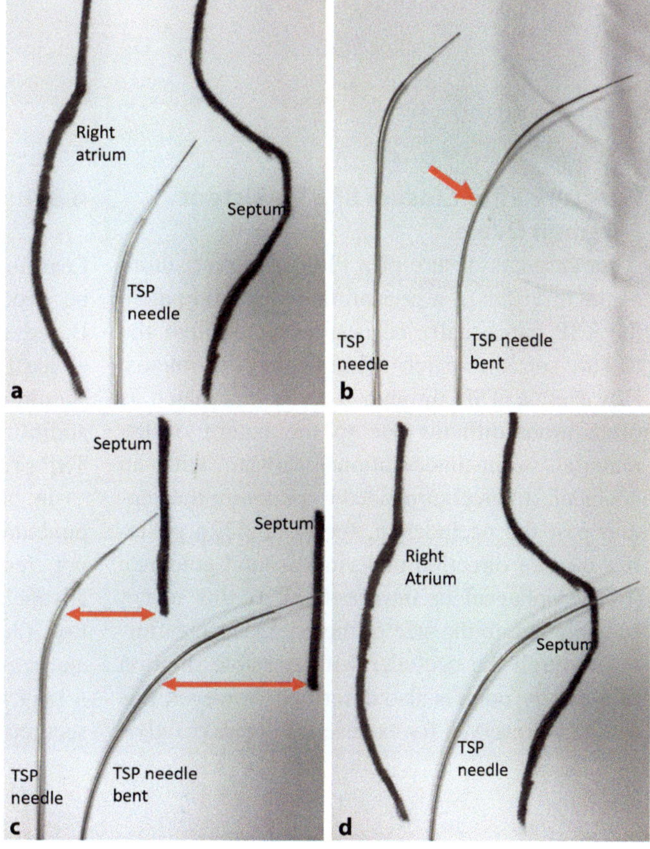

Fig. 4.6 TSP with dilated right atrium. **a** Original pre-bending of the TSP needle is not sufficient to reach the septum. **b** Manual bending of the TSP needle proximal to the original apex (*red arrow*). **c** Reach of the needle tip with original and reinforced bending. **d** TSP with dilated right atrium after manual reinforcement of the TSP needle bend. (From Duncker et al. 2021)

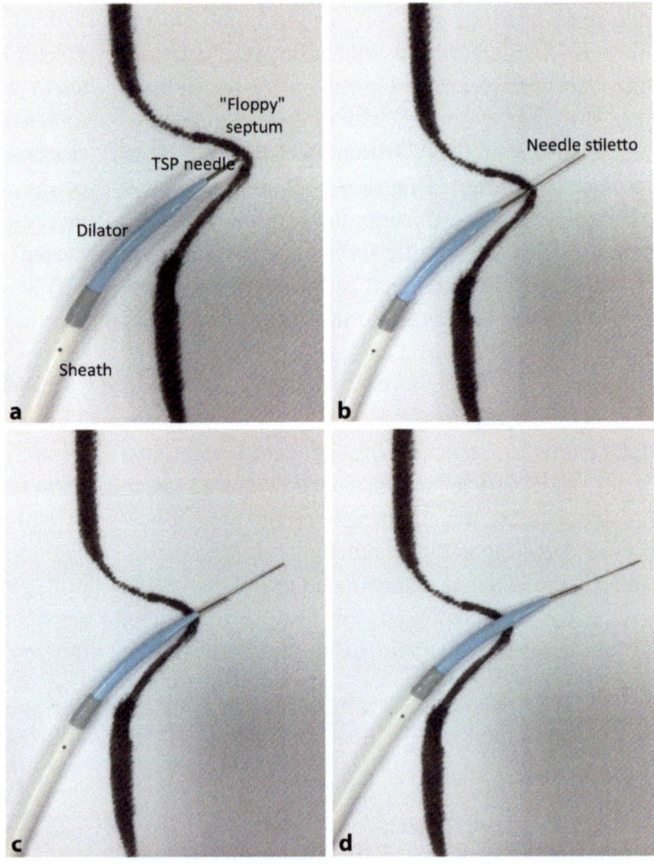

Fig. 4.7 TSP with "floppy" septum using stylet. **a** "Tenting" of the septum using the needle-sheath system. **b** Piercing of the septum using the needle's own stylet. **c** Advancement of the TSP needle into the left atrium over the stylet. **d** Advancement of the dilator and sheath into the left atrium over the TSP needle. (From: Duncker et al. 2021)

Puncture after Closure of a Persistent Foramen Ovale

After surgical closure of a PFO by direct suture or the insertion of a pericardial or Dacron patch, the TSP can usually be performed through the closure or the patch without any problems. However, a TSP through a Gore-Tex patch is often more difficult due to the nature of the material. After interventional closure with an occluder, it is recommended to puncture the septum past the occluder in, for example, a posterior-inferior direction under ultrasound guidance (transesophageal or intracardiac). If this is not possible due to the size of the occluder, puncturing through the occluder with possible dilation of the entry point is also described; however, this should be reserved for experienced centers only.

4.3.4 TSP Training

Learning transseptal puncture should definitely be accompanied by an experienced examiner. Based on our own and published experiences, at least 30 to 50 punctures under supervision should be performed, depending on whether additional imaging (TOE, ICE) is used for the TSP (Yao et al. 2013).

In principle, it should be noted that a mispuncture with the TSP needle alone usually does not result in serious complications, whereas advancing the sheath into an incorrect position (aorta, pericardium) regularly has serious and sometimes fatal consequences. In this case, a long wire should be advanced and the access secured (Chen et al. 2019).

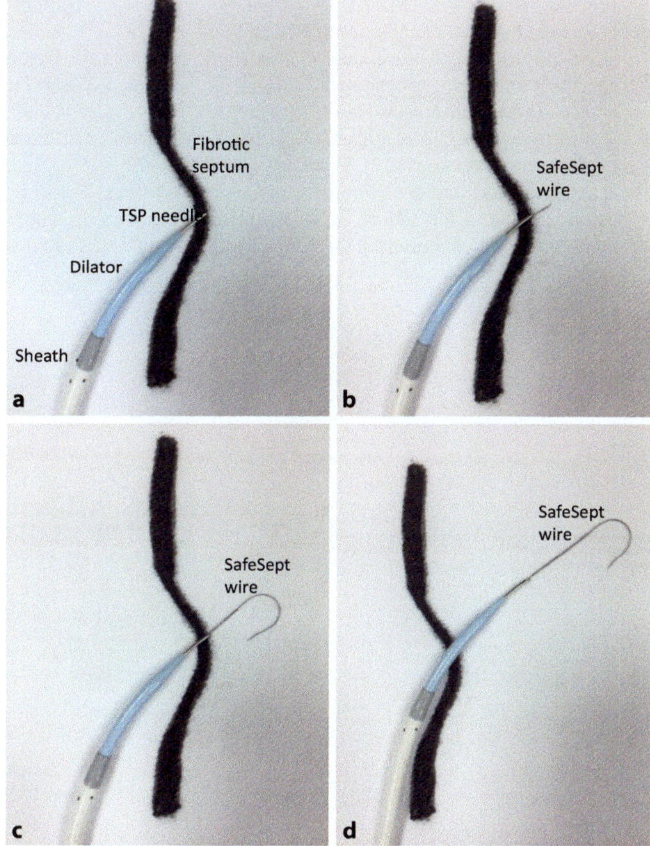

Fig. 4.8 TSP in fibrotic septum using SafeSept wire. **a** "Tenting" of the septum with sheath-needle system. **b** Piercing of the septum with SafeSept wire. **c** Advancing the SafeSept wire into the left atrium with J-shaped deformation. **d** Advancing the TSP needle and dilator over the SafeSept wire into the left atrium. (From Duncker et al. 2021)

▶ Safe access routes are an important element in invasive electrophysiology - after all, the possible complaints due to, for example, hematomas after puncture are something like the "business card" of a clinic. In special clinical situations, alternative access routes such as jugular, subxiphoid, or even transhepatic access may also be necessary. Overall, the safety of the puncture seems to be increased by an ultrasound-supported approach.

References

Ben-Dor I, Sharma A, Rogers T, Yerasi C, Case BC, Chezar-Azerrad C et al (2020) Micropuncture technique for femoral access is associated with lower vascular complications compared to standard needle. Catheter Cardiovasc Interv 129:39. https://doi.org/10.1002/ccd.29330

Brass P, Hellmich M, Kolodziej L, Schick G, Smith AF (2015) Ultrasound guidance versus anatomical landmarks for subclavian or femoral vein catheterization. Cochrane Database Syst Rev. https://doi.org/10.1002/14651858.cd011447

Chen H, Fink T, Zhan X, Chen M, Eckardt L, Long D et al (2019) Inadvertent transseptal puncture into the aortic root: the narrow edge between luck and catastrophe in interventional cardiology. Europace 21:euz42. https://doi.org/10.1093/europace/euz042

Duncker et al (2021) Punktionstechniken in der invasiven Elektrophysiologie. Herzschrittmacherther Elektrophysiol. https://doi.org/10.1007/s00399-021-00761-8

Kupó P, Pap R, Sághy L, Tényi D, Bálint A, Debreceni D et al (2020) Ultrasound guidance for femoral venous access in electrophysiology procedures-systematic review and meta-analysis. J Interv Cardiac Electrophysiol 59:407–414. https://doi.org/10.1007/s10840-019-00683-z

Seldinger SI (2008) Catheter replacement of the needle in percutaneous arteriography. A new technique. Acta Radiol. https://doi.org/10.1080/02841850802133386

Sobolev M, Shiloh AL, Biase LD, Slovut DP (2017) Ultrasound-guided cannulation of the femoral vein in electrophysiological procedures: a systematic review and meta-analysis. Europace 19:850–855. https://doi.org/10.1093/europace/euw113

Ströker E, Asmundis CD, Kupics K, Takarada K, Mugnai G, Cocker JD et al (2019) Value of ultrasound for access guidance and detection of subclinical vascular complications in the setting of atrial fibrillation cryoballoon ablation. Europace 21:434–439. https://doi.org/10.1093/europace/euy154

Tillman B, Debus ES (2012) Anatomie der Gefäße und operativen Zugangswege. Springer, Berlin, Heidelberg

Wang TKM, Wang MTM, Martin A (2019) Meta-analysis of ultrasound-guided vs conventional vascular access for cardiac electrophysiology procedures. J Arrhythmia 35:858–862. https://doi.org/10.1002/joa3.12236

Yao Y, Ding L, Chen W, Guo J, Bao J, Shi R et al (2013) The training and learning process of transseptal puncture using a modified technique. Europace 15:1784–1790. https://doi.org/10.1093/europace/eut078

Leon Iden

5.1 Introduction

In contrast to interventional cardiology, there are several peculiarities in fluoroscopic orientation in electrophysiology. On the one hand, electrophysiological catheters are generally fully visible fluoroscopically even with low-dose programs, and only a few standard projections are used. On the other hand, especially at the beginning of electrophysiological work, orientation and the positional relationship of cardiac structures to each other are often difficult due to the intracavitary location of the catheters.

Here, anatomical-topographical knowledge is indispensable, and it is also helpful to know certain orientation points and to locate them in the respective standard projections.

If a 3D mapping system is used in addition to fluoroscopic catheter localization, there are often overlaps with the frame constructions mounted under the catheter table during extreme angulations. This can, for example, limit the selection of working planes when an intraprocedural coronary angiography is necessary.

Due to the variable heart axes, possible dilation or anatomical variants of the individual

cardiac structures, as well as different physiognomies of the patients, the correlation of certain catheter positions and orientation points to intracardiac electrograms is generally performed. The most common example is the His bundle electrogram, which is an important orientation aid in many constellations and whose position is matched with the fluoroscopic (or 3D mapping system displayed) catheter position. An overview of possible correlation points is provided in Table 5.1.

Occasionally, angiographic verifications of individual structures such as pulmonary vein angiographies are also performed. Furthermore, a complete angiographic representation of the left atrium can also be performed—under adenosine administration or ventricular rapid pacing to slow down the contrast medium flow. Due to the relatively high radiation exposure, this is nowadays only done in exceptional cases.

5.2 Standard Projections and Landmarks

5.2.1 LAO

The LAO ("left anterior oblique") projection is one of the most important standard projections. Here, the detector of the X-ray system is angled approximately 45° to the left side of the patient. This results in a fluoroscopic "view"

L. Iden (✉)
Segeberger Kliniken GmbH, Bad Segeberg, Germany
e-mail: leon.iden@segebergerkliniken.de

Table 5.1 Overview of various landmarks and their correlation with intracardiac electrograms

Landmark	Constellation	Characteristic
His bundle	Ubiquitous landmark, essential in AVNRT, (septal) accessory pathway	Characteristic His bundle signal
Non-coronary aortic cusp	Mapping in the aortic root/LVOT, ablation of septal accessory pathways	Atrial signal in the area of the aortic root possibly with atrial capture
AV valve annuli	Ubiquitous landmark, essential in accessory pathways, left atrial substrate modification, or linear lesions in the atrium	Transition from ventricular near-field signal to ventricular far-field with atrial signal when retracting over the valve
LAA/RAA	Ubiquitous landmark, essential in PVI	Particularly recognizable in atrial fibrillation, high-amplitude, organized atrial signal with a clearly demarcated isoelectric line
Pulmonary veins	Essential in pulmonary vein isolation or choice of ablation line	Characteristic double potential with atrial far-field and near-field from the pulmonary veins
Conduction system (bundle branches/fascicles/Purkinje fibers)	Ablation target in fascicular VTs, Purkinje-associated PVCs	Specific sharp, presystolic potential similar to the His bundle electrogram (but relatively later than the His)

from the apex of the heart perpendicularly onto the AV valve plane. In the LAO projection, the spine is on the right side of the image. The interatrial septum and His bundle are tangential to the viewing axis. With an inserted His or RV apex catheter, the angulation can be adjusted so that the His catheter points directly at the X-ray tube. Then the viewing angle approximately corresponds to the anatomical heart axis. If a 3D mapping system is used, the angulation should be adjusted analogously to fluoroscopy to obtain uniform views (see Fig. 5.1).

▶ The LAO projection is a very frequently used standard projection. Due to the imagined view along the anatomical heart axis through the AV valves into the atria and the tangential view of the interatrial and interventricular septum, it is suitable for a variety of examinations.

Due to the tangential projection of the interatrial septum, the LAO projection is also used in the context of transseptal puncture. The jump of the sheath into the fossa ovalis can be well visualized here.

Furthermore, the LAO projection is helpful for differentiating the wire course in the context of transseptal puncture. If a wire is used, it is advanced through the interatrial septum into the left superior pulmonary vein (LSPV) after passing the sheath tip. Here, advancing the sheath into

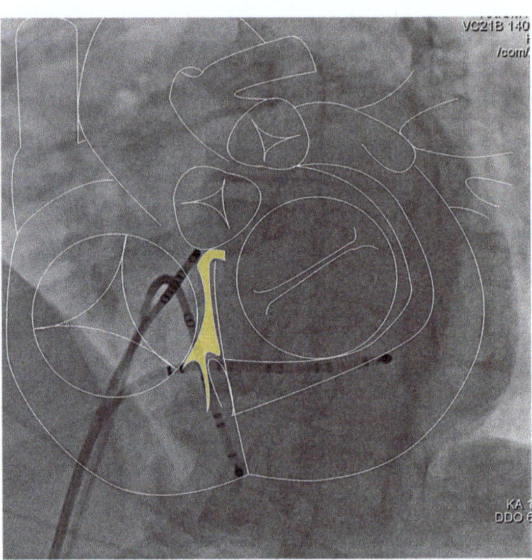

Fig. 5.1 Schematic drawing of the projection of the valve plane, septum, and His bundle in the LAO projection. Note the fully extended course of the CS along the mitral annulus and the His catheter pointing out of the image plane towards the viewer. The RV apex catheter runs towards the viewer along the interventricular septum. (Courtesy of Dr. Stefano Bordignon)

the LAA should be avoided. In the LAO projection, the LAA projects onto the heart boundaries (see above) and does not leave the heart silhouette, so if the wire course extends beyond the boundary of the heart, it is assumed that the wire is positioned in one of the left pulmonary veins..

The LAO projection is also used to place the coronary sinus catheter (CS). This takes advantage of the fact that the CS is maximally stretched along its course along the mitral valve annulus. With an inserted catheter, the CS is an important orientation aid as an approximate marker of the mitral valve plane in all projections.

For ablation targets along the AV valve annuli, such as in the ablation of accessory pathways, the LAO projection is also routinely used, as the AV valve plane is visually spanned here.

Furthermore, the oblique projections are used to visualize the pulmonary vein (PV) ostia of the inferior veins (LAO for the LIPV, RAO for the RIPV), which often point posteriorly at an angle of approximately 45° (see Fig. 5.2).

▶ Due to the oblique course of the inferior pulmonary veins posteriorly, the LAO or RAO projections are preferred over the AP projection for assessing the ostia or, for example, for angiography of the inferior veins.

5.2.2   RAO Projection

In the RAO ("right anterior oblique") projection, the detector of the X-ray tube is angled approximately 45° to the right side of the patient. This causes the line of sight to run tangentially to the AV valve plane, with the ventricles on the right side of the image and the atria on the left side of the image. The spine is located on the left side of the image. The inserted CS catheter runs vertically out of the image plane away from the viewer.

The RAO projection is used during transseptal puncture to check the position of the sheath relative to the CS catheter and to prevent an excessively anterior or posterior position of the transseptal puncture site. By inserting a long wire or a pigtail catheter into the aortic root, the position of the transseptal puncture site relative to the aortic root can be visualized.

The guiding structures of Koch's triangle (CS ostium, tricuspid valve annulus, tendon of Todaro, see Fig. 5.3) with the compact AV node at its

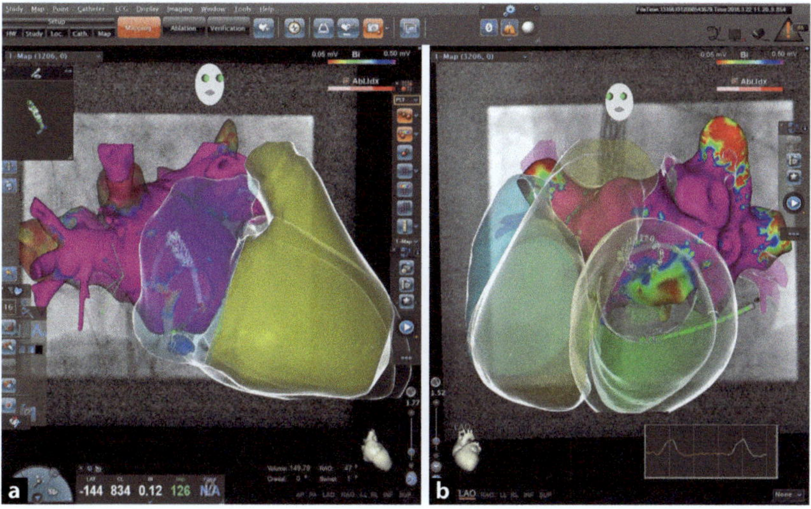

Fig. 5.2 Segmented CT model of the heart with left atrial 3D map in the two standard projections RAO (**a**) and LAO (**b**). Note the position of the AV valve plane, septum, inferior pulmonary veins, and left atrial appendage

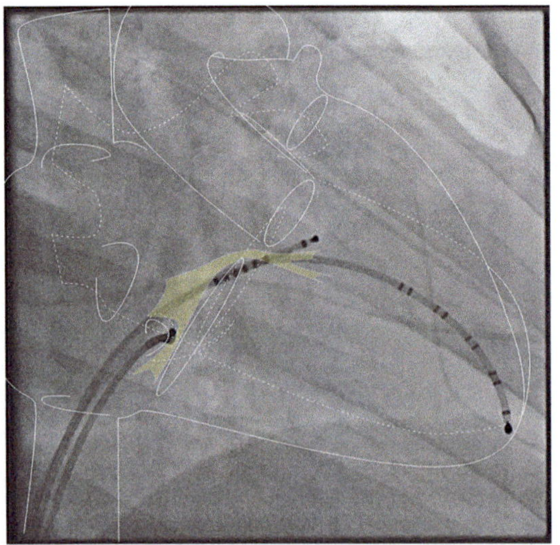

Fig. 5.3 Projection of relevant structures and orientation points onto fluoroscopy in the RAO plane. The inserted CS catheter runs vertically out of the image plane and marks the mitral valve annulus. The CS ostium as a guiding structure of Koch's triangle is also marked. The His bundle is also visualized here as an orientation point by the inserted His catheter, and the compact AV node is projected posteriorly. The RV apex catheter indicates the position of the heart apex.

cranial tip can also be best differentiated in the RAO view due to the marked orientation points.

► In the RAO projection, Koch's triangle is spanned as a guiding structure for the ablation of AVNRT, enabling the precise visualization of the catheter position relative to the CS ostium and the compact AV node.

5.2.3　AP or PA Projection

Here, the X-ray tube or the image intensifier is perpendicular to the sagittal plane. Due to the smaller irradiated volume, this projection is more favorable in terms of radiation exposure for both the patient and the examiner compared to oblique projections. The AP projection is a common working projection for the left atrium, whose posterior wall is usually parallel to the working plane.

► The AP projection is a common working plane for the left atrium, especially during pulmonary vein isolation. It is favorable in terms of radiation exposure due to the small irradiated volume. As a rule of thumb, a 10° higher angulation angle doubles the radiation dose.

Furthermore, the AP plane can serve as a working plane for pericardial puncture, e.g., in the context of complication management to relieve a pericardial effusion or for elective epicardial access, e.g., during VT ablations (see Fig. 5.4).

5.3　Other Landmarks

In patients with prior cardiac procedures, there may be cardiac implants such as valve rings or prostheses, intracardiac devices, etc., which can facilitate fluoroscopic orientation. Thus, mechanical or reconstructed valves naturally mark the respective valve plane and can be helpful landmarks (see Fig. 5.5).

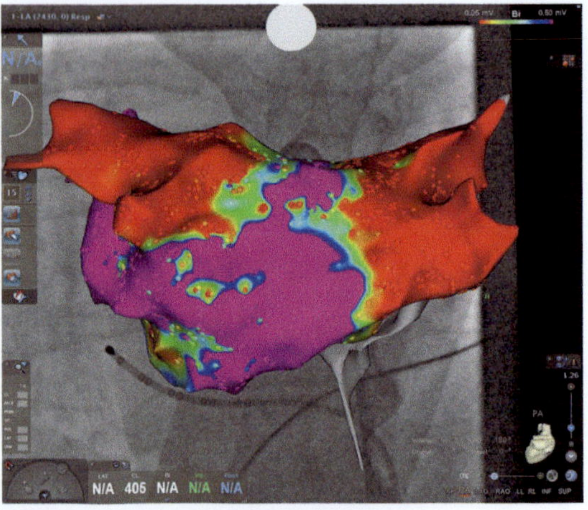

Fig. 5.4 Example of a voltage map of a left atrium in the PA view. Note the nearly symmetrical position of the pulmonary veins with the oblique course of the CS catheter along the AV valve plane.

Electrophysiological procedures are often performed in patients with implanted pacemaker or ICD or CRT systems.

While the chosen position of the RV lead in the right ventricle varies depending on the implantation technique, the atrial lead is routinely implanted in the area of the right atrial appendage. Knowledge of this position can be used as a landmark for further fluoroscopic orientation.

In the case of an implanted CRT system, the LV lead marks the course of the coronary sinus and serves as an orientation aid (see Fig. 5.6).

Coronary stents or coronary calcifications are rarely visible fluoroscopically, especially when fluoroscopy programs with higher dose rates are used. This can be an important orientation aid, particularly in procedures in the outflow tract or in the area of the ventricles, especially in epicardial ablations.

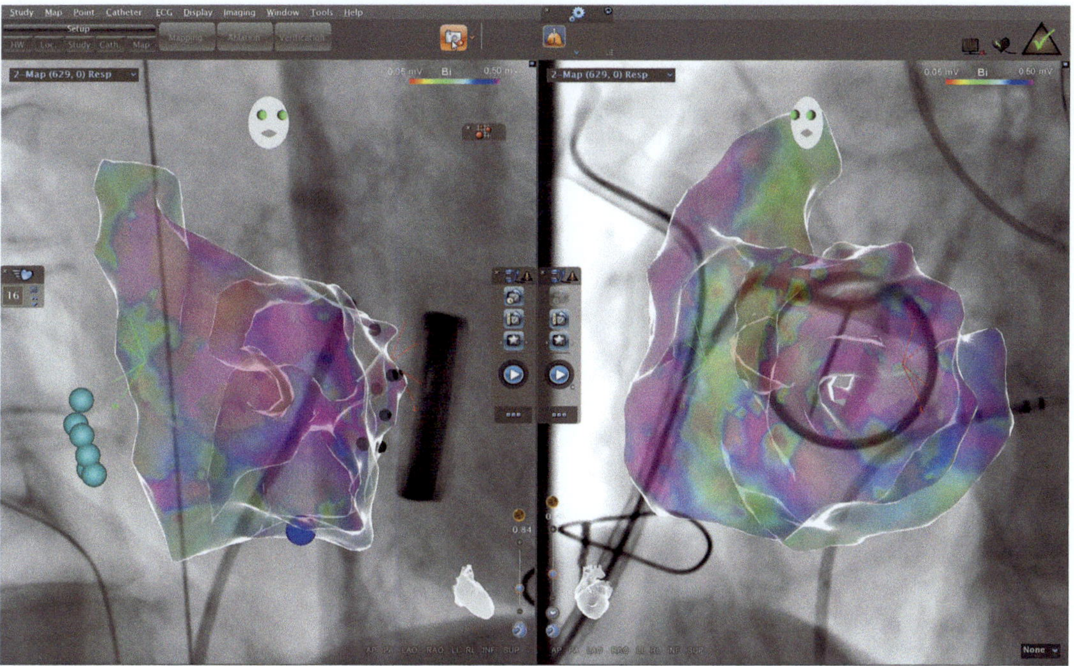

Fig. 5.5 Example of a mechanical tricuspid valve prosthesis with a CS catheter in place and a 3D map of a right atrium in RAO and LAO views. The *black dots* in the RAO view mark the catheter positions with metal artifacts due to contact with the mechanical valve

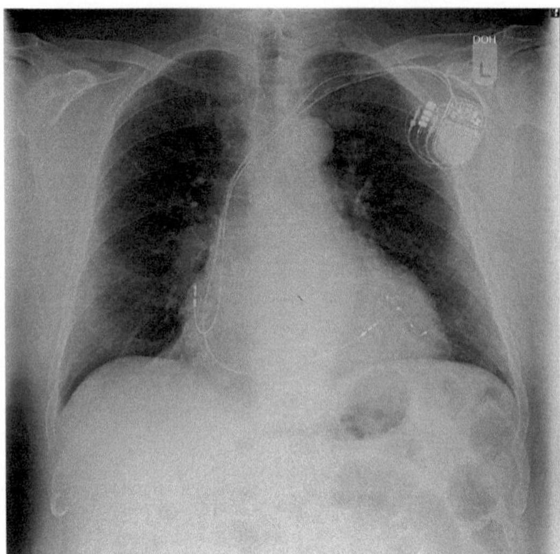

Fig. 5.6 Example of the lead course with an implanted CRT pacemaker. Note the course of the quadripolar LV lead along the coronary sinus (with a subsequent bend into a posterolateral ventricular vein) and the projection of the atrial lead onto the right atrial appendage

Basis Principles of 3D Mapping Systems

6

Martin Borlich and Philipp Sommer

6.1 Introduction

The interventional therapy of cardiac arrhythmias is an indispensable component of modern cardiological treatment. The development in the field of three-dimensional mapping systems and catheter technology has led to high-resolution visualization of electroanatomical information due to precise catheter localization. Furthermore, the new cardiac mapping systems significantly contribute to the reduction of fluoroscopy time and radiation exposure. The following will present the functionalities and applications of the CARTO, EnSite Precision, and Rhythmia systems.

6.2 CARTO

CARTO 3 is a third-generation electroanatomical mapping system from Biosense Webster (Biosense Webster Inc., Diamond Bar, CA, USA), currently available in software version v8. This system operates with three separate coils, each generating a weak magnetic field ($5 \cdot 10^{-6}$ to $5 \cdot 10^{-5}$ T). These magnetic coils are attached under the examination table to a "location pad." Together with six patches on the patient's upper body, mapping catheters with embedded magnetic location sensors, a graphic display, and a data processing unit, the system enables precise real-time electroanatomical mapping with high spatial resolution and an accuracy of less than 1 mm in space. CARTO uses both impedance-based and magnetic information for catheter localization and map creation. The catheter localization is calculated by a triangulation algorithm, similar to the functionality of a GPS. The catheter tips move through the three magnetic fields generated by the coils, allowing conclusions about the catheter's position and orientation. The accuracy of position determination is highest in the center of the magnetic field; therefore, it is important to position the "location pad" under the patient's chest (Fig. 6.1). The accuracy is increased by incorporating current-based information into the calculation of catheter localization. For this purpose, a small current is sent through each catheter electrode and registered and processed by the six patches attached to the upper body.

Each electrode emits a current of low intensity and specific frequency. By measuring the current at each point, a current ratio is determined for each coordinate, allowing the system

M. Borlich (✉)
Segeberger Kliniken GmbH, Bad Segeberg, Germany
e-mail: martin.borlich@segebergerkliniken.de

P. Sommer
Herz- und Diabeteszentrum NRW, Bad Oeynhausen, Germany
e-mail: psommer@hdz-nrw.de

L. Iden et al. (eds.), *Invasive Electrophysiology for Beginners*, https://doi.org/10.1007/978-3-662-70158-4_6

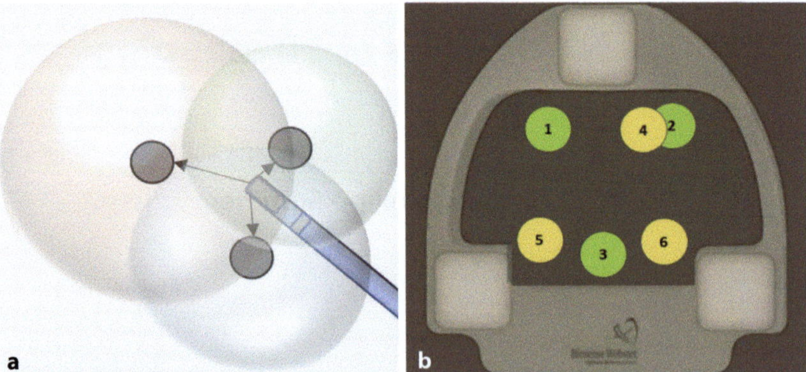

Fig. 6.1 **a** Illustration of catheter position detection by the CARTO-3 system. The emitted ultra-weak magnetic fields of the three coils (*black*), which are attached to the "location pad," are shown in color. The field strength of the three electromagnets is measured by the sensor element of the catheter tip and used for position determination by means of a triangulation algorithm. **b** The "location pad" of the CARTO system with the three built-in magnetic coils (*white*) and display of the six patches that are attached to the patient's upper body (*green*= dorsal, *yellow*= ventral)

to adjust the information obtained from the magnetic data. CARTO can display six degrees of freedom (forward/backward, up/down, left/right, yaw, pitch, roll) and a color-based visualization of the catheter's current position, rotation, deflection, and movement direction in real-time. Artifacts caused by patient movement, heart activity, system movement, and breathing are compensated for by using the back pads and the "Location pads" as a position reference (body coordinate system). Additional information about breathing through the use of the ACCURESP module can further minimize inaccuracies caused by respiratory artifacts (Borlich and Sommer 2019).

For the ablation of cardiac arrhythmias with the CARTO system, a variety of diagnostic and therapeutic catheters are available. These steerable uni- or bidirectional therapeutic catheters are available in three sizes: 4 mm, 8 mm (closed tips), and 3.5 mm (irrigated tip) as well as various curve sizes. The Surround-Flow (SF) technology, available for irrigated catheters, allows for the reduction of fluid for cooling the catheter tip without compromising signal resolution and performance. Numerous diagnostic catheters can be used for the derivation of intracardiac signals. Catheters from other manufacturers can be partially used with CARTO with a special connector. However, only five catheters can be displayed simultaneously.

The development of numerous modules in recent years has shortened procedure duration, improved clinical outcomes, and reduced the need for fluoroscopy. With the introduction of CARTO 3, fast anatomical mapping ("fast anatomical mapping" = FAM) became possible. The creation of the 3D model during the continuous movement of the mapping catheter shortened the examination duration and improved the map resolution. The CONFIDENSE module offers the electrophysiologist a high-density mapping solution with automatic data acquisition. Simultaneous electroanatomical data acquisition via multi-electrode catheters is possible. HD COLORING has further improved the interpolation and resolution of high-resolution maps. The 3D model is generated as a triangular mesh and converted into a grid of congruent cubic voxels (voxelization of a mesh). The Laplace interpolation for calculating additional voxels and the representation of a high-resolution map have increased spatial resolution and accuracy. Abbott's new EnSite X system also uses this calculation via voxels. The extended version of the CONFIDENSE module with a continuous pattern-matching filter allows users to selectively capture specific ventricular signals to quickly and effectively treat PVC or complex ventricular tachycardias (VT). Ripple mapping enables the dynamic representation of activation patterns, including compensation for inaccuracies in electrogram annotation or incorrectly set window of interest (WOI). It allows cardiologists to recognize the dominant direction of tachycardia propagation.

The PASO module allows the morphology of the recorded VES or part of the tachycardia to be compared with a morphology generated by focal stimulation. This is particularly useful in cases with rare VES or non-inducible tachycardias. The crucial component for reducing fluoroscopy was the introduction of CARTOUNIVU. This image integration technology allows physicians to integrate a static fluoroscopy image into the electroanatomical reconstruction after the initial registration. Dynamic sequences such as a coronary angiography can also be integrated. The use of CARTOUNIVU led to a significant reduction in total fluoroscopy time and average radiation dose without affecting the procedure duration or ablation success rate. Another tool for image integration is called CARTOSeg. The system can fuse CT datasets with the 3D map and calculate the ideal fusion of both models. Centers with access to intracardiac ultrasound (ICE) can perform left atrial interventions without fluoroscopy. CARTO combines multiple ECG-guided 2D ultrasound cross-sections from a navigated SOUNDSTAR catheter to create a 3D model using the CARTOSound image integration module (den Uijl et al. 2008).

With its integrated algorithm and standard workflow, the CARTOVISITAG module allows electrophysiologists to focus on the ablation index value, which combines stability, contact force, time, and power, thus objectifying lesion quality. The catheters of the Smarttouch series, which feature contact force measurement, are used for ablation index (AI)-guided ablation. These 3.5 mm catheters with irrigated catheter tips measure the contact force (*"contact force"* = CF) via a small spring in the catheter shaft. The CF calculation is based on the change in distance between the magnetic transmitter coil and three location sensors with a known spring

constant. With this equipment, the CARTO system offers sufficient capabilities for the ablation of all arrhythmias.

CARTO 3, Version 7 includes innovations such as the COHERENT-MAP module. A computed color-based LAT map with directional vectors enables the visualization of electrical impulse propagation as well as zones of slow conduction or a conduction block (SNO-Zones, Slow-or-no-conduction-Zones). The CARTOFINDER-4D-LAT algorithm is being investigated for faster identification of ablation targets in patients with persistent atrial fibrillation. CARTOFINDER collects electrical signals from multi-electrode catheters. VT tools allow the simultaneous capture of the morphology of multiple entities in the sense of an extended pattern comparison (Bertagnolli et al. 2018).

On the catheter technology side, the new QDOT-MICRO catheter enables ablation with high power and short duration (90 W for 4 s), which improves lesion formation and shortens examination time. The technology is based on the Smarttouch-SF catheter, contains 66 irrigation holes and 6 thermosensors (Fig. 6.2). The sensors allow very fast and precise feedback of the local tissue temperature. The catheter can operate in temperature-controlled or temperature-limited mode. A special generator (NGEN RF generator) is used for this purpose. With the VARIPULSE catheter and the TRUPULSE generator, the use of PFA technology ("pulse field ablation") will be enabled via the CARTO platform in the future. An upgrade to CARTO 4 is expected in a few years. The new system could possibly be equipped with its own EP workstation.

6.3   EnSite Precision

The EnSite Precision Cardiac Mapping System (Abbott, IL, USA) has been available since 2016 and uses hybrid impedance and magnetic field technology for precise localization of diagnostic and ablation catheters in the body. The resolution, accuracy, and stability of this system are significantly higher compared to the previous

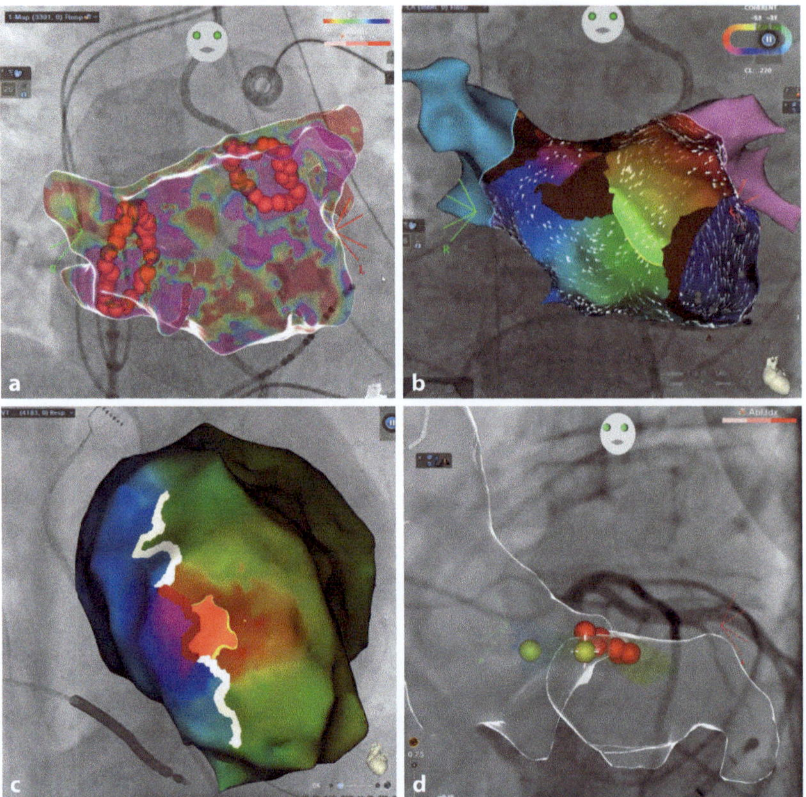

Fig. 6.2 Illustration of the use of the CARTO-3 mapping system for the treatment of various arrhythmias. **a** 3D reconstruction and voltage map of a left atrium with visualization of a pulmonary vein isolation. **b** Visualization of the local activation time (LAT) in atypical left atrial flutter. **c** 3D map of the left ventricle and visualization of the local activation time (LAT) in ventricular tachycardia. The critical isthmus on the anterior wall is recognizable. **d** Ablation of PVC from the LCC with visualization of a sufficient distance to the left coronary arteries using CARTOUNIVU

models EnSite NavX and EnSite Velocity. EnSite Precision enables high-resolution mapping with its HD Grid catheter. The system consists of the following components:

- the EnSite amplifier, which converts the patient's physiological signals into digital signals processed by the workstation,
- the EnSite Precision "Field Frame",
- the display workstation, and
- eight surface electrodes (three transthoracic pairs for three orthogonal axes and two patient reference sensors).

Compared to other systems, it is an open platform compatible with almost all catheters. For impedance-based localization of the catheters, the EnSite NavX navigation and visualization technology of the earlier EnSite systems is used. A 5.7 kHz low-current signal of 350 mA is alternately sent through each of the three pairs of surface electrodes to create a voltage gradient in all three spatial axes. The voltage is measured via the electrodes of the catheter used, adjusted to the gradient created by the 5.7 kHz signal in the x, y, and z axes. Additionally, EnSite Precision increases the accuracy of localization by < 1 mm by adding magnetic field-based localization data to refine impedance-based tracking in real-time (Issa et al. 2018).

Catheters with this hybrid technology are marked with the addition "Sensor Enabled, SE". The EnSite Precision™ Field Frame is mounted under the patient bed and generates a weak magnetic field in which the position of a Sensor Enabled™ catheter can be detected. The magnetic field-based localization data are also used by the EnSite Stability Monitor to maintain localization accuracy in the event of unexpected changes in the impedance field. With these technical capabilities, an accurate electroanatomical reconstruction of the respective heart chamber can be created. In addition to a large number of possible catheters, the Advisor FL is often used as a circular mapping catheter. "Sensor Enabled" ablation catheters are available without contact force (CF) measurement (FlexAbility) or with this technology (TactiCath Quartz). This 3.5 mm irrigated catheter consists of a thermocouple for temperature measurement and a CF sensor. This triaxial fiber optic sensor consists of three optical fibers, and the CF measurement is not affected by the angle of the applied force, resulting in high accuracy of CF visualization during ablation (Bourier et al. 2017).

To objectify the lesion characteristics, the EnSite Precision Mapping System works with several indices that provide feedback on lesion quality. The FTI Index (Force Time Integral) was tested and introduced by Shah in 2010, and its significance as an independent predictor for the outcome after ablation was demonstrated in the TOCCATA study. The combination of this information with the Lesion Index (LSI), the contact force (CF), and the duration of the high-frequency application could further improve the quality of lesion formation. Therefore, an EnSite CF module was integrated into the EnSite systems. The CF technology and the use of lesion assessment tools are currently essential components of a modern ablation strategy. In addition to this catheter technology and the tools for lesion assessment, EnSite Precision is capable of quickly and automatically annotating and visualizing arrhythmias. For this purpose, automation tools such as EnSite AutoMap, TurboMap, or SparkleMap are used. For the creation of high-density maps, the multipolar mapping catheter "Advisor HD Grid SE" (Abbott, MN, USA) is available. This diagnostic catheter allows for bipolar recordings parallel and perpendicular to the splines over 16 electrodes. The catheter is successfully used endocardially and epicardially.

EnSite Precision also offers tools for image integration. With the "EnSite Fusion" module, magnetic resonance imaging (MRI) or computed tomography (CT) data can be fused with electro-anatomical maps using corresponding reference points. The EnSite Verismo segmentation tool enables the segmentation and 3D reconstruction of heart models from layer-based MRI or CT data.

The system is capable of working with non-fluoroscopic catheter tracking systems such as MediGuide to enable nearly fluoroscopy-free treatment of cardiac arrhythmias (Sommer et al. 2018).

At the beginning of 2022, the new cardiac mapping platform "EnSite X EP" was approved. This system includes the proprietary EnSite Omnipolar Technology (OT), which enables 360° mapping to generate better and "true" electrograms (EGM) with the Advisor HD Grid catheter. In a series of triangles between three electrodes, the omnidirectional electrical signals flowing through them are captured. Additionally, the speed and direction of the electrical signals are quantitatively evaluated and visualized using colors and arrows. This provides very detailed images, regardless of the orientation of the inserted catheter. The 360° sampling of EGMs by the EnSite X EP system (see Fig. 6.3) allows the representation of 1 million points with local information, which can help identify precise ablation targets. The EnSite X system with EnSite OT technology combines unipolar and bipolar measurement principles to maximize data acquisition.

6.4 Rhythmia

The Rhythmia HDx Mapping System (Boston Scientific, MA, USA) is one of the latest high-resolution three-dimensional (3D) mapping systems. It consists of four main components: the signal station, the software, the IntellaMap Orion catheter, and the localization system.

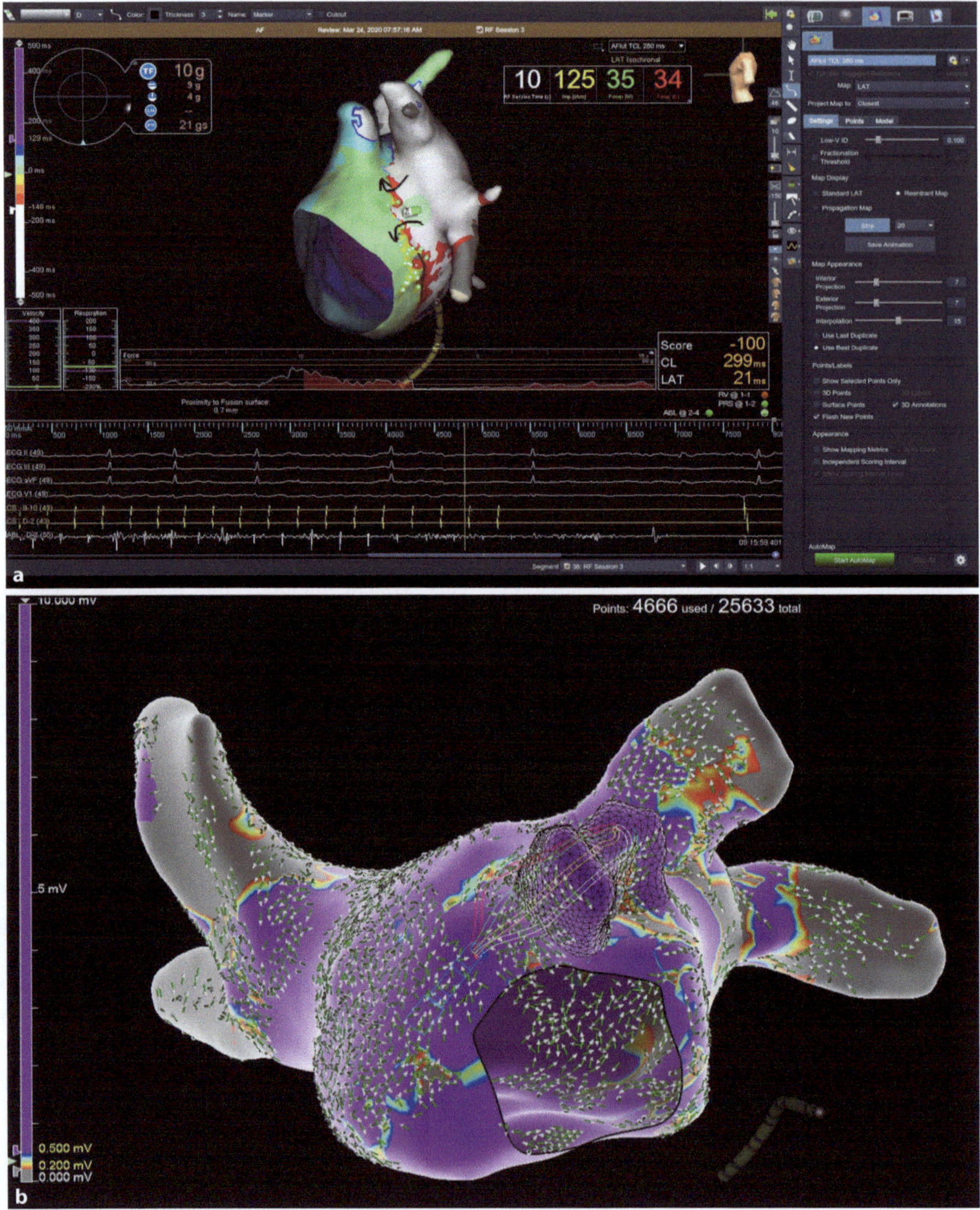

Fig. 6.3 EnSite Precision and EnSite X EP. **a** LAT map of atypical left atrial flutter using EnSite Precision with termination under ablation. View from the left lateral. **b** 3D and voltage map of the left atrium using EnSite X EP with omnipolar technology (OT) and the Advisor HD Grid mapping catheter

The signal station offers advanced signal processing with filters that enable the recording of clear signals with low noise and reduced artifacts. Up to 200 intracardiac channels are supported. It provides easy connectivity to the IntellaMap Orion catheter as well as to other compatible third-party electrophysiological catheters. Rhythmia uses a hybrid tracking technology similar to CARTO and EnSite Precision, which combines both impedance-based and magnetic field data. A special electrode is applied as a patch on the patient's back and serves as a reference electrode. The IntellaMap Orion catheter is used for creating high-resolution maps. This bidirectional 8.5″ 8-spline basket catheter is designed for the rapid acquisition and visualization of intracardiac signals. Attached to these splines are 64 flat, low-noise, iridium oxide-coated microelectrodes with an area of 0.4 mm² each and a spacing of 2.5 mm. Each electrode can be located based on impedance, and an additional magnetic field sensor at the catheter tip allows the localization of the catheter with an accuracy of < 1 mm in space (Sohns et al. 2016). The diameter of the 23 mm long catheter can be varied between 3 and 22 mm, allowing adaptation to the respective anatomical conditions. The catheter can be used with both non-steerable and steerable sheaths for better maneuverability. The Rhythmia HDx 0.01 mV noise floor has a very favorable signal-to-noise ratio. Low background noise allows for very good processing of low-amplitude signals, thus facilitating the differentiation of electrical tissue properties (Ellermann et al. 2018).

In high-density mapping, numerous local electrograms are recorded and processed in a short time. For Rhythmia, there is no upper limit on collected points. The surface geometry of the heart chamber is continuously created based on the position of the outermost electrodes, adjusted for movements due to the respiratory and cardiac cycles. The Rhythmia system offers an efficient algorithm for automatic annotation. This annotation is based on four defined trigger and seven beat acceptance criteria. The trigger criteria determine which electrograms need to be analyzed and which need to be filtered out. The acceptance criteria ensure a distinction between a specific arrhythmia and other rhythm disturbances. All criteria must be met for recording.

This continuous automatic mapping is very accurate. Mantziari published in 2015 that 99.98% of all points were correctly annotated (Mantziari et al. 2015). To determine the temporal activation, the Rhythmia system combines the acquisition of unipolar and bipolar signals, thus enabling the elimination of far-field signals. The electrogram timing is based on the maximum negative $\mathrm{d}V/\mathrm{d}t$ of the unipolar electrograms or the maximum amplitude of the bipolar signals. For fractionated signals, the temporal activation component of the surrounding signals is included in the calculation. However, manual annotation is possible. After successful ablation, the Rhythmia HDx validation mapping (vMap™) can create validation maps in a short time, which help in assessing the ablation, detecting gaps, and confirming the procedural endpoints.

Hindricks et al. demonstrated in the TRUE-HD study that both the rate of ablation-related complications and the success with the use of Rhythmia correspond to the range of adverse events reported in the literature for endocardial ablation of arrhythmias (Bollmann et al. 2018). The acute success rate depends on the type of arrhythmia and ranged between 64 and 96%. In direct comparison with another high-resolution mapping system, CARTO, there is no difference in terms of procedure duration and acute success in pulmonary vein isolation (PVI), only the time required for mapping was slightly extended. There are no data for a direct comparison with the EnSite Precision system.

The advantages of HD mapping for differentiating the electrical tissue properties and the dynamics of ongoing arrhythmias are obvious, and it does not seem to matter whether a map is created with an Orion, a Pentaray, or an HD Grid catheter or other high-resolution mapping catheters.

Unique to the Rhythmia system is the Directsense technology. The electrode design of the IntellaNav MIFI (MicroFidelity) ablation catheter with open irrigation is used to enable local impedance measurement at the tip of the catheter and incorporate this data into the ablation information. This allows the investigator to monitor the effects of the radiofrequency ablation in real-time (Sulkin et al. 2018). This technology distinguishes the catheter from the IntellaNav-ST catheter.

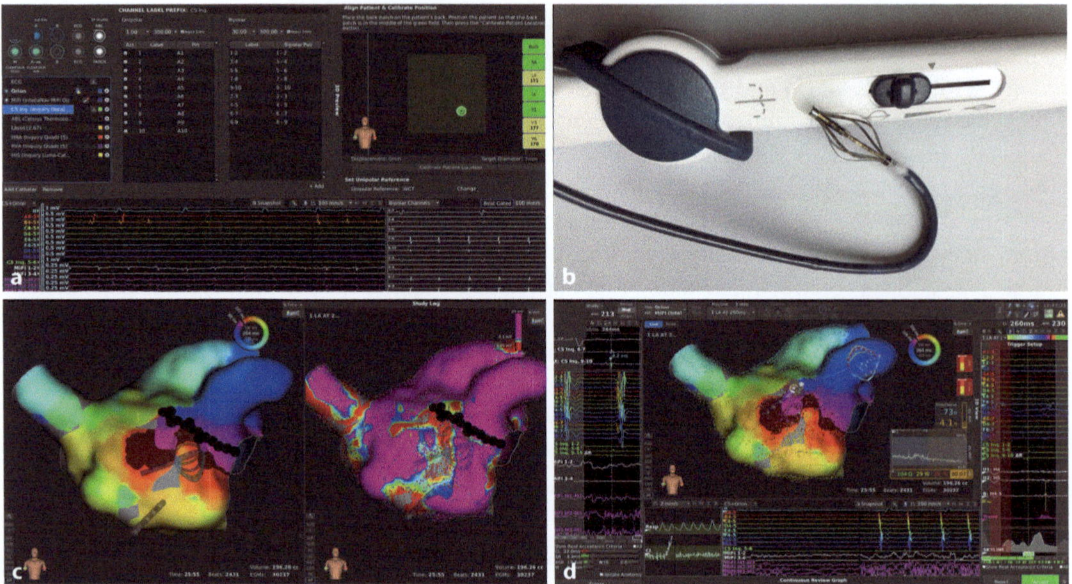

Fig. 6.4 Rhythmia HDx mapping system. **a** User Interface. **b** Orion catheter. **c** Ablation of atypical left atrial flutter. The electroanatomical reconstruction of the left atrium and the mapping of the local activation time (LAT) as well as the corresponding visualization of the local signal amplitude (Voltage Map) show areas with low signal amplitude on the anterior wall and the ablation line that leads to the termination of this tachycardia (**d**)

The IntellaNav-Stablepoint catheter with DIRECTSENSE technology is a navigable CF catheter on a Total-Tip-Cooling platform (see Fig. 6.4). In 2018, the Lumipoint software module for Rhythmia HDx was released, a first suite of tools for automatic map analysis, enabling quick and reliable interpretation of maps.

▶ The modern 3D mapping systems and the current catheter technology enable increasing accuracy and automation of electroanatomical reconstruction, annotation of intracardiac signals, and high-quality lesion formation. This increases the success of ablation with high safety for patients while simultaneously reducing the need for fluoroscopy. Intensive research in the field of invasive electrophysiology and the rapid introduction of innovative technologies have made this treatment method indispensable in cardiology in recent years. In this very dynamic area of technological development, further innovations are to be expected, which are likely to contribute to even higher effectiveness and safety of the procedures.

References

Bertagnolli L, Torri F, Richter S, Dinov B, Müssigbrodt A, Arya A, Hilbert S (2018) Three-dimensional mapping : special aspects and new features of CARTO. Herzschrittmacherther Elektrophysiol 29(3):259–263. https://doi.org/10.1007/s00399-018-0583-x

Bollmann A, Hindricks G, Maury P, Tung R, Raciti G, Weiner S, Mounsey JP (2018) 527Safety and acute effectiveness of the 3D RHYTHMIA mapping system for ablation of arrhythmias: results of the TRUE-HD study. Europace 20(suppl_1):i101–i101. https://doi.org/10.1093/europace/euy015.294

Borlich M, Sommer P (2019) Cardiac mapping systems: rhythmia, topera, ensite precision, and CARTO. Card Electrophysiol Clin 11(3):449–458. https://doi.org/10.1016/j.ccep.2019.05.006

Bourier F, Gianni C, Dare M, Deisenhofer I, Hessling G, Reents T, Al-Ahmad A (2017) Fiberoptic contact-force sensing electrophysiological catheters: how precise is the technology? J Cardiovasc Electrophysiol 28(1):109–114. https://doi.org/10.1111/jce.13100

Ellermann C, Frommeyer G, Eckardt L (2018) High-resolution 3D mapping : opportunities and limitations of the Rhythmia™ mapping system. Herzschrittmacherther Elektrophysiol 29(3):284–292. https://doi.org/10.1007/s00399-018-0580-0

Issa Z, Miller JM, Zipes DP (2018) Clinical arrhythmology and electrophysiology E-book: a companion to Braunwald's heart disease. Elsevier

Mantziari L, Butcher C, Kontogeorgis A, Panikker S, Roy K, Markides V, Wong T (2015) Utility of a novel rapid high-resolution mapping system in the catheter ablation of arrhythmias: an initial human experience of mapping the atria and the left ventricle. JACC Clin Electrophysiol 1(5):411–420. https://doi.org/10.1016/j.jacep.2015.06.002

Sohns C, Saguner AM, Lemes C, Santoro F, Mathew S, Heeger C, Metzner A (2016) First clinical experience using a novel high-resolution electroanatomical mapping system for left atrial ablation procedures. Clin Res Cardiol 105(12):992–1002. https://doi.org/10.1007/s00392-016-1008-7

Sommer P, Bertagnolli L, Kircher S, Arya A, Bollmann A, Richter S, Hindricks G (2018) Safety profile of near-zero fluoroscopy atrial fibrillation ablation with non-fluoroscopic catheter visualization: experience from 1000 consecutive procedures. Europace. https://doi.org/10.1093/europace/eux378

Sulkin MS, Laughner JI, Hilbert S, Kapa S, Kosiuk J, Younan P, Bollmann A (2018) Novel measure of local impedance predicts catheter-tissue contact and lesion formation. Circ Arrhythm Electrophysiol 11(4):e5831. https://doi.org/10.1161/CIRCEP.117.005831

den Uijl DW, Tops LF, Tolosana JM, Schuijf JD, Trines SA, Zeppenfeld K, Schalij MJ (2008) Real-time integration of intracardiac echocardiography and multislice computed tomography to guide radiofrequency catheter ablation for atrial fibrillation. Heart Rhythm 5(10):1403–1410. https://doi.org/10.1016/j.hrthm.2008.07.020

Supraventricular Tachycardias

Daniel Steven and Lars Eckardt

7.1 Introduction

Catheter ablation for the treatment of cardiac arrhythmias began in the mid-1980s with the therapy of accessory pathways (atrioventricular reentrant tachycardias, AVRT) using direct current treatment. This was followed by the therapy of AV node reentrant tachycardias (AVNRT) and focal atrial tachycardias. Today, due to the similar or even identical clinical symptoms, all AV node-dependent tachycardias (AVNRT/AVRT) as well as focal atrial tachycardias are collectively referred to as paroxysmal supraventricular tachycardias (SVT), which are predominantly prognostically benign rhythm disorders.

Supplementary Information The online version contains supplementary material available at https://doi.org/10.1007/978-3-662-65797-3_7. The videos can be accessed individually by clicking the DOI link in the accompanying figure caption or by scanning this link with the SN More Media App.

D. Steven (✉)
Abteilung für Elektrophysiologie, Herzzentrum der Uniklinik Köln, Köln, Germany
e-mail: daniel.steven@uk-koeln.de

L. Eckardt
Klinik für Kardiologie II: Rhythmologie, Universitätsklinikum Münster, Münster, Germany
e-mail: Lars.eckardt@ukmuenster.de

In most cases, a narrow QRS complex is found in the surface ECG of these patients, as ventricular activation occurs antegradely via the AV node. Exceptions such as an AV reentrant tachycardia with antegrade ventricular activation via the accessory pathway (antidromic AVRT) and a pre-existing or frequency-dependent bundle branch block can also lead to a wide QRS complex in the surface ECG in the case of an SVT.

In addition to the characteristic findings in the surface ECG, it is primarily the anamnesis details, such as age at first manifestation, type and frequency of occurrence, duration, and termination, that characterize an SVT. Moreover, patients with an SVT usually do not have structural heart disease. We will address typical anamnesis indications in the further course. However, it is important in this context that in the case of an unclear wide complex tachycardia, a ventricular tachycardia should always be assumed first, and that in the case of hemodynamic instability, rhythmization should be performed immediately, if necessary, using electrical cardioversion.

▶ AV node-dependent tachycardias (AVNRT/AVRT) as well as focal atrial tachycardias are collectively referred to as paroxysmal supraventricular tachycardias (SVT). These are predominantly prognostically benign rhythm disorders.

7.2 Mechanisms

The details of the SVT mechanisms are discussed in more detail in the following Chap. 8 –10. In summary, AV node-dependent tachycardias are based on a reentrant excitation. This occurs within the AV node in AV node reentrant tachycardia. In AV reentrant tachycardia, the atrium, ventricle, AV node, and an accessory pathway are involved in the reentrant excitation. Focal atrial tachycardias are focal tachycardias where increased automaticity of a group of atrial myocardial cells leads to a focal cardiac arrhythmia originating from the atrial myocardium. The two main mechanisms are therefore reentry and increased automaticity (Delacrétaz 2006). Reference is made here to Chap. 1, where the mechanisms of cardiac arrhythmias are described in detail.

7.3 Patient Selection and Preliminary Examination

Patients with an SVT usually present as emergency patients or consult their general practitioner or cardiologist due to complaints. These typically include a long-standing history of regular palpitations. Patients often report a sudden onset and equally sudden end of episodes (so-called "on-off" phenomenon) with sometimes very high pulse rates up to 250/min. Many patients report successfully terminating the palpitations using vagal maneuvers, which suggests the presence of AVNRT/AVRT. In the case of AVNRT, patients often notice a pounding in the neck (*"frog sign"*), which can be explained by venous reflux during atrial contraction against closed AV valves. In addition to these classic symptoms, episodic nonspecific complaints such as chest tightness, dizziness, dyspnea, or similar may also occur.

The anamnestic differentiation between AVNRT/AVRT and focal atrial tachycardias is difficult. Atrial tachycardias often occur repetitively at shorter intervals. Vagal maneuvers often lead to no changes. In contrast to AVNRT/AVRT, patients sometimes report a gradual onset and subsiding of SVT episodes (*"warming-up/cooling-down"*).

The indication for an electrophysiological study usually arises from the patient's desire for a non-pharmacological and curative therapy. A purely diagnostic electrophysiological study is a rarity in this context. An electrophysiological study (EPS) should always be performed with readiness for ablation. An ECG documentation is desirable. In the case of frequent, relatively short episodes, an external event recorder or a smartwatch can be helpful in attempting documentation. If documentation is not possible due to short or rare episodes, an EPS should not be omitted in the case of a typical anamnesis. Given the low complication rate, the threshold for an EPS and ablation is low nowadays.

7.4 ECG Differentiation

In principle, the presence of the SVT mechanism can only be estimated from the surface ECG; the actual definitive differentiation occurs in the invasive examination. Nevertheless, the episode ECG provides important information that is crucial for procedure planning (e.g., use of a 3D mapping system).

The classification is based on the visibility or distinguishability of the P-waves in relation to the QRS complex into short-RP and long-RP tachycardias. A short-RP tachycardia is present when the P-wave falls before the imaginary midline between two QRS complexes, meaning the RP interval is shorter than the PR interval (RP < PR). The short-RP tachycardias are further subdivided into very short RP (< 90 ms) and short RP > 90 ms.

In very short-RP tachycardias or if no P-waves are visible at all (and an overlap by the QRS complex is assumed), the presence of a typical AVNRT – also due to its more frequent occurrence – is to be assumed.

In short-RP tachycardias > 90 ms, a typical AVNRT is unlikely; an orthodromic AVRT, an atypical (i.e., fast-slow or slow-slow) AVNRT, or a focal atrial tachycardia may be present.

In long-RP tachycardias , the presence of a focal atrial tachycardia is most likely; rarer differential diagnoses here are AVRT or atypical AVNRT.

Furthermore, it is true that in a (typical or atypical) AVNRT, the excitation of the atrium occurs from the AV node, so the P-wave in the inferior leads II, III, and aVF has a negative polarity. Positive P-waves in the inferior leads exclude an AVNRT.

Furthermore, in any ECG constellation, the presence of a focal atrial tachycardia is theoretically possible, as the AV node is passively excited here and is not part of the tachycardia cycle. The RP or PR interval here depends on the distance of the focus from the AV node as well as the conduction properties of the atrial myocardium and the AV node.

7.5 Significance of the EPS

The goal of an EPS is to identify the exact cause of an SVT and to perform targeted therapy. The main differential diagnoses here, in addition to AVNRT/AVRT, include FAT, atrial flutter, and atrial fibrillation. The individual entities and their specific aspects are discussed in further chapters of this book. According to the authors, there is only a place for a purely diagnostic EPS in individual cases today, e.g., in suspected ventricular tachycardia in a patient with a previous infarction with syncope or documented non-sustained ventricular tachycardias with moderately impaired LV function (LV-EF between 35 and 40%).

7.6 Conducting an EPS

In most electrophysiological laboratories, a total of three to four sheaths are positioned for the examination, for example, 2–3 in the left femoral vein (e.g., 4–8 Fr) and 1–2 in the right femoral vein. Catheters for diagnostics are then positioned through these sheaths. On the one hand, a 2- to 4-pole catheter is positioned in the right atrial appendage (alternatively a multipolar

catheter in the coronary sinus), and another 2- to 4-pole catheter is placed in the right ventricle. For localization and diagnostics, a multipolar catheter (so-called His catheter) is also positioned septally in the area of the His or AV node. The position ideally results in a proximal atrial signal and a distal ventricular signal being recorded in addition to the His signal. In the presence of a left-sided rhythm disorder, e.g., an accessory pathway along the mitral valve annulus or a left atrial tachycardia, the positioning of a multipolar catheter in the coronary venous sinus may also be required.

The management of anticoagulation varies significantly between centers. Controlled data do not exist. In many cases, heparin is administered during procedures in the right atrium. Typically, 2500–5000 I.U. of heparin is administered intravenously after the placement of the sheaths. For mapping/ablation in the left atrium (left atrial tachycardia, left-sided accessory pathway), heparin administration should be ACT-controlled. Here, an activated clotting time (*"activated clotting time"*, ACT) of 250–300 s is recommended. Sedation is performed depending on the center, e.g., with propofol and fentanyl, possibly additionally with midazolam. Continuous monitoring of oxygen saturation, blood pressure, and heart rhythm is mandatory and required throughout the entire procedure. All membrane-active antiarrhythmics as well as beta-blockers and calcium antagonists should be discontinued at least two half-lives before the EPS, if necessary even under inpatient conditions.

7.6.1 Basic EPS

In principle, there are internally established protocols for conducting a basic EPS. At this point, the step-by-step procedure is described as an example:

1. Determination of intracardiac baseline intervals (AH, HV, possibly intra-atrial conduction HRA to His-A) in sinus rhythm.
2. Retrograde conduction (IVP = incremental ventricular pacing, retrograde Wenckebach):

Starting from CL 600 ms, shortening the CL in 10 ms steps until the loss of VA conduction. Question of concentric or eccentric atrial activation (Fig. 7.1).

3. Programmed retrograde stimulation: Stimulation with baseline cycle length, e.g., 600 ms, coupling of an S2 at e.g., 450 ms with a decrease of the S2 intervals by 10 ms per cycle. Determination of VA conduction, question of decremental conduction, possibly retrograde dual conduction (VA jump).

4. Antegrade conduction (IAP = incremental atrial pacing, atrial Wenckebach). Stimulation with baseline cycle length 600 ms, shortening in 10 ms steps, determining the atrial Wenckebach point. Question of preexcitation (HV time, QRS morphology) (Fig. 7.2).

5. Programmed antegrade stimulation with a basic cycle length of, e.g., 600 ms; coupling of S2 (up to S4); shortening by 10 ms per cycle, question of dual AV conduction (jump, electrical longitudinal dissociation) with prolongation of the AH time by $\geq$ 50 ms with shortening of the S2 interval by 10 ms and, if necessary, induction of tachycardia (Figs. 7.3 and 7.4).

6. If necessary, repeat after pharmacological provocation (atropine, isoprenaline, orciprenaline, adenosine), especially in the case of VA block under baseline conditions.

▶ The standardized procedure of an electrophysiological study should be internalized and its execution should not be neglected in favor of a quick start of ablation.

7.6.2 Intracardiac Findings

In the case of inducibility of clinical tachycardia, the assessment of the temporal sequence of atrial and ventricular activation can already provide a clue to the genesis of the rhythm disorder. For example, if the atrium is excited late at the septum during tachycardia in an SVT with a narrow QRS complex, a typical AV nodal reentrant tachycardia is unlikely. Other indications often arise from the AV nodal conduction properties. In AV nodal reentrant tachycardia, dual AV nodal conduction properties are usually detectable. Here, extrastimulation with an

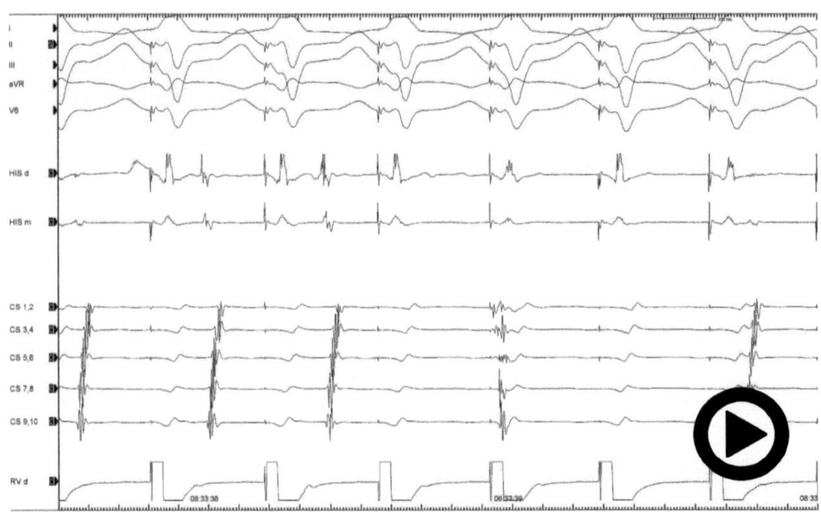

Fig. 7.1 IVP/retrograde Wenckebach stimulation: Stimulation at the RV apex with gradual shortening of the stimulated cycle length until the loss of 1:1 VA conduction. Note/determine the retrograde Wenckebach point or frequency. Incidentally, after the loss of 1:1 VA conduction, a left atrial extrasystole (CS 1,2 leading) is found (https://doi.org/10.1007/000-d2k)

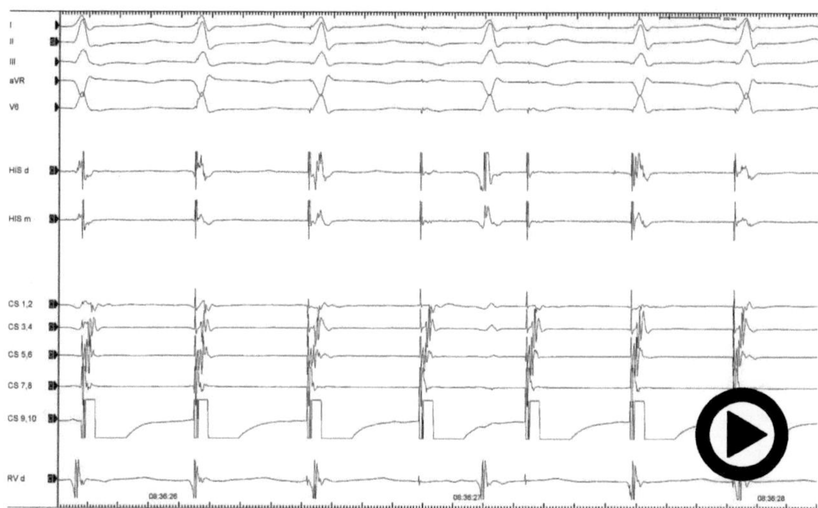

Fig. 7.2 IAP/antegrade Wenckebach stimulation: Stimulation in the proximal CS (alternatively HRA) until the loss of antegrade 1:1 AV conduction. Note/determine the antegrade Wenckebach point or frequency (https://doi.org/10.1007/000-d2j)

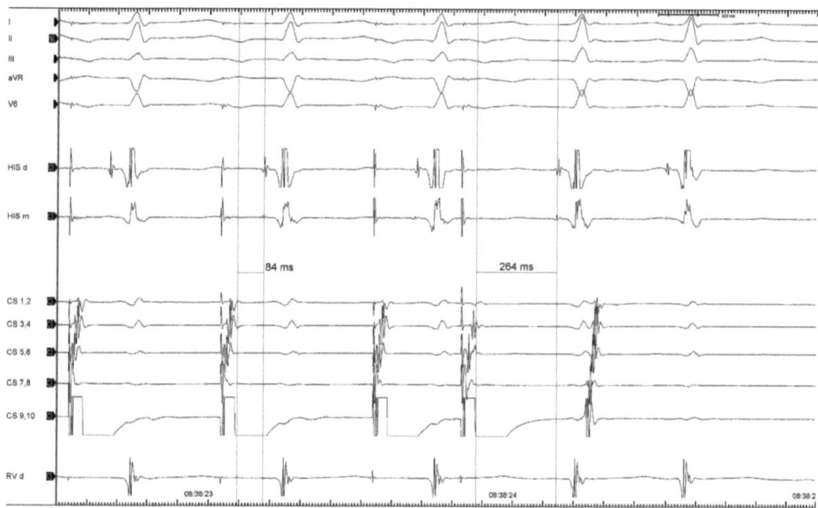

Fig. 7.3 AH jump: Exemplary representation of the AH jump: Under baseline conditions (S1 stimulation from the proximal CS), an AH time of 84 ms is found. After shortly coupled S2, an extension of the AH time to 264 ms is found. An AH jump (*jump*) is spoken of if the AH time increases abruptly from one stimulation cycle to the next with a 10 ms shorter coupling of S2 by at least 50 ms (not shown here, see video)

extrastimulus coupled 10 ms shorter leads to an abrupt increase in AH time by more than 50 ms (AH jump, "jump"). This so-called dual AV nodal conduction property is a prerequisite for the presence of AV nodal reentrant tachycardia. If the tachycardia occurs simultaneously with the presence of this AH jump, the presence of AV nodal reentrant tachycardia is very likely.

Just as a short VA interval (< 70 ms) during tachycardia very likely indicates AVNRT, a long VA interval (> 70 ms) must primarily suggest the involvement of an accessory pathway. Here, various stimulation maneuvers, primarily ventricular entrainment, can be used to investigate the differential diagnosis. This will be explained in detail in subsequent articles of this book. If

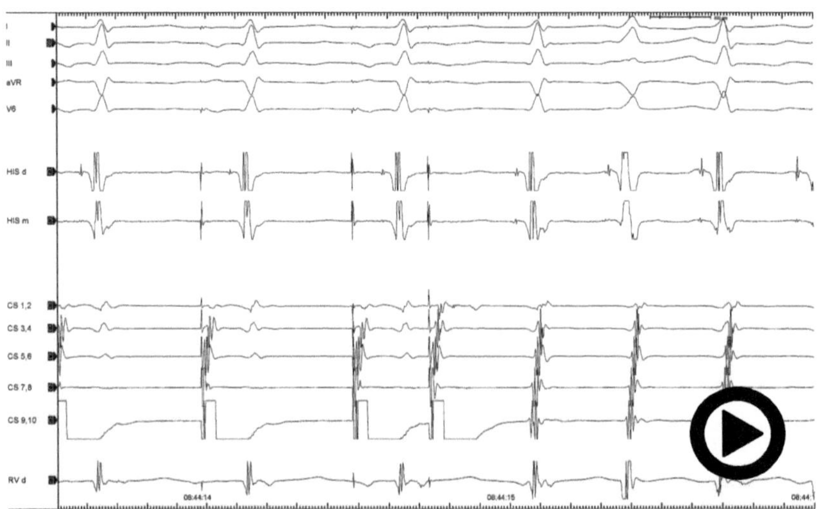

Fig. 7.4 Induction: With further shortening of the S2 coupling interval, antegrade conduction via the *slow pathway* (long AH time) leads to the induction of a typical (slow-fast) AVNRT with a short HA time and thus retrograde conduction via the *fast pathway* (see also video "Induction") (https://doi.org/10.1007/000-d2h)

an SVT with a long VA interval is induced, the placement of a multipolar CS catheter is recommended. In the case of eccentric atrial activation, AVNRT is excluded, and tachycardia via a posterior accessory pathway is very likely (DD focal left atrial tachycardia). The occurrence of VA dissociation in SVT excludes AVRT. Often, stimulation maneuvers are also required for the differential diagnosis of reentry tachycardia versus atrial tachycardia. If focal atrial tachycardia is detected (e.g., with varying AA intervals where ventricular activations follow atrial signals, gradual increase or decrease in cycle lengths ["*warming up*" and "*cooling* down"]), localization is determined using early mapping (so-called activation map, LAT map). Unlike reentry tachycardias, where ablation treatment is mostly performed during sinus rhythm, this requires ongoing tachycardia. Therefore, with difficult induction, the success rate of ablation for focal atrial tachycardia is lower. During the mapping of a FAT, the earliest origin of the tachycardia can be conventionally determined with the ablation catheter by measuring the temporal relationship to a reference. The latter can be chosen individually (e.g., the beginning of the P wave in the surface ECG or intra-atrial signal, such as the atrial appendage or CS ostium) but should be as stable as possible. Nowadays, a 3D mapping

system should always be part of the localization diagnostics. The details of the differential diagnosis are also presented in the specialized chapters of this section (Figs. 7.5 and 7.6).

An overview of the differentiation maneuvers is provided in Table 7.1 .

The SVT visual diagnoses are shown in Tab. 7.2.

In the case of accessory pathways located immediately at the His, some investigators favor focal cryoablation over the radiofrequency ablation otherwise favored in SVT. The success rates for ablation of SVT are up to 98%. Only in focal atrial tachycardias must a recurrence rate of 10-15% be expected depending on mapping conditions.

In principle, for the ablation of an SVT, with generally very good prognosis, a special risk assessment is required. If, for example, there is an increased risk of AV block during the ablation of the SVT (accessory pathway located immediately at the His, complex anatomy, or unusual location of the "*slow pathway*") or a lesion of the phrenic nerve (origin of an atrial tachycardia in the area of the crista terminalis), this should be explicitly discussed with the patient, the procedure possibly aborted, and/or a staged approach or referral to a particularly experienced clinic considered.

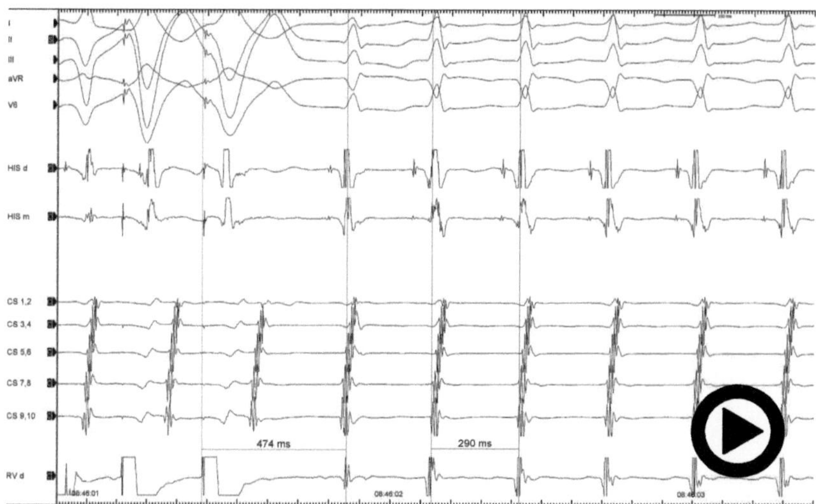

Fig. 7.5 PPI RV: Ventricular *Overdrive pacing* during ongoing typical AVNRT: After the end of ventricular stimulation, a VV interval of 474 ms is found with a tachycardia cycle length of 290 ms. The difference of 184 ms argues against AVRT (PPI-TCL > 115 ms). Furthermore, after the end of stimulation, a VAV sequence is found, which argues against FAT (then VAAV sequence) (https://doi.org/10.1007/000-d2m)

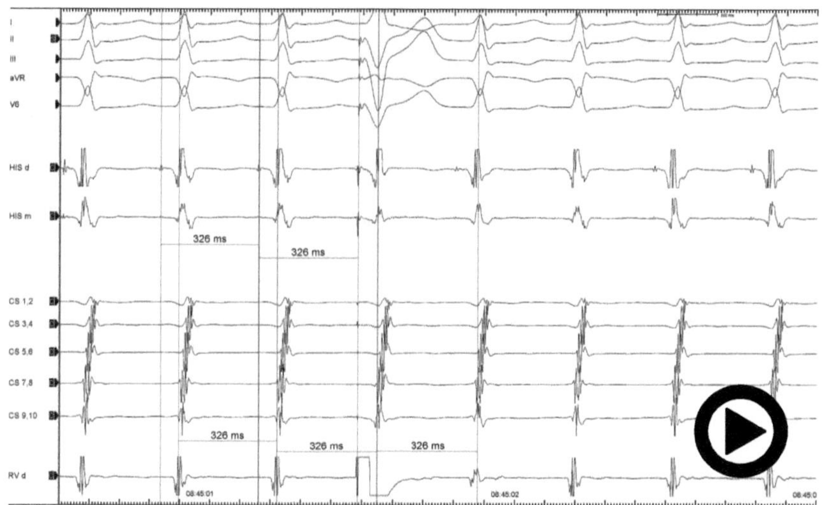

Fig. 7.6 PVC on His with marker/*Preceding*: During ongoing tachycardia, a stimulus is delivered via the His catheter with a refractory His bundle. Here, attention must be paid to ventricular capture (recognizable by the deformed QRS complex in the surface ECG). The AA intervals before and after the stimulus are determined. Here, no advancement of the next atrial activation is found (during ongoing typical AVNRT). This is referred to as negative preceding (see also video "Preceding") (https://doi.org/10.1007/000-d2n)

Tab. 7.1 Differentiation maneuvers

Name	Question	Procedure	Difficulties	**Findings**
Ventricular *Overdrive Pacing*/Ventricular Entrainment/Michaud I	What is the tachycardia sequence if the tachycardia continues?	Stimulation in the RV-A about 20 ms faster than TCL. Pay attention to atrial entrainment. Stop stimulation and record the sequence	Termination of tachycardia possible	VAV in AVNRT, AVRT VAAV in FAT
Ventricular Overdrive Pacing/Ventricular Entrainment/Michaud II	Is the ventricular myocardium part of the excitation circuit?	Like VOP. After stopping the stimulation, measure the interval from stimulus to ventricular excitation (= PPI). Subtract PPI-TCL	Termination of tachycardia possible	PPI-TCL < 115 ms in AVRT PPI-TCL > 115 ms in AVNRT, FAT (ventricle not part of the reentry)
Ventricular Overdrive Pacing/Ventricular Entrainment/Michaud III	Are atrium and ventricle activated in parallel or sequentially?	Like VOP. Determine the intervals between stimulus (S) and atrium (A) and native ventricular excitation (V) and A and subtract: SA-VA	Termination of tachycardia possible. Not possible if retrograde conduction is absent	SA-VA > 85 ms in AVNRT SA-VA < 85 ms in AVRT
Preceding/PVC on His	Is the ventricular myocardium part of the excitation process?	During ongoing tachycardia, deliver V-stimulus during His refractoriness. Determine A-A intervals	Termination possible. False positive if stimulus is delivered too early (before His refractoriness)	Advancement (= Preceding) of the next atrial excitation positive in AVRT. Negative in AVNRT, FAT
Parahisian pacing	Is there a septal accessory pathway?	Stimulation at the His (in SR) with different output and generation of 2 QRS morphologies: narrow (His+V capture) & wide (V capture only). Determine VA intervals	Distorted by fusion beats or extrasystoles	VA(His+V) ≪ VA(V) argues against septal pathway VA(His+V) = VA(V) in septal pathway

Tab. 7.2 Visual diagnoses in SVT

Distal CS is activated before proximal CS during tachycardia (or V-pace) (eccentric CS sequence, occasionally *"bracketing"*)	Proof of left-sided accessory pathway
Eccentric atrial activation during tachycardia (HRA is activated before the A on the His catheter)	Excludes AVNRT
Lack of conduction of a beat to the ventricles	Excludes AVRT
Non-decremental (retrograde) conduction	Suggestive of accessory pathway
Change in AA interval precedes a corresponding change in VV interval *"AA predicts VV"*	Suggestive of FAT
P waves with inferior axis	Excludes AVNRT
Increase in cycle length > 30 ms with the occurrence of a bundle branch block (or decrease with cessation of the block) = Coumel phenomenon	Suggestive of ipsilateral accessory pathway

7.6.3 Empirical Slow-Pathway Modulation

Even with documented, symptomatic tachycardia, corresponding rhythm disturbances are not always inducible during the EPU. In such a situation, the question arises whether a slow-pathway modulation should be performed with the – albeit small – risk of an AV block. Frequently, this is done according to the guidelines when there is typical documentation and dual conduction properties, even if the control conditions are difficult. In the absence of documentation of tachycardia and the presence of dual AV node physiology but with a typical history, it must be decided on a case-by-case basis whether AV modulation appears justified (Pott et al. 2015).

7.6.4 Ablation of an Accessory Pathway

In patients with pre-excitation and tachycardias (WPW syndrome) or tachycardia-conducted atrial fibrillation involving an accessory pathway (FBI tachycardia; *Fast-Broad-Irregular*), the indication for ablation of an accessory pathway is clearly given. The situation is different for patients with an asymptomatic accessory pathway. Here, the prognostic benefit of ablation is controversial (Obeyesekere and Klein 2014). Current data show that in the long-term (median follow-up: 8 years), 1.5% of all patients with an accessory pathway develop significant, potentially dangerous arrhythmias and ventricular fibrillation. However, this had no impact on mortality in a study of 2169 patients (Pappone et al. 2014). Due to the low periprocedural risk, ablation is often considered today in asymptomatic patients. While traditionally non-invasive stress tests (ergometry) were used to assess the conduction properties of accessory pathways, the reliability of this determination is moderate and the results often variable over time. Therefore, invasive risk stratification is currently recommended to determine the refractory period. In the case of high-risk features such as a refractory period ≤ 250 ms; the identification of multiple accessory pathways or the inducibility of tachycardias, ablation treatment should then be performed. Here, the location and thus the estimated procedural risk as well as the experience of the investigators should be taken into account. In the case of low-risk features, clinical follow-up is recommended. Alternatively, direct catheter ablation can be considered (Brugada et al. 2020).

However, it should always be noted that the conduction properties of the accessory pathway can vary. In case of doubt (e.g., in the presence of atrial fibrillation), ablation of the accessory pathway should always be performed.

7.7 Complications

The complications of the examination are primarily in bleeding at the puncture site. Since patients with SVT are much less frequently anticoagulated than patients with atrial fibrillation or atrial flutter, these are rare. The same applies to the occurrence of pericardial tamponade, which can be reported in this cohort with a frequency of $< 0.5\%$. The frequency of an AV block requiring subsequent pacemaker implantation is less than 1%, as is the incidence of phrenic nerve lesions with consequent diaphragmatic paralysis. In the case of left-sided ablation, neurological complications should also be discussed, although these are overall very rare given the described ablation and time effort.

7.8 After the Ablation

Following a successful ablation, depending on the control conditions and the course of the ablation, a waiting period and, if necessary, control stimulation of 15–30 minutes should be observed. During this waiting period, the sustained success of the ablation should be monitored. In patients with AV node reentrant tachycardia, this seems to be unnecessary (Steven et al. 2009). The administration of isoproterenol after ablation to verify the success of the ablation is often performed. Post-procedure follow-up in most clinics also includes echocardiographic exclusion of pericardial effusion. Some centers recommend taking aspirin for several weeks after SVT ablation to prevent thrombotic deposits at the ablation site. However, there are no controlled data on this.

References

Brugada J et al (2020) 2019 ESC Guidelines for the management of patients with supraventricular tachycardia. Eur Heart J 41:655–720

Delacrétaz E (2006) Clinical practice. Supraventricular tachycardia. N Engl J Med 354:1039–1051

Obeyesekere MN, Klein GJ (2014) The asymptomatic Wolff-Parkinson-White patient: time to be more proactive. Circulation 130:805–807

Pappone C et al (2014) Wolff-Parkinson-white syndrome in the era of catheter ablation. Circulation 130:811–819

Pott C, Wegner F, Bögeholz N (2015) Outcome predictors of empirical slow pathway modulation: Clinical and procedural characteristics and long-term follow-up. Clin Res Cardiol 104:946–954

Steven D et al (2009) Favorable outcome using an abbreviated procedure for catheter ablation of AVNRT: results from a prospective randomized trial. J Cardiovasc Electrophysiol 20:522–525

Diagnosis and Therapy of AV Nodal Reentrant Tachycardia

Christian von Bary and Charalampos Kriatselis

8.1 Epidemiology and Clinic

The AV nodal reentrant tachycardia (AVNRT) is the most common regular supraventricular tachycardia in clinical practice. The cardiac arrhythmia with a typical heart rate between 150–220/min occurs particularly in middle-aged women (ratio f:m 2:1), but it can also occur in other age groups (Liuba et al. 2006; Steven et al. 2015). Clinically, the AVNRT is characterized by a sudden onset and a sudden end (On/Off phenomenon). Valsalva maneuvers or the administration of adenosine can terminate the cardiac arrhythmia.

▶ In the diagnosis of AVNRT, a precise medical history is of essential importance.

8.2 Pathophysiology

The AVNRT is pathophysiologically based on dual AV nodal conduction with a slow (so-called "Slow Pathway" = SP) and a fast conducting

C. von Bary (✉)
Klinik für Innere Medizin I – Kardiologie und Pneumologie, Rotkreuzklinikum München, München, Germany
e-mail: christian.vonbary@swmbrk.de

C. Kriatselis
Klinik für Innere Medizin – Kardiologie, Angiologie, Nephrologie und konservative Intensivmedizin, Vivantes Klinikum Neukölln, Berlin, Germany
e-mail: charalampos.kriatselis@vivantes.de

component (so-called "Fast Pathway" = FP). Anatomically, the SP is located in the inferior septum near the coronary sinus (CS) ostium, and the FP is located in the area of the superior septum at the compact AV node. Both structures are located in the Koch's triangle, which is defined by the following structures: ostium of the CS, septal tricuspid valve, and tendon of Todaro (extension of the Eustachian valve towards the AV node). Precise knowledge of the anatomical structures is mandatory for the successful ablation of AVNRT (see Fig. 8.1).

Electrophysiologically, the SP exhibits a reduced conduction velocity with a relatively short refractory period, while the FP exhibits a higher conduction velocity with a relatively long refractory period. Dual AV node conduction is more about functional conduction properties than specific conduction pathways. The functional duality is explained, among other things, by the phenomenon of "anisotropy." Anisotropy is defined as different conduction velocities in the same tissue, depending on the direction of the electrical excitation front in relation to the orientation of the myocardial fibers. If the electrical excitation runs parallel to the myocardial fibers, the conduction velocity is higher than in a transverse course. Similarly, the refractory period is longer with parallel excitation than with transverse excitation (Kotadia et al. 2020; Spach and Josephson 1994). The extent of anisotropy depends on various factors, such as the expression of gap junction proteins.

L. Iden et al. (eds.), *Invasive Electrophysiology for Beginners*, https://doi.org/10.1007/978-3-662-70158-4_8

Immunohistochemical studies have shown that the gap junction protein CX43 is expressed to varying degrees in the AV node region. Low expression of this "cell-connecting" protein in the area of the inferior parts causes a conduction delay (in the area of the SP), whereas high expression of CX43, for example, in the area of so-called "transitional cells," promotes rapid conduction (in the area of the FP) (Katritsis and Efimov 2019; see Fig. 8.1).

The mentioned conduction properties form the pathophysiological substrate of AVNRT. However, triggers are required to induce an AVNRT. In sinus rhythm, the ventricle is usually excited via the fast conduction pathway. In the case of dual AV node conduction, there is an additional depolarization of the SP, which reaches the His bundle with a delay. Since the His bundle and the FP are refractory due to the preceding depolarization, the excitation front from the SP is blocked here (Fig. 8.1d, *a –c*).

An early atrial extrasystole cannot be conducted due to the longer refractory period in the FP (depolarization of the FP by the preceding sinus action), and only the antegrade depolarization of the SP occurs (Fig. 8.1c, *d*). This results in a sudden prolongation of AV conduction, referred to as an AH jump ("jump"). With slow conduction, the excitation can now be conducted via the His bundle into the ventricle and retrogradely into the atrium via the FP after the refractory period has elapsed. The SP is now excited antegradely again. Thus, the reentry in the sense of a slow-fast AVNRT (typical AVNRT) is closed (see Fig. 8.1c, *e, f*). If such a short circuit occurs only once, it is referred to as an AV nodal echo.

Approximately 6% (Heidbüchel and Jackman 2004; Katritsis et al. 2015) of AVNRTs exhibit an activation pattern that differs from the excitation pattern of "typical" AVNRT (slow-fast). In "atypical" AVNRT, the **retrograde** conduction does not occur via an FP but via an SP. This results in a longer HA interval (> 70 ms). The **antegrade** conduction can occur either via an FP (AH interval < 200 ms, so-called "fast-slow" AVNRT) or via another SP (AH interval $\geq$ 200 ms, so-called "slow-slow" AVNRT). The earliest **retrograde** atrial activation in atypical AVNRT is usually located near the CS ostium(atrial insertion of the SP). In very rare cases, there are also left atrial insertions of the SP, which can only be successfully ablated in the inferoseptal left atrium (Heidbüchel and Jackman 2004; Katritsis et al. 2015).

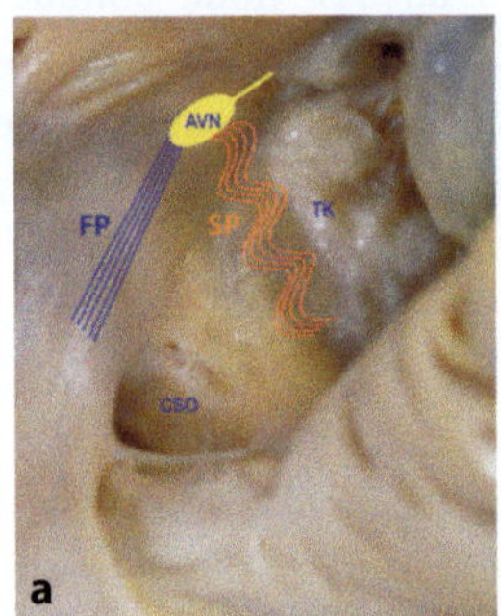

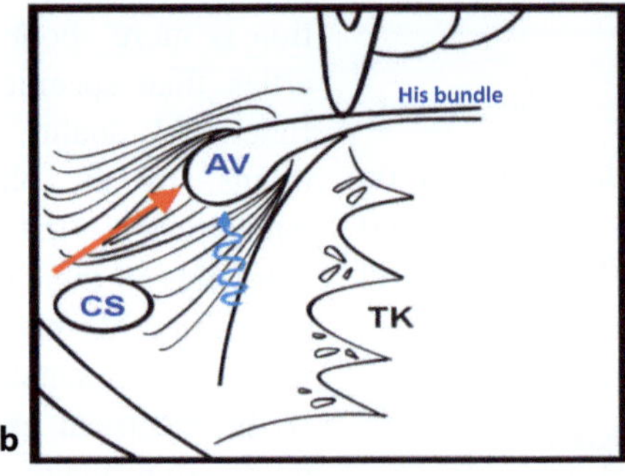

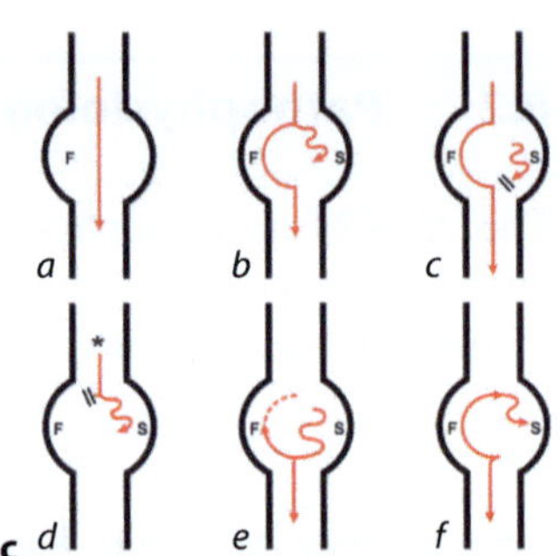

Fig. 8.1 **a** Anatomy of the Koch's triangle, which is defined by the following structures: ostium of the CS (CSO), septal tricuspid valve (TV), and tendon of Todaro (extension of the Eustachian valve towards the compact AV node = AVN). Here, the anatomical location of the FP (*blue*) as well as the SP (*red*) is also shown. **b** Anisotropy in the AV node. The electrical excitation parallel to the fiber orientation (*red arrow*) occurs quickly with a long refractory period, transverse to the fiber orientation (*blue arrow*) slowly with a short refractory period. AV = AV node, CS = coronary sinus, TV = tricuspid valve. **c**a shows a depolarization without AV node duality during sinus rhythm. *b* and *c* with dual conduction pathway in sinus rhythm. *d* to *f* show the induction of slow-fast reentry tachycardia, triggered by an extrasystole. * = extrasystole. F = FP. S = SP. The induction mechanism is explained in detail in the text

▶ In AVNRT, the typical (slow-fast) form is distinguished from the atypical form (slow-slow or fast-slow).

8.3 ECG Criteria

Electrocardiographically, slow-fast AVNRT presents as a regular narrow complex tachycardia with typical frequencies between 150–220/min. In V1, a supposed r′ often appears, which is caused by the retrograde atrial excitation. Also, in the inferior leads, atrial excitation with a superior axis is often visible immediately at the end of the QRS complex. With the termination of the AVNRT, the r′ or the inverse atrial excitation disappears, and the regular P wave is again visible before the QRS complex. In atypical AVNRT, a "long-RP tachycardia" also appears with negative P waves in the inferior leads, which are now clearly distinguishable from the QRS complex and can often be located after the T wave (see Fig. 8.2).

8.4 Electrophysiological Diagnostics and Therapy

The indication for electrophysiological diagnostics in readiness for ablation is given in symptomatic patients with corresponding ECG documentation. However, even in the absence of ECG documentation, an EPU can be pursued in symptomatic patients with characteristic clinical presentation (Aliot et al. 2003; Brugada et al. 2020; Lauschke et al. 2015).

8.4.1 Electrophysiological Study

Differential Diagnoses

The AVNRT exhibits certain characteristics in the EPS, which are explained below. It is necessary to distinguish between the typical and atypical forms. Additionally, the AVNRT must be differentiated from an orthodromic AVRT with an accessory pathway or an atrial tachycardia originating from the inferoseptal atrium or the non-coronary aortic cusp (NCC-AT) using specific stimulation maneuvers (Chokr et al. 2021; Iesaka et al. 1997). A rare differential diagnosis is junctional ectopic tachycardia (JET), which has its focal origin in the His region (Alasti et al. 2020).

▶ The differential diagnoses of AVNRT must be known and excluded during the EPU using specific stimulation maneuvers. A standardized scheme should be followed in this process.

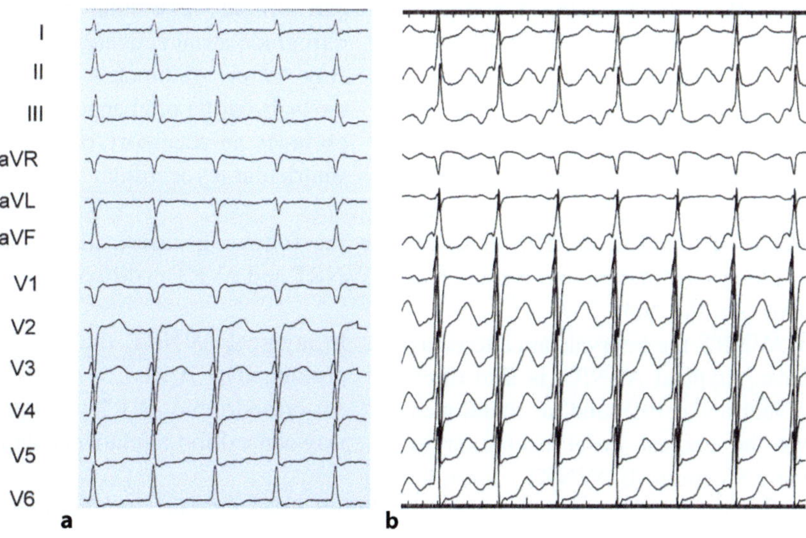

Fig. 8.2 The figure shows a typical (**a**) and an atypical (**b**) (fast-slow) AVNRT. The ECGs are explained in detail in the text

Electrophysiological Findings in AVNRT

In general, during the EPS for suspected AVNRT, diagnostic catheters are positioned in the right ventricular (RV) apex, in the His region, in the high right atrium (high right atrium = HRA) and/or in the CS (see Fig. 8.3; Steven et al. 2015).

First, programmed electrical stimulation (PES) in the ventricle (e.g., S1 500 ms, S2 450 ms, shortening interval S2 by 10 ms each) should be started. The following parameters are assessed: presence of a VA conduction (not infrequently, a VA dissociation is present due to increased vagotonia, which can be resolved by administering adrenergic substances), earliest atrial excitation in the CS (early atrial excitation in the distal CS proves an accessory conduction pathway), decrementality of the VA conduction (conduction delay with shortening of the coupling interval; indicative of retrograde conduction via the AV node), and retrograde Wenckebach point. Subsequently, the anterograde Wenckebach point and atrial PES (e.g., S1 500 ms, S2 450 ms, shortening interval S2 by 10 ms each) are assessed. The following parameters are evaluated by measuring the AH interval: decrementality of the anterograde AV conduction, evidence of an anterograde "jump" (abrupt increase in AH time > 50 ms and thus evidence of dual AV node physiology), and possibly AV nodal echoes. Ideally, an AVNRT with "jump" and typical intracardiac excitation pattern can be induced. Characteristically, typical AVNRT presents with synchronous excitation of the atrium and ventricle and a fusion of atrial and ventricular signals at the His, with the earliest atrial excitation found in the HIS catheter. Additionally, a long AH interval and a short HA interval < 70 ms (see Fig. 8.4).

In atypical AVNRT, the intervals are altered as described above. Atypical AVNRT is also often inducible via ventricular PES and, as mentioned earlier, shows the earliest atrial excitation in the area of the CS ostium. If AVNRT cannot be induced, the following measures can be taken:

1. Administration of orciprenaline/isoprenaline and possibly atropine i.v. (goal: shortening of the retrograde refractory period to < 400 ms)
2. Burst stimulation in the atrium at the Wenckebach point (goal: repetitive blocking of the FP)
3. Additional (S3) or triggered extrastimulus
4. PES in the ventricle

Differentiation of AVNRT vs. orthodromic AVRT with accessory pathway

In most cases, the differentiation between AVNRT and AVRT is simple:

1. Approximately 70% of accessory pathways are located posteriorly (mitral valve annulus, approximately 2–4 o'clock in an LAO projection). In these cases, the earliest retrograde atrial activation is detectable in the distal CS. This may only become visible in sinus rhythm during rapid ventricular stimulation (sequence change in the CS).
2. In typical AVNRT, the HA interval is short (≤ 70 ms), as the His is excited antegradely and the FP retrogradely in quick succession. In AVRT, the earliest atrial activation occurs at the insertion site of the accessory pathway (AP). This extends the HA interval to more than 70 ms, as the excitation first depolarizes part of the ventricular myocardium before retrograde atrial activation can occur.
3. Any AV or VA block without interruption of the tachycardia or change in cycle length (CL) excludes an accessory pathway, as atrial and ventricular myocardium are part of the reentry.

In the following cases, differentiation between AVNRT and AVRT is difficult:

1. In atypical AVNRT, the HA interval is also prolonged (> 70 ms).
2. An orthodromic AVRT via a parahisian pathway can exhibit a relatively short VA interval.

In this case, specific stimulation maneuvers such as "atrial preceding" or the Michaud maneuver

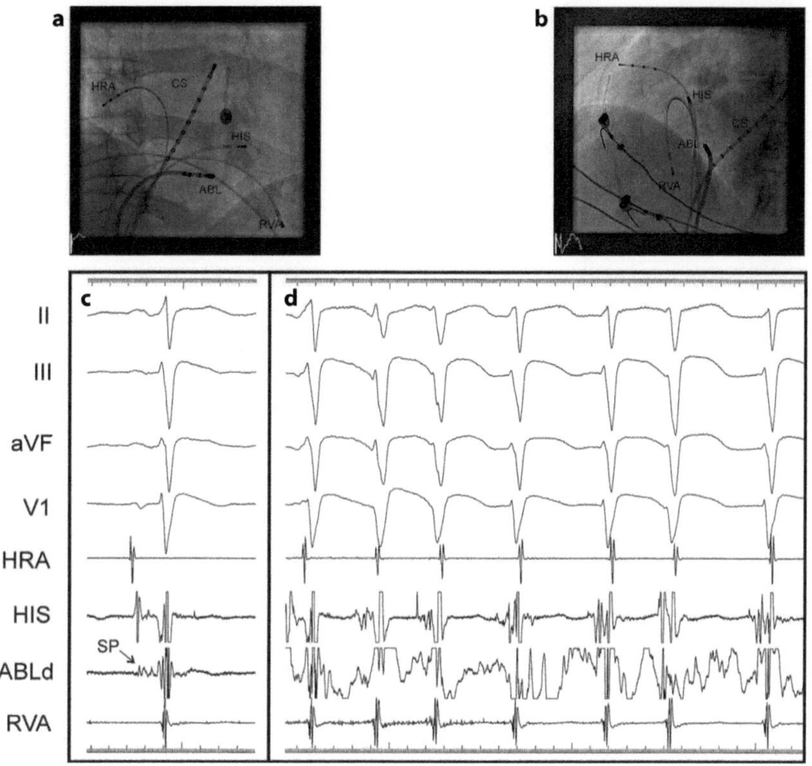

Fig. 8.3 **a,b** Positioning of the diagnostic catheters. HRA = high right atrium, HIS = His bundle, RVA = right ventricular apex, CS = coronary sinus, ABL = ablation catheter (at the typical site for slow pathway ablation). **a** corresponds to an RAO projection, **b** image of an LAO projection. **c** shows a typical fractionated slow pathway potential (SP) in the mapping catheter before ablation. **d** demonstrates junctional beats during RF energy delivery in the area of the slow pathway. HRA = high right atrium, HIS = His bundle, ABLd = distal ablation catheter, RVA = right ventricular apex

(also ventricular overdrive pacing, ventricular entrainment) are available for further differentiation (Michaud et al. 2001).

1. **Atrial Preceding**: If a ventricular extrasystole (VES) is generated in the RV apex simultaneously with the anterograde excitation of the His during ongoing tachycardia, this does not change the cycle length of the atrium in the presence of an AVNRT. Since the reentry in the context of AVNRT occurs above the His and the His is refractory at the time of the delivered VES, the retrograde excitation caused by the VES cannot be transmitted to the atrium (no atrial "preceding/reset"). In contrast, in the case of an AVRT, the atria are prematurely excited via the accessory pathway after a VES is delivered during His

refractoriness, leading to a shortening of the AA interval during the VES delivery (positive atrial "preceding/reset") (see Fig. 8.5).

2. **Maneuver according to Michaud**: During tachycardia, the ventricle is stimulated with a CL that is 20–40 ms shorter. The stimulation should be continued until the atrial CL corresponds to the stimulated ventricular CL (atrial entrainment). After the stimulation ends and provided the tachycardia does not terminate, the ventricular post-pacing interval (PPI) is determined between the last RV stimulus (S) and the first spontaneous ventricular action (V). If this interval is more than 115 ms longer than the CL of the tachycardia (i.e., PPI - TCL > 115 ms), then the stimulation site is far from the reentry and the ventricle is not part of the reentry. This indicates the presence of an

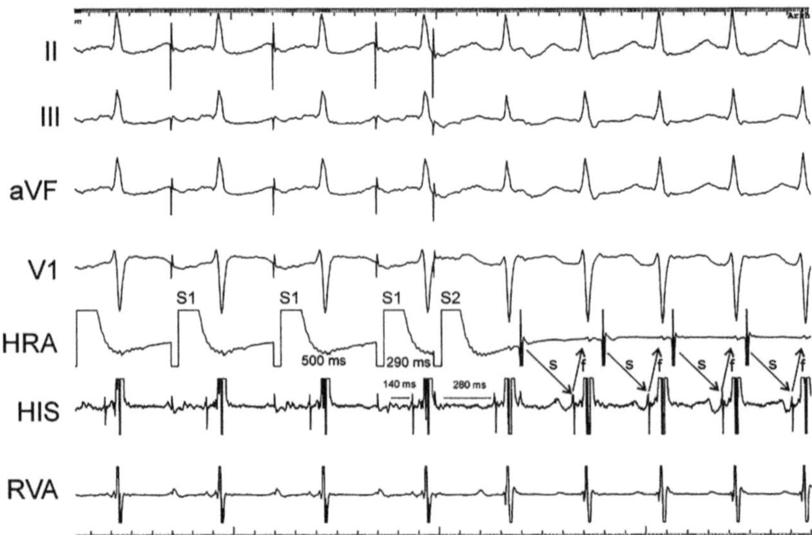

Fig. 8.4 Induction of a typical AVNRT by programmed atrial stimulation. Baseline stimulation with S1S1 of 500 ms. With a coupling interval S1S2 of 290 ms, a significant increase in the AH interval from 140 to 280 ms and the onset of tachycardia ("slow-fast" type: anterograde conduction via the "slow" [s] and retrograde conduction via the "fast" [f] pathway). HRA = high right atrium, HIS = His bundle, RVA = right ventricular apex

AVNRT (see Fig. 8.5). In a second step, after entrainment, the interval between the last RV stimulus (S) and the first spontaneous atrium (A) as well as the interval between intrinsic ventricular excitation (V) and the subsequent first spontaneous atrium (A) during ongoing tachycardia is determined. If this interval is more than 85 ms due to the retrograde decremental conduction properties of the AV node (i.e., SA − VA > 85 ms), an AVNRT is also to be assumed. Important: this maneuver can only succeed if a VA conduction is present.

Differentiation AVNRT vs. Focal Atrial Tachycardia (FAT)

In most cases, the differentiation between AVNRT and FAT is well possible. The following criteria should be considered:

1. An eccentric atrial excitation generally excludes an AVNRT. This is the case when the HRA electrogram is recorded earlier than the atrium at the His catheter or the distal CS is recorded earlier than the proximal CS.
2. In the case of a FAT originating from the inferoseptal right or left atrium, the atrium

at the His is also recorded earlier than in the HRA or distal CS, similar to an AVNRT. After termination of the tachycardia, it is advisable to perform ventricular stimulation with the CL of the tachycardia. If a VA block can be demonstrated, an AVNRT or AVRT (which require retrograde conduction for their maintenance) as a differential diagnosis is very unlikely. Ventricular stimulation should be performed immediately after termination of the tachycardia, as increasing vagotonia after termination of the tachycardia can lead to VA block.

3. During the tachycardia, the ventricle is stimulated with a CL that is 20–40 ms shorter. If 1. VA dissociation occurs without a change in the atrial activation sequence and 2. the tachycardia continues unchanged after the termination of V-stimulation, a focal atrial tachycardia is likely, as VA dissociation has been demonstrated (Knight et al. 1999).
4. During the tachycardia, the ventricle is stimulated with a CL that is 20–40 ms shorter until a 1:1 VA conduction is achieved (the AA interval shortens from the CL of the tachycardia to the CL of the V-stimulation with a

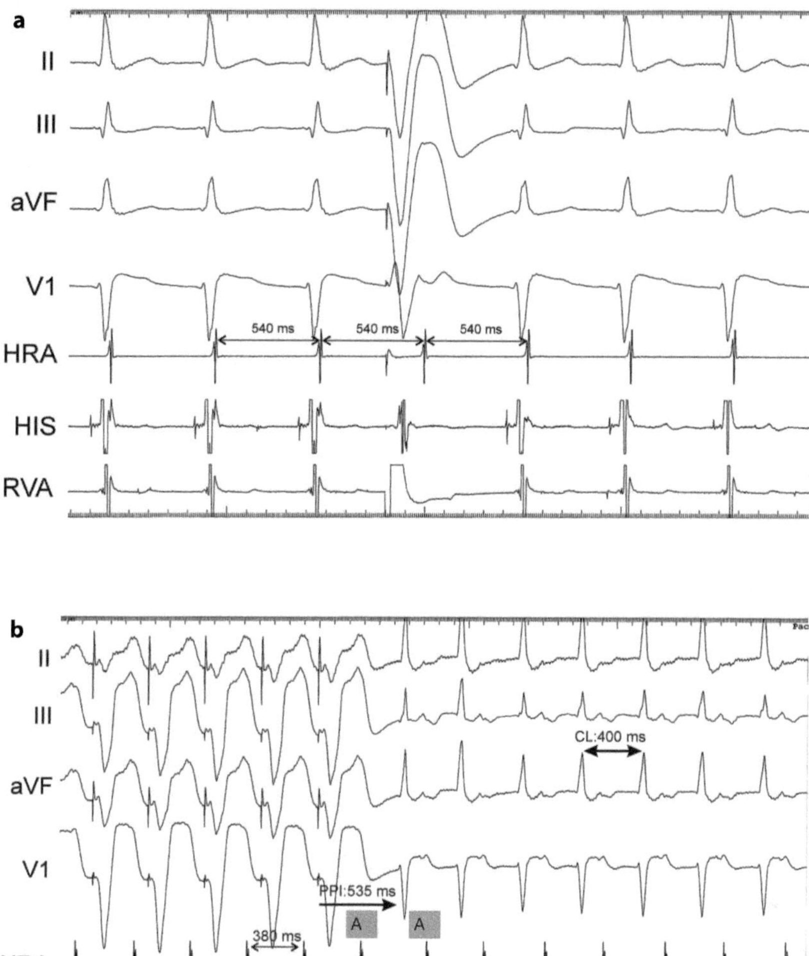

Fig. 8.5 **a** Negative atrial preceding (explanation see text). HRA = high right atrium, HIS = His bundle, RVA = right ventricular apex. **b** Michaud maneuver (further explanation also see text). During tachycardia (CL 400 ms), the ventricle is stimulated with a CL of 380 ms. After the end of the stimulation, the ventricular post-pacing interval (PPI) between the last stimulus and the first spontaneous ventricular action is determined. This interval is 535 ms, 135 ms (> 115 ms) longer than the CL of the tachycardia. In this case, it is an atypical AVNRT. Congruently, the electrogram shows a VAV sequence after the end of the stimulation. HRA = high right atrium, HIS = His bundle, RVA = right ventricular apex

stable VA interval). If two consecutive atrial excitations occur without a ventricular excitation (V-A-A-V) after ventricular stimulation during ongoing tachycardia, a FAT is highly likely (Knight et al. 1999; see Fig. 8.6).

5. In the case of an AVNRT, a V-A-V configuration is observed (see Fig. 8.5).
6. If a PVC terminates the tachycardia without retrograde conduction to the atrium, a focal atrial tachycardia can be excluded.

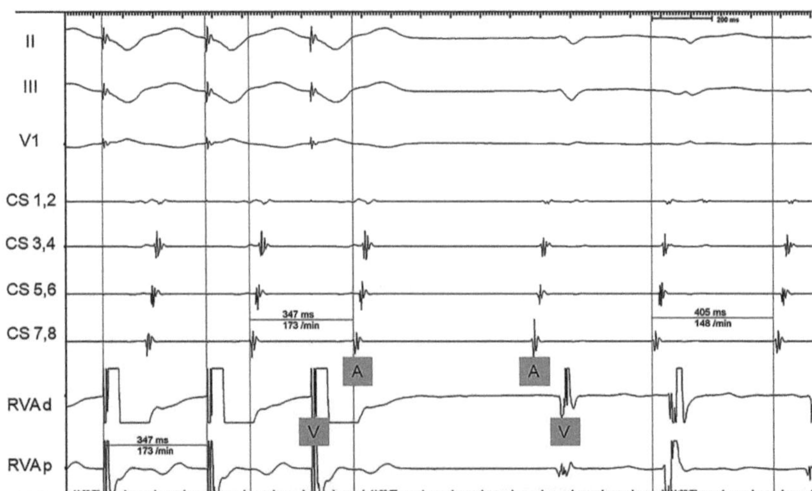

Fig. 8.6 Differentiation AVNRT vs. FAT (see text for explanation). After the termination of ventricular stimulation, two consecutive atrial actions are visible before the next ventricular excitation occurs (V-A-A-V). Thus, a FAT is likely. CS = coronary sinus, RVAd = distal RV apex

8.4.2   Ablation in AVNRT

Indication and Success Prospects

The ablation or modulation of the SP represents, according to current guideline recommendations, the therapy of choice for the treatment of symptomatic AVNRT (typical and atypical form) (Class IB) (Brugada et al. 2020). Generally, ablation is performed after the induction of an AVNRT and the exclusion of relevant differential diagnoses within the framework of the preceding EPU. In cases of non-inducibility, empirical ablation can also be performed if dual AV node physiology with typical history and the presence of characteristic SVT documentation is proven (Aliot et al., 2003; Lauschke et al. 2015). The sole presence of dual AV node physiology without documentation of an AVNRT does not justify ablation treatment.

During the ablation of the SP, the duality of the AV node is completely eliminated. In modulation, it is preserved, but the tachycardia is no longer inducible. Catheter ablation shows a high success rate and a low complication rate. The probability of recurrence after successful RF ablation is < 2%, and approximately 9% for (focal) cryoablation. Although a higher-grade AV block is the most feared complication, it occurs in less than 0.3% of cases in experienced centers, with the risk of an AV block being slightly increased in the presence of a pre-existing AV conduction disorder (Brugada et al. 2020; Deisenhofer et al. 2010).

Ablation Technique

Orientation to anatomical structures in combination with local electrograms enables the localization and successful ablation of the SP. The use of an electroanatomical mapping system is not mandatory.

Typically, diagnostic catheters are placed in the His region or the coronary sinus during an EPU. These anatomical landmarks outline the aforementioned structures of the Koch's triangle fluoroscopically in AP projection, RAO 30°, or LAO 40–60° projection. The ablation/modulation of the SP is anatomically guided in the area between the CS ostium and the tricuspid valve in the inferoseptal region of Koch's triangle in LAO projection (see Fig. 8.3).

Additionally, a typical intracardiac electrogram of the SP can be derived in sinus rhythm when the ablation catheter is correctly positioned. This is characterized by a relatively low-amplitude, fractionated atrial electrogram followed by a ventricular signal in an A:V ratio of approximately 1:4. This signal is typically relatively delayed compared to the atrial signal in the His (see Fig. 8.3). In **atypical** AVNRT, the site of the earliest atrial activation during ongoing tachycardia corresponds to the atrial insertion of the SP.

Usually, an uncooled ablation catheter with a 4-mm long tip and a temperature-controlled generator setting of 30–50 W for a maximum duration of 90 seconds is used. During effective ablation, junctional beats are characteristically induced during energy delivery (see Fig. 8.3). It is essential to continuously monitor AV/VA conduction with particular attention to atrial activation, as atrial activation during junctional beats represents conduction over the FP. If there is a delay or loss of the atrial component, ablation should be immediately interrupted to prevent an impending AV block. The authors recommend performing ablation in sinus rhythm. Energy delivery during ongoing tachycardia or burst atrial extrasystoles should not be performed, as AV conduction cannot be adequately assessed.

The endpoint of ablation is the non-inducibility of tachycardia, which should be tested under adrenergic provocation depending on the initial inducibility. If no anterograde "jump" can be detected under programmed stimulation after ablation, complete ablation of the SP is assumed. If tachycardia is non-inducible but a "jump" is still detectable, the SP has been modulated. In this case, a maximum of one AV nodal echo can be accepted, which does not increase the recurrence rate (Deisenhofer et al. 2010). Ablation should also be discontinued in the event of pathological prolongation of AV conduction to avoid a higher-grade AV block due to further ablation measures.

Techniques for Difficult Ablation

If ablation is difficult, the following strategies/questions are recommended:

1. Is the diagnosis of AVNRT correct?
2. Ensure sufficient contact pressure by rotating the ablation catheter against the septum (beware of dislocation into the CS). If necessary, use long (steerable) sheaths.
3. If necessary, switch to an electroanatomical mapping system or cryotechnology.
4. If necessary, ablate a left atrial insertion of the SP in the left inferoseptal atrium.

References

Alasti M, Mirzaee S, Machado C et al (2020) Junctional ectopic tachycardia (JET). J Arrhythm 36:837–844

Aliot EM, Kuck KH, Alpert JS et al (2003) ACC/AHA/ESC guidelines for the management of patients with supraventricular arrhythmias

Brugada J, Katritsis DG, Arbelo EE et al (2020) 2019 ESC Guidelines for the management of patients with supraventricular tachycardia. Eur Heart J 41:655–720

Chokr M, Moura LG, Sousa IBDS, Pisani CF et al (2021) Catheter ablation of focal atrial tachycardia with early activation close to the his-bundle from the non coronary aortic cusp. Arq Bras Cardiol 116:119–126

Deisenhofer I, Zrenner B, Yin YH, Pitschner HF et al (2010) Cryoablation versus radiofrequency energy for the ablation of atrioventricular nodal reentrant tachycardia (the CYRANO Study): results from a large multicenter prospective randomized trial. Circulation 122:2239–2245

Heidbüchel H, Jackman WM (2004) Characterization of subforms of AV nodal reentrant tachycardia. Europace 6(4):316–329

Iesaka Y, Takahashi A, Goya M et al (1997) Adenosine-sensitive atrial reentrant tachycardia originating from the atrioventricular nodal transitional area. j Cardiovasc Electrophysiol 8:854–864

Katritsis DG, Sepahpour A, Marine JE et al (2015) Atypical atrioventricular nodal reentrant tachycardia: prevalence, electrophysiologic characteristics, and tachycardia circuit. Europace 17:1099–1106

Katritsis DG, Efimov IR (2019) Cardiac connexin genotyping for identification of the circuit of atrioventricular nodal re-entrant tachycardia. Europace 21:190–191

Knight BP, Zivin A, Souza J et al (1999) A technique for the rapid diagnosis of atrial tachycardia in the electrophysiology laboratory. J Am Coll Cardiol 33:775–781

Kotadia I, Whitaker J, Roney C et al (2020) Anisotropic cardiac conduction. Arrhythm Electrophysiol Rev 9:202–210

Lauschke J, Schneider J, Schneider R et al (2015) Electrophysiological studies in patients with paroxysmal supraventricular tachycardias but no electrocardiogram documentation: findings from a prospective registry. Europace 17:801–806

Liuba I, Jonsson A, Safstrom K, Walfridsson H (2006) Gender-related differences in patients with atrioventricular nodal reentry tachycardia. Am J Cardiol 97:384–388

Michaud GF, Tada H, Chough S et al (2001) Differentiation of atypical atrioventricular node reentrant tachycardia from orthodromic reciprocating tachycardia using a septal accessory pathway by the response to ventricular pacing. j Am Coll Cardiol 38:1163–1167

Spach MS, Josephson ME (1994) Initiating reentry: the role of nonuniform anisotropy in small circuits. J Cardiovasc Electrophysiol 5:182–209

Steven D, Bonnemeier H, Deneke T et al (2015) How to approach the patient with supraventricular tachycardia in the EP lab: a systematic overview. Herzschrittmacherther Elektrophysiol 26:167–172

Melanie Gunawardene and Stephan Willems

9.1 Introduction

Atrial tachycardias belong to the group of supraventricular tachycardias and are found in 5–15% of electrophysiological studies conducted due to suspected supraventricular tachycardia (Roberts-Thomson et al. 2006a).

The general prevalence of focal atrial tachycardias (FAT), synonymously ectopic atrial tachycardia (EAT), is 0.34% (Brugada et al. 2020). They are defined according to their underlying mechanism, which can be either macroreentry, microreentry, localized reentry, or a focal mechanism. Previously, FAT and microreentry tachycardias were grouped together as one entity. Nowadays, however, they are clearly defined separately, although it can be difficult to differentiate them in electrophysiological studies.

Supplementary Information The online version contains supplementary material available at https://doi.org/10.1007/978-3-662-65797-3_9. The videos can be accessed individually by clicking the DOI link in the accompanying figure caption or by scanning this link with the SN More Media App.

M. Gunawardene (✉) · S. Willems
Abteilung für Kardiologie und Internistische Intensivmedizin, Asklepios Klinik St. Georg, Hamburg, Germany
e-mail: Melanie.gunawardene@gmail.com

S. Willems
e-mail: s.willems@asklepios.com

▶ In the context of further diagnostics of a supraventricular tachycardia, an atrial tachycardia is found in 5–15% of cases in the electrophysiological study. Excluded from this are atrial tachycardias that occur after previous atrial fibrillation ablations (possibly with prior substrate modification).

9.2 Definition

The FAT is defined by an atrial activation that spreads centrifugally from a small, well-defined spot (a so-called "focus") in the atrium and from there electrically excites the rest of the atrium (Brugada et al. 2020; Fig. 9.1). In contrast to a macroreentry (a circulating excitation over the atrium), the entire cycle length of the atrial tachycardia does not have to be detectable in the atrium (Roberts-Thomson et al. 2006a). The mechanism of FAT can be due to increased (abnormal) automaticity or triggered activity of the myocardial cells. The mechanism of microreentry and the mechanism of localized reentry should be considered separately (see Chap. 12).

▶ The term "atrial tachycardia (AT)" initially does not define the exact cardiac arrhythmia as a generic term. In the context of narrow complex tachycardias in patients without structural heart disease, it is often used synonymously with focal atrial tachycardia. After left atrial ablations, AT is often referred to until the mechanism of the tachycardia has been clearly identified and named during the invasive study. This can therefore also involve various forms of atypical atrial flutter.

The origin of FAT is often in the right atrium (approx. 80%), but can also be identified in the left atrium (approx. 20%) (Türkmen et al. 2020). The origins of FAT are not randomly distributed. Typical locations in the right atrium are the crista terminalis, the ostium of the coronary sinus, areas of the tricuspid valve annulus, the right atrial appendage, the transition to the superior vena cava, and right-septal. In the left atrium, the origin is usually found in one of the pulmonary veins or at the mitral valve annulus, less frequently left-septal or in the area of the left atrial appendage (Schmitt et al. 2006). Rarer entities are FAT from the area of the non-coronary cusp of the aortic sinus (Ouyang et al. 2006) (Figs. 9.2 and 9.4).

Since it is an atrial tachycardia, it can often be diagnosed already in the surface ECG . Usually, there is an isoelectric line between the P waves, unlike, for example, in typical atrial flutter. However, the distinction from a macroreentry can be difficult and ultimately not clearly separable.

By determining the P-wave morphology, conclusions can be drawn about the location of the tachycardia (see Sect. 9.4.1). The P wave is monomorphic during tachycardia, unlike in atrial fibrillation (Brugada et al. 2020). The distinction from other supraventricular tachycardias can be difficult in the ECG, so an electrophysiological study may be necessary to confirm the diagnosis.

► Focal atrial tachycardias have a discretely defined origin and show a centrifugal spread of excitation. They mostly originate from the right atrium but can also arise from the left atrium or the non-coronary cusp in the aortic root.

9.3 Epidemiology and Clinical Picture

Symptoms of patients affected by FAT can vary greatly. Typically, symptomatic patients experience palpitations, tachycardia, dyspnea, chest pain,

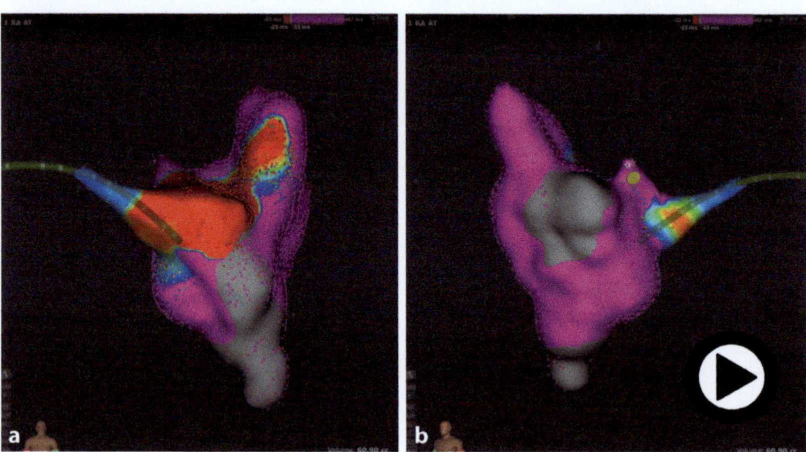

Fig. 9.1 Ultra-high-resolution 3D anatomy of a right atrial focal tachycardia. Shown is a high-resolution three-dimensional activation map of a focal atrial tachycardia of the right atrium (**a** posterior view ["PA"], **b** left-anterior-oblique view ["LAO"]). The origin of the focal atrial tachycardia is shown right-septal at the roof of the ostium of the coronary sinus. From there, the atrial activation spreads centrifugally and excites the rest of the atrium from here. The catheter shown in *green* indicates the diagnostic catheter in the coronary sinus (https://doi.org/10.1007/000-d2p)

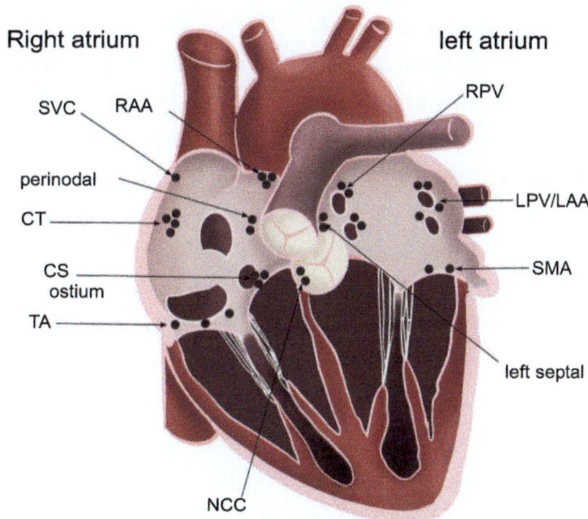

Fig. 9.2 Intracardiac locations of focal atrial tachycardias. The figure shows the typical locations of focal atrial tachycardia in the right and left atrium and in the non-coronary cusp of the sinus of Valsalva. CS ostium = ostium of the "CS" (= coronary sinus); CT = crista terminalis; LAA = left atrial appendage; LPV = left pulmonary veins; NCC = non-coronary cusp aortic sinus = RAA = right atrial appendage; RPV = right pulmonary veins; SMA = superior mitral annulus; TA = tricuspid valve

dizziness, or occasionally syncope. In rare cases, tachycardiomyopathy may also occur (Bhasin et al. 2021). FAT affects all age groups and can be diagnosed even in newborns. The data on gender distribution are inconsistent. Most studies report no difference between genders. In more recent studies, there is an increase in FAT in females (Türkmen et al. 2020; Brugada et al. 2020).

The atrial rate is usually between 130 and 250/min but can also deviate from this (Roberts-Thomson et al. 2006a). In a large study with 487 patients with FAT, the atrial cycle length was on average 375 ± 82 ms (women) and 384 ± 106 ms (men).

Clinically, the phenomenon of "warming up and cooling down" occasionally appears. This means that with the onset of the rhythm disorder, the cycle length steadily decreases due to adrenergic stimulation, making the tachycardia faster. The end of the episode is also not sudden but gradually slows down until termination. This frequency behavior can also be recognized in frequency profiles of long-term ECGs. Such a history can thus already provide a clue to the entity of the rhythm disorder. In these cases, the mechanism of abnormal automaticity is often underlying (Hirao 2018).

The peculiarity of FAT also lies in the fact that it is not always sustained. Sustained tachycardias were found more frequently in men than in women (22 vs. 5%) (Türkmen et al. 2020). In the case of non-sustained episodes, this can complicate both the diagnosis and the mapping and thus the ablation treatment. To enable the diagnosis of only rare and/or short-lasting episodes, so-called "wearables" like smartwatches are increasingly used. The implantation of an event recorder can also be used as a diagnostic tool.

▶ Focal atrial tachycardias can present with the phenomenon of "warming up and cooling down" and in a non-sustained form. In the case of rare and/or non-sustained episodes, the use of so-called "wearables" can help secure the diagnosis.

9.4 Diagnostics

9.4.1 P-Wave Morphology

As already mentioned, the diagnosis of FAT can often be made from the ECG. Since atrial tachycardia can originate in various locations in the atrium, the morphology of the P-wave in the 12-lead ECG can provide information about the intracardiac localization of the rhythm disorder. As early as 2006, a P-wave algorithm was identified that could predict the localization of FAT in the heart with 93% accuracy (Kistler et al. 2006). This algorithm was updated in 2021 by the same authors (Kistler et al. 2021).

▶ The intracardiac localization of the origin of focal atrial tachycardia can be narrowed down based on the P-wave morphology in the 12-lead ECG.

In the updated algorithm of 2021, FATs originating in the area of the CS ostium, right septal, perinodal (related to the AV node), left septal, the non-coronary cusp, and the superior mitral valve annulus were summarized as paraseptal FATs. The reason for this is the limitation in the spatial resolution of the P-wave morphology in the surface ECG due to the anatomical proximity of these structures to each other (Kistler et al. 2021). The algorithm is shown in Fig. 9.3. The morphology of the P-wave in lead V1 plays a central role here. A distinction is made between purely positive, negative, or isoelectric P-wave morphology, but also between an initially positive and then negative (+/−) or initially negative (−/+) or isoelectric (iso/+) and then positive P-wave. According to the algorithm, 93% of the localizations could be predicted in the original publication (Kistler et al. 2021).

In some cases, it can be difficult in clinical practice to determine the P-wave morphology in the surface ECG, depending on whether it coincides with the T-wave, for example (Fig. 9.4). For tips on better visualizing the P-wave in electrophysiological studies, see Sect. 9.4.2.

▶ In particular, the P-wave morphology in lead V1 in the 12-lead ECG is crucial for determining the intracardiac location of the focal atrial tachycardia.

In the case of sinus node-near FAT (e.g., from the area of the superior crista terminalis), the

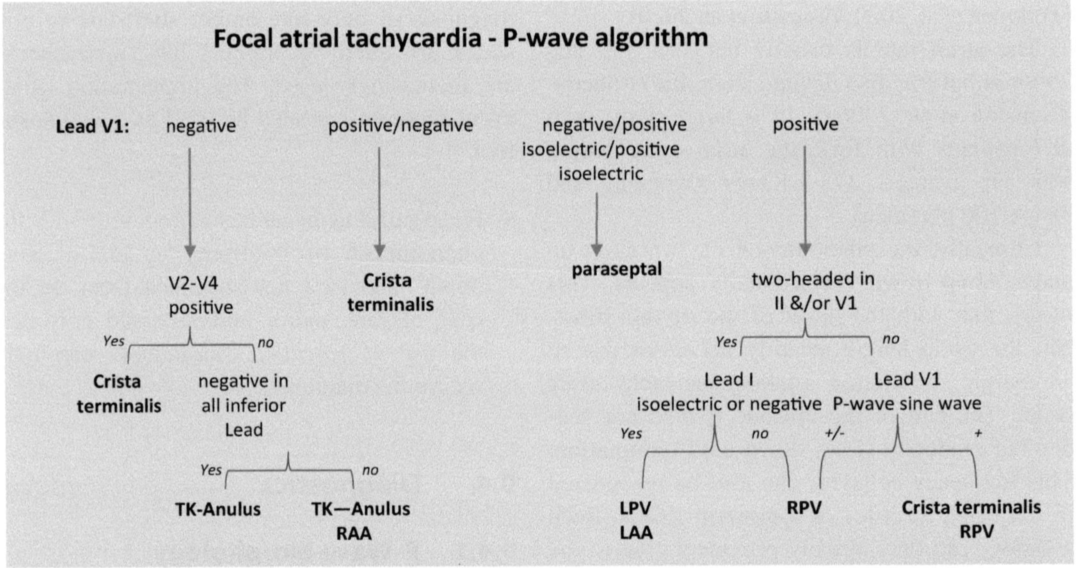

Fig. 9.3 P-wave morphologies in atrial tachycardias. The figure shows the P-wave algorithm, adapted from Kistler et al. (2021), for determining the intracardiac location of the tachycardia origin. TK = tricuspid valve; LPV = left pulmonary vein; RAA = right atrial appendage; RPV = right pulmonary vein

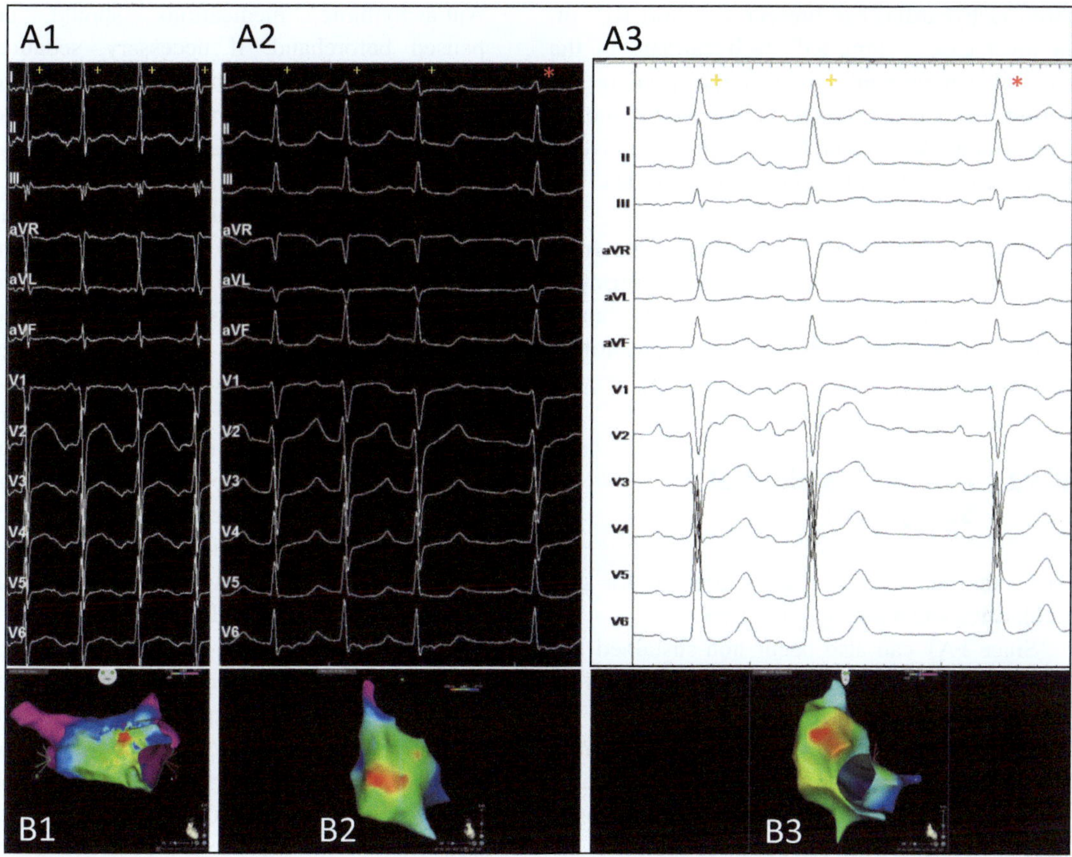

Fig. 9.4 12-lead ECG of different focal atrial tachycardias with 3D mapping. Three examples of focal atrial tachycardias in the 12-lead ECG (row A) with the respective intracardiac location in three-dimensional mapping (row B: activation maps are shown: red = early activation, purple = later activation of the electrical excitation propagation). A1-B1: 12-lead ECG of a focal atrial tachycardia (50 mm/s). The P-wave is predominantly positive in lead V1 and negative to isoelectric in lead I. In the 3D mapping, the location is found anterior to the left atrial appendage in the anatomy of the left atrium shown here. A2-B2: 12-lead ECG of a non-sustained focal atrial tachycardia (*yellow plus*, 75 mm/s) with termination into sinus rhythm (*red star*). This example highlights the difficulty of distinguishing the P-wave during tachycardia and the differential diagnosis of AV node reentry tachycardia. In the three-dimensional mapping, the focal atrial tachycardia originates in the inferior region of the crista terminalis (B3: right lateral (RL) view of the right atrium). A3-B3: 12-lead ECG of a non-sustained focal atrial tachycardia (*yellow plus*, 50 mm/s) with termination into sinus rhythm (*red star*). The P-waves in tachycardia show similarities to the P-waves in sinus rhythm. On closer inspection, it is noticeable that the P-wave in leads II, III, avR, avF differs slightly from that in sinus rhythm. Lead V1 even shows a different polarity of the P-wave. The focal atrial tachycardia originates from the high lateral right atrium and is thus located near the sinus node (B3: right anterior oblique [RAO] view of the right atrium, the tricuspid valve is cut out)

P-wave morphology can correspond to that of the sinus node (II, III, aVF positive, aVR negative) and thus cannot be distinguished from an inappropriate sinus tachycardia in the surface ECG (Fig. 9.4). This can complicate diagnostics and therapy in such cases. The challenge in these cases is to differentiate these entities from all findings, the medical history, and the invasive electrophysiological examination and to establish an adequate therapy (e.g., ablation or medication therapy, such as with ivabradine).

On the other hand, differentiation between an AV node reentry (AVNRT) or AV reentry tachycardia (AVRT) and an FAT can also be difficult based on the 12-lead ECG (Fig. 9.4). Depending on the conduction properties of the AV node, atrial tachycardias can present as "short-RP" or, in most cases, "long-RP" tachycardias. In the case of a paraseptal origin of the atrial tachycardia, the P-wave morphology can be similar to that of an AVNRT or AVRT, being negative in the inferior leads and having a superior axis.

▶ Differentiating focal atrial tachycardia from sinus tachycardia or another supraventricular tachycardia such as AVNRT or AVRT can be difficult before the invasive electrophysiological examination.

9.4.2 Electrophysiological Study (EPS)

The examiner should already prepare for particularities when planning the EPS.

Since FAT can also occur non-sustained and thus both the diagnostic and mapping conditions can be challenging, it is important to ensure the best possible examination conditions in advance.

FAT, which arise from abnormal automaticity, also depend on the activity of the autonomic nervous system. This can result in the tachycardia possibly not being inducible on the day of the examination.

This also means that all antiarrhythmic medications, especially beta-blockers, which could potentially suppress the arrhythmia, should be tapered off several days before the planned EPS. In some cases, sedation is also avoided for the same reason (Hirao 2018).

For better induction and provocation of the tachycardia, medications such as isoproterenol and atropine can be used in the EPS. These can especially induce tachycardias with the mechanism of abnormal automaticity. Attention should also be paid to the "wash-out" phase of isoproterenol. Additionally, handgrip maneuvers can be used for adrenergic stimulation. Unlike triggered activity, tachycardia due to abnormal automaticity often cannot be induced by programmed stimulation (Hirao 2018).

▶ The preparation and execution of the EPS in FAT require some particularities.

Antiarrhythmic medications should be paused beforehand. If necessary, sedation must be reduced or even stopped during the EPS, and medication provocation should be performed to induce the arrhythmia.

The differentiation of various types of supraventricular tachycardias can also pose a challenge in the EP study. It is difficult to confirm the presence of atrial tachycardia with just a single diagnostic maneuver, so all recorded intracardiac tracings must be interpreted in a common context. The following provides tips and assistance for differentiating the entities. Additionally, Chap. 7 can be used for the differentiation of supraventricular tachycardias. However, since this topic is very extensive, only the most clinically relevant aspects will be addressed below (Roberts-Thomson et al. 2006a; Schmitt et al. 2006; Hirao 2018):

- The P wave in tachycardia usually differs from that in sinus rhythm. To make the P wave more visible in the EP study, a brief ventricular stimulation can be performed, after which the P wave can be assessed (since the ventricle is temporarily refractory due to the last activation, allowing the P wave to be assessed without the QRS complex) or by administering adenosine, which unmasks the P wave. An inferior axis of the P wave (i.e., the origin of the tachycardia is superior in the atrium) excludes AVNRT.
- A "long-RP" sequence (the RP interval is longer than the PR interval, meaning the P wave appears *before* the QRS complex) can indicate atrial tachycardia. However, an atypical AVNRT or an accessory pathway located far left can also exhibit a "long-RP" sequence.
- Absence of "VA linking": Unlike AVRT or AVNRT, there is no fixed connection between the atrium (A) and ventricle (V) in atrial tachycardia, as the ventricle is not part of the tachycardia mechanism. A different VA interval or different post-pacing intervals after atrial stimulation can thus indicate the absence of VA linking.
- "V-A-A-V" response during ventricular entrainment. The AV node is refractory for

antegrade conduction due to the last retrograde atrial activation by ventricular stimulation, so in ongoing atrial tachycardia, a "V-A-A-V" (or also described as "A-A-V") response occurs (see Chap. 7).

- A positive "preceding" (with refractory His) excludes atrial tachycardia. If the ventricle is stimulated sporadically during tachycardia while the His is refractory at that time, then premature excitation of the atrium, i.e., a "pulling" of the atrial signal, is only possible if an additional conduction pathway is present in the heart and the tachycardia mechanism involves the ventricle.
- VA dissociation: the absence of atrial (A) capture during rapid ventricular stimulation (V) has a positive predictive value of 80% for the presence of atrial tachycardia.
- Termination of tachycardia by adenosine does not allow differentiation between the various entities of supraventricular tachycardias. However, if the tachycardia continues despite adenosine administration and AV block at the atrial level, atrial tachycardia can be differentiated (Glatter et al. 1999).
- Under the administration of isoproterenol, the region of the sinus node may migrate superiorly during mapping, as the sinus node region responds to the autonomic nervous system. In contrast, a FAT from the area of the crista terminalis does not migrate and remains localized at this site. Thus, a distinction between sinus tachycardia and FAT is possible.
- A 2:1 or 3:1 conduction of the tachycardia does not necessarily confirm the presence of atrial tachycardia, as an infra-Hisian block can also occur in AVNRT (while the AVNRT continues to circulate in the AV node and only further inferiorly does not leave the conduction system and thus cannot excite the ventricle).

9.5 Therapy Management

9.5.1 Acute Therapy

Large multicenter studies on the acute and chronic therapy of the rather rare FAT are still lacking, so there is no class-A evidence-grade recommendation for this condition in the current guidelines. In the acute situation, medications that delay conduction to the ventricle and thus control the heart rate (e.g., beta-blockers or calcium channel blockers) can be used. Antiarrhythmic drugs of class Ia, Ic, or III, as well as adenosine (triggered tachycardias), can also terminate the tachycardias but are generally less effective. Electrical cardioversion can usually successfully terminate the current episode, but the tachycardia can spontaneously reinitiate afterward (Brugada et al. 2020).

9.5.2 Long-term Therapy

Here too, the study situation regarding drug therapy is very thin, so no clear recommendations are given in the current guideline. Beta-blockers, calcium antagonists, class Ic antiarrhythmics, and ivabradine, combined with a beta-blocker, can be used here (Brugada et al. 2020). The best therapy option for treating recurrent FAT is catheter ablation with success rates between 75–100% (Class IB recommendation) (Brugada et al. 2020).

▶ Catheter ablation is the best therapy option for recurrent focal atrial tachycardias.

9.5.3 Mapping and Catheter Ablation

Nowadays, atrial tachycardias are usually localized and then ablated using three-dimensional mapping techniques. Regardless of the system used, an activation map is created by locating the earliest activation during the FAT. There is the possibility to either map the tachycardia point-by-point with the ablation catheter itself or to use multipolar mapping catheters. With high-resolution mapping catheters, the spatial resolution of the electrodes and thus the measurement accuracy is greatest. During ongoing FAT, the inside of the right and/or left atrium (or even the aorta) is scanned, and the collected electrograms are summarized in an activation map (Fig. 9.5).

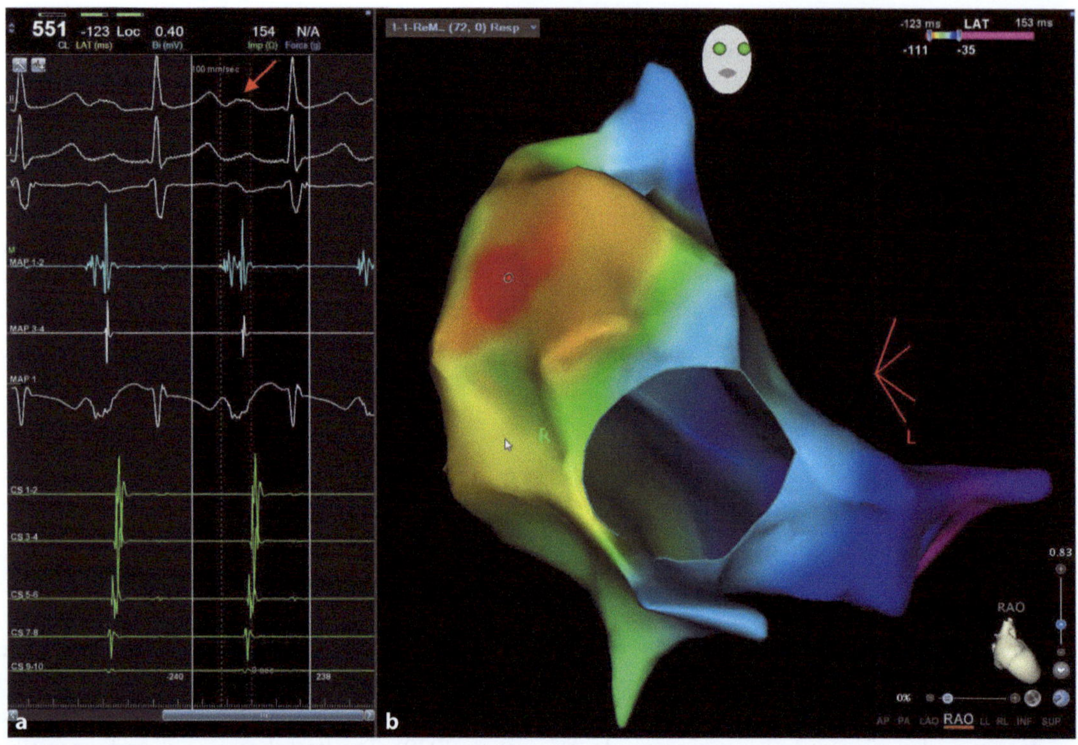

Fig. 9.5 Ablation signal of a focal atrial tachycardia. **a** Focal atrial tachycardia with a cycle length of 554 ms. Shown is the surface ECG and intracardiac electrograms of the ablation catheter (MAP) and the 10-pole diagnostic catheter in the coronary sinus (CS) (100 mm/s). The bipolar signal (Map 1-2, distal ablation electrodes) shows the earliest activation of the focal atrial tachycardia at the ablation site. The signal is fractionated and begins before the P-wave in the 12-lead ECG (*red arrow*) and is 123 ms before the intracardiac CS reference. **b** Shown is the 3D activation map of the focal right atrial tachycardia with localization of the earliest origin and centrifugal spread of excitation (regarding activation, red means early and purple late; view from oblique right (RAO) to the right atrium). The origin is shown in the high lateral right atrium

Using these high-resolution mapping catheters, an even earlier activation sequence can be measured compared to point-by-point mapping, and the mapping and procedure times can be significantly shortened (Chieng and Lee 2020). The use of so-called "post-processing" algorithms of the various mapping system software can also help to better localize the earliest activation (Yagishita et al. 2019). The use of high-resolution mapping systems could also increase the acute procedural success (Kellnar and Estner 2022).

As already mentioned, it is important that the examiner ensures good mapping conditions. Especially in the case of non-sustained FAT, mapping can be difficult, and drug provocation with, for example, isoprenaline may be necessary. Under isoprenaline, the cycle length of the tachycardia can change, but not the localization. However, higher doses or vulnerability during isoprenaline administration can lead to atrial fibrillation during the procedure. This can not only make further mapping difficult but also result in the tachycardia no longer being inducible.

During mapping, the tachycardia can also be mechanically terminated (i.e., by the movement of the mapping catheter within the heart), which can also pose a challenge in mapping FAT.

In rare cases where FAT is difficult to induce, non-invasive mapping, for example, by wearing a special vest with 252 electrodes (CardioInsight™, Medtronic, MN, USA) can help to localize FAT.

However, this is not a routine examination in clinical practice and is reserved for certain centers (Yamashita et al. 2018). Another alternative is the so-called "non-contact" mapping, to avoid mechanical terminations or to map only short-lasting episodes. Here, the mapping catheter is merely placed in the atrium but does not need to have wall contact to capture the electrical information (Roberts-Thomson et al. 2006b). Depending on the technology, theoretically, one tachycardia beat is sufficient to represent an activation (Willems et al. 2019).

A rarely used option for very difficult-to-induce FATs, similar to the mapping of ventricular extrasystoles, is the possibility of pace mapping. Here, stimulation is performed at various points in the atria, and the P-wave generated is compared with the P-wave morphology. If the intracardiac activation sequence of the diagnostic catheters also matches, the origin of the AT can be identified in this way (Hayashi et al. 2016).

Once the earliest activation of the FAT has been found, ablation can be performed. The signal at the origin of the tachycardia itself may or may not be fractionated. It should be located at least approximately 30 ms before the onset of the P wave (Fig. 9.5). If this is not the case, the origin of the FAT may be in the other atrium, and a transseptal puncture from the right to the left atrium may become necessary. If the P wave is difficult to delineate in the ECG, an intracardiac reference (e.g., the CS catheter) can alternatively be used. At the site of the earliest activation, a purely negatively deflected unipolar signal (QS) with an initially steep drop can be an additional indication for the localization of the AT origin (Roberts-Thomson et al. 2006b). Typically, the FAT is ablated with cooling. In the case of parahisian localization, ablation can also be performed without cooling.

▶ Catheter ablation of focal atrial tachycardia is nowadays performed with a 3D mapping system. As a rule of thumb: the ablation signal should be at least 30 ms before the onset of the P wave.

9.6 Special Entities

9.6.1 Acoronary Pocket of the Sinus Valsalva

Especially septally located FAT can pose a challenge for the electrophysiologist. If the earliest activation is near the His signal, an aortic origin of the FAT should be considered. The prevalence of FAT from the acoronary pocket of the Sinus Valsalva is 4.1–8.8% and is therefore rare. The acoronary pocket is located near the superior portion of the AV node, directly adjacent to the atrial myocardium of the intra-atrial septum. Histopathologically, myocardial extensions can be found in the aortic root and be held responsible for the development of FAT from the acoronary pocket. Ablation of this particular FAT is performed via puncture of the femoral artery and retrograde access to the aortic root (Beukema et al. 2015).

9.6.2 Localized Reentry

In the era of high-resolution mapping, the differentiation of "localized reentry" is becoming increasingly well-defined. The so-called "localized reentry" is defined by the fact that at least 85% of the tachycardia cycle length is found in the area of the earliest activation of the AT, within a circumscribed area smaller than 2 cm^2. Compared to FAT, a "localized reentry" can be successfully entrained (post-pacing interval < 20 ms) to secure the diagnosis. In contrast to the myocardial origin of FAT, the origin of "localized reentry" is more frequently associated with areas of "slow conduction" and electrical signal paucity, summarized with scar areas (Sanders et al. 2005). Further explanations can be found in Chap. 12.

References

Beukema RJ et al (2015) Ablation of focal atrial tachycardia from the non-coronary aortic cusp : case series and review of the literature. Europace 17:953–961

Bhasin D et al (2021) Incessant focal atrial tachycardia leading to tachycardiomyopathy. Cureus 13(1):1–6

Brugada J et al (2020) 2019 ESC Guidelines for the management of patients with supraventricular tachycardia. Eur Heart J 41(5):655–720

Chieng D, Lee G (2020) Multipolar mapping with the high density grid catheter compared with conventional point by point mapping to guide catheter ablation for focal arrhythmias. J Cardiovasc Electrophysiol 31(9):2288–2297

Glatter KA et al (1999) Electrophysiologic effects of adenosine in patients with supraventricular tachycardia. Circulation 99:1034–1040

Hayashi K et al (2016) Pace mapping for the identification of focal atrial tachycardia origin. Circ Arrhythm Electrophysiol 9:e3930

Hirao K (2018) Catheter ablation – A current approach on cardiac arrhythmias. Springer Nature, Singapore

Kellnar A, Fichtner A, Mehr M, Czermak T, Sinner MF, Lackermair K, Estner HL (2022) Single-center experience of ultra-high-density mapping guided catheter ablation of focal atrial tachycardia. Clin Cardiol 45:291–298

Kistler PM et al (2006) P-wave morphology in focal atrial tachycardia development of an algorithm to predict the anatomic site of origin. J Am Coll Cardiol 48(5):1010–1017

Kistler PM et al (2021) P-wave morphology in focal atrial tachycardia. JACC Clin Electrophysiol 7:1547–1556

Ouyang F et al (2006) Focal atrial tachycardia originating from the non-coronary aortic sinus. J Am Coll Cardiol 48(1):122–131

Roberts-Thomson KC, Kistler PM, Kalman JM (2006a) Focal atrial tachycardia I : clinical features , diagnosis , mechanisms , and anatomic location. Pacing Clin Electrophysiol 29:643–652

Roberts-Thomson KC, Kistler PM, Kalman JM (2006b) Focal atrial tachycardia II. Management 29:769–778

Sanders P et al (2005) Characterization of focal atrial tachycardia using high-density mapping. J Am Coll Cardiol 46(11):2088–2099

Schmitt C, Deisenhofer I, Zrenner B (2006) Catheter ablation of cardiac arrhythmias. Springer

Türkmen Y et al (2020) Focal atrial tachycardia-the localization differences between men and women: a study of 487 consecutive patients. Anatol J Cardiol 24:405–409

Willems S et al (2019) Targeting nonpulmonary vein sources in persistent atrial fibrillation identified by noncontact charge density mapping. Circ Arrhythmia Electrophysiol 12(7):e7233

Yagishita A et al (2019) Utility of a ripple map for the interpretation of atrial propagation during atrial tachycardia. J Interv Cardiac Electrophysiol 56(3):249–257

Yamashita S et al (2018) High-density contact and non-invasive mapping of focal atrial tachycardia: evidence of dual endocardial exits from an epicardial focus. Pacing Clin Electrophysiol 41(6):666–668

AVRT

10

Jakob Lüker

10.1 Introduction

Atrioventricular reentrant tachycardias (AVRT) are enabled by congenital accessory pathways (AP). The atrial myocardium, the ventricular myocardium, and the AV node are other critical structures of the reentry mechanism.

The conduction properties of AP determine which arrhythmias occur in these patients and whether the presence of the AP is evident in the resting ECG. The phenomenon of preexcitation depends on the anterograde conduction properties of the AP, which acts as an electrical connection between the atrium and ventricle. Ventricular myocardium in the area of the ventricular insertion is prematurely depolarized during anterograde conduction originating from the atria, so that—depending on the anterograde conduction properties and location of the AP, as well as AV node conduction properties—a more or less pronounced delta wave appears instead of the isoelectric line between the P wave and QRS complex (Fig. 10.1). The polarity of the delta wave can be positive, negative, or isoelectric, determined by the location of the AP and the vectors generated during the depolarization of the ventricular myocardium in the Cabrera circle. The most common location of the AP is in the area of the mitral valve (60% of cases), followed by a septal location (25% of cases) and rarely along the tricuspid valve (15% of cases).

The ability of an AP to conduct retrogradely is a prerequisite for the development of orthodromic AV reentrant tachycardia. Anterograde activation occurs via the AV node and the specific conduction system, so that in the absence of a bundle branch block, it presents as a narrow complex tachycardia, usually with visible, mostly inferior negative atrial depolarizations between the QRS complexes. Rarely, in the presence of an AP with both anterograde and retrograde conduction properties, an antidromic AVRT can occur (about 5% of cases). This presents as a wide complex tachycardia due to the electrical activation of the ventricles via the AP. The common discrimination algorithms between SVT with bundle branch block and VT cannot distinguish between antidromic AVRT and VT, as the conduction system is not involved in the excitation of the ventricular myocardium.

In the case of exclusively retrograde conduction properties (about 1/3 of all AP), patients become symptomatic only in the case of AVRT. The genesis in this case, unlike with additionally present anterograde conduction properties, is

Supplementary Information The online version contains supplementary material available at https://doi.org/10.1007/978-3-662-65797-3_10. The videos can be accessed individually by clicking the DOI link in the accompanying figure caption or by scanning this link with the SN More Media App.

J. Lüker (✉)
Abteilung für Elektrophysiologie, Herzzentrum der Uniklinik Köln, Köln, Germany
e-mail: jakob.lueker@uk-koeln.de

not evident in the resting ECG due to the lack of preexcitation. This is referred to as "concealed" AP (Katritsis et al. 2017).

10.2 Preexcitation, WPW Syndrome, and ECG Algorithms

The prevalence of preexcitation in the resting ECG is about 0.1%, and about half of those affected become symptomatic due to arrhythmias, especially the occurrence of AVRT, in the further course (Brugada et al. 2020; Zhang and Li 2020). Intermittent preexcitation is possible and depends on the refractory period of the AP (Fig. 10.1).

The combination of preexcitation in the ECG with the occurrence of symptomatic tachycardias is summarized as WPW syndrome after the first describers Wolf, Parkinson, and White.

▶ The term WPW syndrome encompasses the combination of overt preexcitation (visible delta wave in the ECG) and tachycardias. In the case of delta waves in the resting ECG without the occurrence of tachycardias, it is referred to as the "WPW pattern." In the case

of a concealed, exclusively retrogradely conducting accessory pathway ("concealed pathway"), orthodromic AVRT can occur. In this case, however, no delta wave is present in the resting ECG. Colloquially, this is sometimes referred to as a concealed WPW, although this term is not formally correct.

There are various algorithms that predict the location of the AP based on the preexcitation in the ECG. The algorithms of Arruda et al., Xie et al. (also: "St. George's algorithm"), and D'Avila et al. have comparable predictive accuracy (Arruda et al. 1998; Xie et al. 1994; D'Avila et al. 1995). Both for planning an ablation and for informing about complications and success rates, it is advisable to perform this localization diagnostics in advance. This is particularly relevant in the case of septal AP due to the risk of AV block or in the case of left-sided AP for planning a transseptal puncture (Exemplary: Arruda algorithm, Fig. 10.2).

An algorithm based on maximal preexcitation (Pambrun algorithm) enables an equally accurate and reproducible localization of manifest accessory pathways. Since a localization of the ALB is desired before the start of the electrophysiological study, instead of examining the QRS polarity

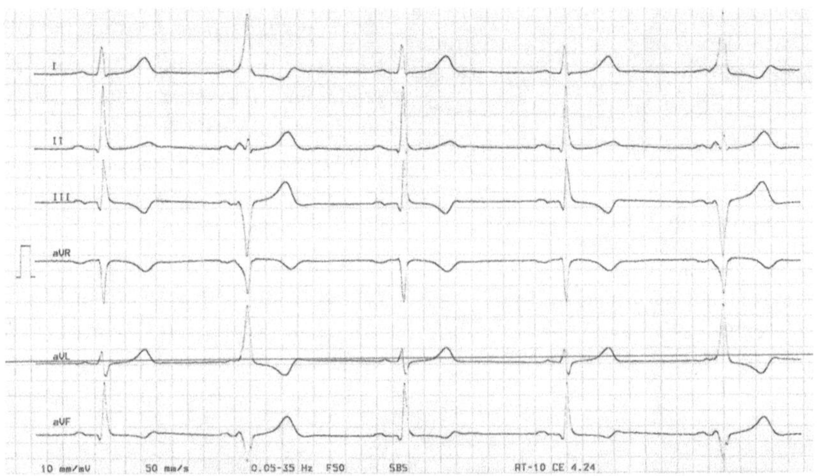

Fig. 10.1 Intermittent preexcitation. Normal AV conduction exclusively through the specific conduction system in QRS complexes 1, 3, and 4. QRS complexes 2 and 5 show positive preexcitation in I and aVL and negative preexcitation in III and aVR. Writing speed 50 mm/s

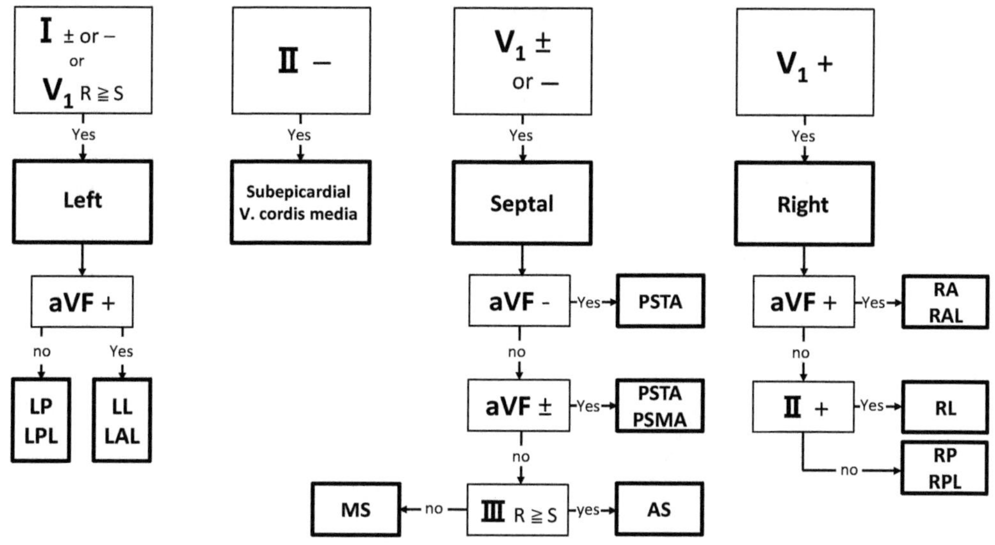

Fig. 10.2 Arruda ECG algorithm for the localization of accessory pathways. Assessment of the polarity of pre-excitation 20 ms after onset. + = pre-excitation positive, − = pre-excitation negative, ± = pre-excitation isoelectric. AS = antero-septal, MS = mid-septal TK annulus, PSTA = postero-septal TK annulus, PSMA = postero-septal MK annulus, RA = right anterior, RAL = right antero-lateral, RL = right lateral, RPL = right postero-lateral, RP = right posterior. (According to Arruda et al. 1998)

at maximal preexcitation, the polarity of the delta wave in the individual leads can be examined more simply (Pambrun et al. 2018; Fig. 10.3).

10.3 Risk of Malignant arrhythmias in Patients with accessory Pathway

Patients with AP have an increased risk of developing atrial fibrillation, with about half experiencing episodes of paroxysmal atrial fibrillation (Gemma et al. 2013; Nicolai et al. 1981).

Depending on the anterograde conduction properties, these episodes can be rapidly conducted to the ventricles. Due to the varying degree of fusion from conduction via the AV node with conduction via the AP, an irregular tachycardia with a variably wide QRS complex occurs, up to beats with maximal preexcitation (Fig. 10.4—**FBI tachycardia**).

Such episodes can, in the worst case, lead to ventricular tachycardias or ventricular fibrillation.

The risk for this is difficult to objectify and is reported, depending on the source, as 2.4/1000 patient-years or a 4% lifetime risk (Pappone et al. 2014; Katritsis et al. 2017). A clear association of preexcitation with increased mortality has not yet been confirmed, but it has been described in cohort studies (Skov et al. 2017).

While there is a clear recommendation for ablation in patients with symptomatic AVRT, the indication for ablation in asymptomatic patients with preexcitation is less clear. Due to the risk of malignant arrhythmias, the guidelines recommend risk stratification. Essentially, this consists of attempting to objectify the anterograde conduction properties of the AP during an EPS to estimate the risk of rapid conduction of atrial arrhythmias to the ventricles (increased risk with a refractory period ≤ 250 ms). The non-invasive risk stratification, which was frequently performed in the past, for example, during an ergometry, has proven to be unreliable and poorly reproducible.

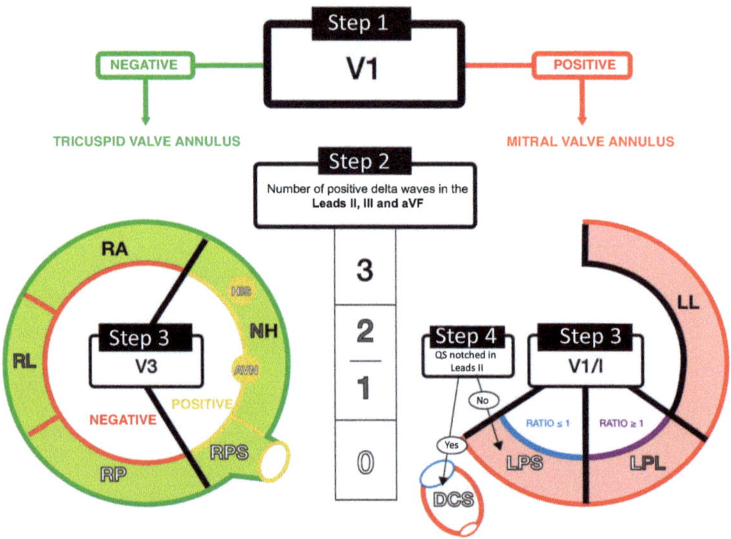

Fig. 10.3 Modified Pambrun algorithm, depicted as an anatomical schema. The locations of the accessory pathways are green if they are right-sided and red if they are left-sided. The font color of the AP locations is white if there is no positive polarity in the inferior leads (II, III, aVF), gray if a positive polarity is observed in 1 or 2 inferior leads, and black if all 3 inferior leads show a positive polarity. Right-sided AP are framed in orange or yellow if the V3 lead is negative or positive, respectively. Left-posterior AP are framed in blue if the V1/I ratio > is less than 1, or violet if the V1/I ratio ≥ is greater than 1. Abbreviations: right anterior (RA), right lateral (RL), right posterior (RP), right paraseptal (RPS), nodo-Hisian (NH), deep coronary sinus (DCS), left paraseptal (LPS), left posterolateral (LPL), and left lateral (LL). In the original, the polarity of the QRS morphology at maximal preexcitation in the inferior leads is examined. For the localization of the ALB in the 12-lead ECG before the start of the EPS, the number of positive delta waves in the inferior leads is examined here in step 2. (Mod. after Pambrun et al. 2018)

10.4 Electrophysiological Study and Differential Diagnosis of AVRT

While in patients with pre-excitation the presence of an accessory pathway (AP) is already confirmed by the surface ECG, the differential diagnosis of regular narrow complex tachycardia requires an electrophysiological study (EPS) with various diagnostic measurements and maneuvers.

The assessment of antegrade and retrograde conduction properties before tachycardia induction should be part of the standard procedure for SVT diagnostics. Here, the presence of an AP can often be excluded or confirmed early on. The demonstration of retrograde non-decremental conduction properties is indicative of a retrogradely conducting AP. The positioning of a multipolar catheter in the coronary sinus can quickly confirm a retrogradely conducting AP along the mitral annulus by demonstrating a so-called "bracketing" phenomenon (retrograde atrial activation presents eccentrically or in the form of a bracket in the CS catheter) during ventricular stimulation (Fig. 10.5).

In cases of questionable pre-excitation on the surface ECG, the investigation of the antegrade Wenckebach point (= loss of 1:1 conduction from the atrium to the ventricle) through atrial stimulation and measurement of the HV interval (shortened in antegradely conducting AP) can usually demonstrate the antegrade conduction of an AP.

Sometimes, tachycardia induction occurs repeatedly before or during these maneuvers, so the diagnosis must be made based on the tachycardia. An orthodromic AVRT is characterized by a long (> 70 ms) VA interval. However, this also applies to atypical AVNRT and atrial tachycardias (AT). Various spontaneous observations

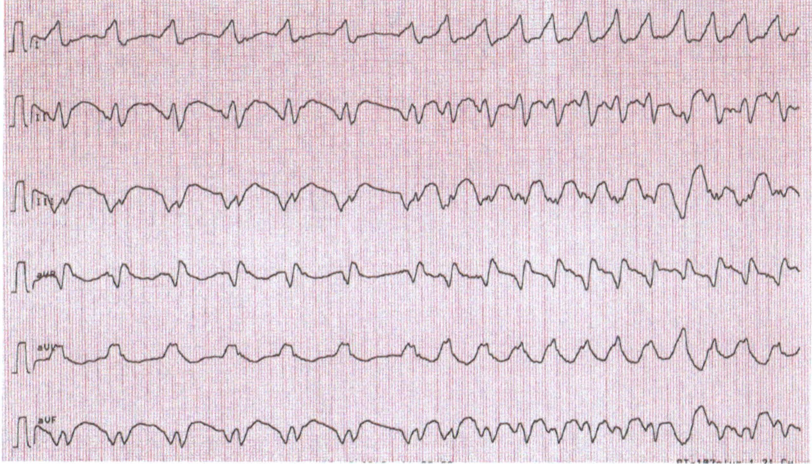

Fig. 10.4 Atrial fibrillation with tachycardic conduction via an accessory pathway, presenting as an FBI ("fast, broad, irregular") tachycardia

and active stimulation maneuvers during tachycardia are suitable for the differential diagnosis of AVRT vs. AVNRT vs. AT.

10.4.1 Observations Indicative of the Presence of AVRT

If there is an increase or decrease in the tachycardia cycle length, attention should be directed to the VA interval. An unstable, variable VA interval argues against a coupling of atrial and ventricular activity, as is the case with AVRT. Particularly if a change in the A-A interval precedes a similar change in the V-V interval (so-called "A-A predicts V-V"), this is indicative of an AT.

A bundle branch block during tachycardia is helpful in diagnosis. The increase in the VA interval by > 30 ms with the occurrence of a bundle branch block suggests an AVRT with an accessory pathway on the ipsilateral side of the block (i.e., a left-sided accessory pathway in the case of an increase in VA with a left bundle branch block) and is referred to as the Coumel phenomenon (not to be confused with Coumel tachycardia, see below).

Conclusions can also be drawn from the spontaneous termination of tachycardia by an AV block. AVRT and AVNRT are AV node-dependent tachycardias. An AV block would terminate both tachycardias. However, since AT is not dependent on the AV node in its mechanism, an AV block should not lead to the termination of AT. Such an observation is a strong, though not conclusive, indication of the presence of AT. However, it should be ensured that there was no change in the tachycardia cycle length or an atrial extrasystole before the occurrence of the AV block, as this can also lead to termination in the case of AT.

10.4.2 Stimulation Maneuvers for the Differential Diagnosis of Long VA Tachycardia

There are a number of maneuvers that can differentiate AVRT from atypical AVNRT and AT with varying sensitivity and specificity. Typically, certain maneuvers have become standard in different EP labs, and it is advisable to become familiar with the maneuvers used in your lab.

Two of the commonly used maneuvers (1. Ventricular Overdrive Pacing or "V-Entrainment" and 2. "VPD-Scanning" or "Preceding" maneuver) are presented below. A detailed presentation of all maneuvers with explanatory illustrations would exceed the scope of this work. Therefore, reference is made to the publications mentioned below, particularly

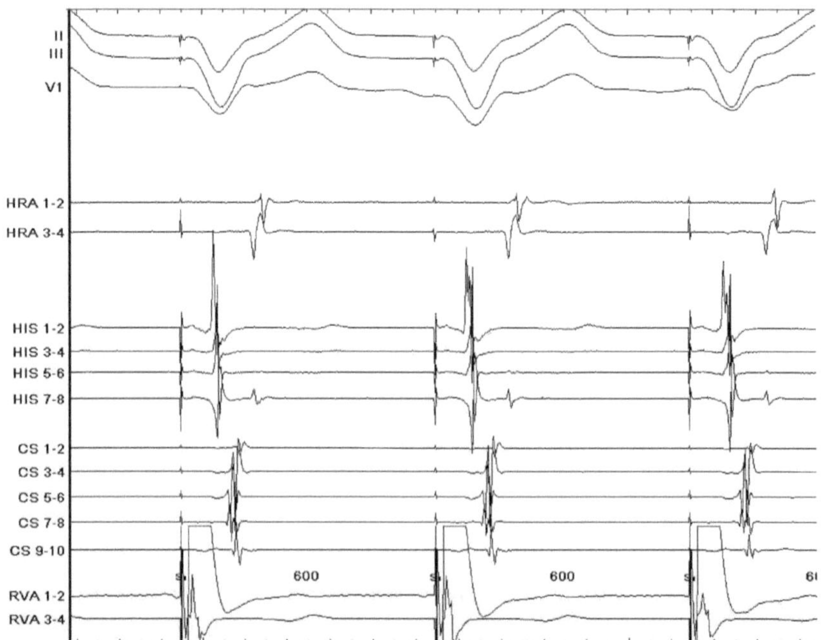

Fig. 10.5 Bracketing. The phenomenon of "bracketing" is shown during retrograde atrial activation via an accessory pathway during fixed-rate ventricular stimulation. The earliest retrograde atrial activation is visible in lead CS 5–6 of the diagnostic catheter in the coronary sinus. In leads CS 3–4 and CS 7–8, a later atrial activation is seen, creating the suggested shape of a bracket. This is not compatible with retrograde conduction via the AV node, given the appropriate position of the CS catheter. CS = 10-pole catheter in the coronary sinus, HRA = 4-pole catheter in the RA, HIS = 8-pole His catheter, RVA = 4-pole catheter in the right ventricle

the EHRA consensus document and the excellent two-part publication by Veenhuyzen (Veenhuyzen et al. 2011, 2012; Katritsis et al. 2017; Knight et al. 2000).

Ventricular Overdrive Pacing (VOP) (Fig. 10.6)

During tachycardia, stimulation is performed via a ventricular catheter with the aim of taking over atrial activation. If successful, the stimulation is stopped and the further behavior of the tachycardia is assessed. It is important that atrial activation was taken over during ventricular stimulation; otherwise, this maneuver leads to false conclusions.

A so-called V-A-V response of the tachycardia as shown in Fig. 10.6 excludes the presence of an AT. Differentiation of an AVRT from an AVNRT is usually achieved by subtracting the TCL from the post-pacing interval (PPI). A PPI-TCL < 110 ms is indicative of an AVRT. The stimulus-to-A (SA) interval and VA interval can also be considered. An SA-VA < 85 ms is indicative of an AVRT (Michaud et al. 2001; Ho et al. 2013; González-Torrecilla et al. 2006).

In the event of termination of the tachycardia during the VOP, the aforementioned measurements are not possible; however, the so-called transition zone can be considered to still draw conclusions from the maneuver (= phase of increasing ventricular fusion through stimulation during ongoing tachycardia. The transition zone ends with complete takeover of the QRS complex by V stimulation, after which the QRS morphology remains stable). A change in the A-A interval of the tachycardia already within the transition zone is indicative of an AVRT (AlMahameed et al. 2010).

Ventricular-Premature-Beat (VPB) Scanning (also: "Preceding Maneuver")

By appropriately setting the stimulator, His-synchronous stimuli are applied in the ventricle during tachycardia. If, after the ventricular stimulus ("sensed stimulus"), there is a preceding of the subsequent atrial action, an AVRT is to be assumed. It is important that the ventricular stimulus is delivered during refractory His to exclude retrograde conduction via the AV node. If the His signal is not clearly visible, the occurrence of an initial fusion of the QRS complex can be used as a surrogate (Figs. 10.7 and 10.8).

10.5 Ablation Therapy

The successful ablation of an AP is significantly dependent on the precise placement and stabilization of the ablation catheter. The choice of catheter and sheath also depends on the location. While an AP in the area of the CS ostium can be reached without a long sheath, ablation along the mitral and tricuspid valves generally requires a long sheath for sufficient catheter stabilization. A steerable sheath may be particularly necessary for AP in the area of the superior tricuspid valve annulus. The use of a 3D mapping system can be advantageous to reduce radiation exposure.

Mapping and ablation of AP along the mitral valve require a transseptal or retrograde aortic approach. The ablation is performed here analogously to atrial fibrillation ablation and VT ablation, mostly using cooled ablation.

10.5.1 Mapping Strategy Before Ablation

The positioning of the ablation catheter on the AP is based on the local potential. Here, a potential with fusion of the atrial and ventricular signals is sought, as an expression of the immediate conduction through the AP at this point. To achieve positioning along the annulus, a ratio of approximately 1:4 from atrial to ventricular amplitude is also aimed for. In the case of retrograde conduction of the AP, this can be done during fixed-rate stimulation via a ventricular catheter or during

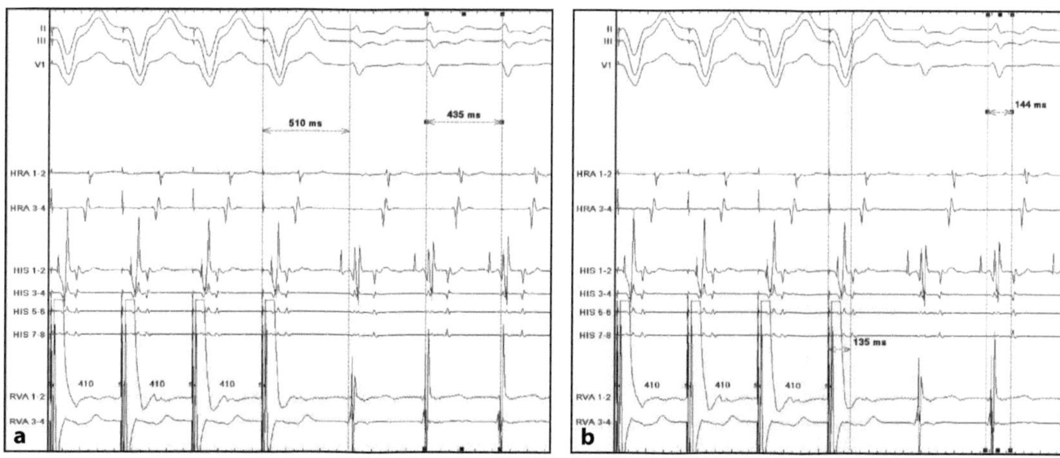

Fig. 10.6 Ventricular Overdrive Pacing (VOP) maneuver. Fixed-rate stimulation with 410 ms via the ventricular RVA catheter, taking over atrial activation. The tachycardia persists after stopping the stimulation. **a** A V-A-V response is observed after the end of the stimulation. Additionally, measurement of the post-pacing interval (PPI) from the last stimulus in the RVA catheter to the so-called "return cycle," the next tachycardia beat in the RVA catheter (here 510 ms), and measurement of the tachycardia cycle length (here 435 ms). **b** Measurement of the stimulus-to-atrium interval during the VOP maneuver (SA interval, measurement from the RVA stimulus to the earliest atrial signal. Here 135 ms) and the ventricle-to-atrium interval during tachycardia (VA interval, measurement from the earliest ventricular signal [surface ECG] to the earliest atrial signal [here 144 ms]). HRA = 4-pole catheter in the RA, HIS = 8-pole His catheter, RVA = 4-pole catheter in the right ventricle

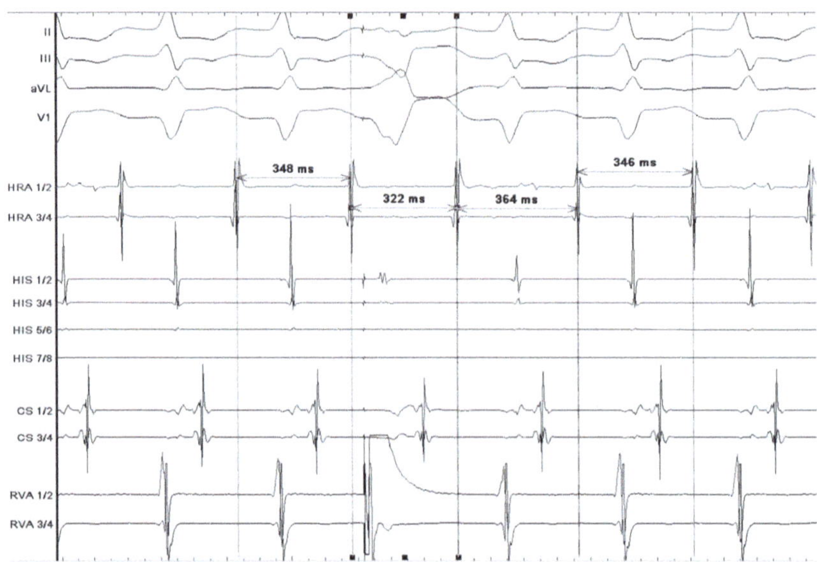

Fig. 10.7 VPB Scanning/Preceding. It shows a narrow complex tachycardia with a long VA interval (not measured here) and a tachycardia cycle length (TCL) of about 348 ms (measured here at 346 and 348 ms). A single ventricular stimulation via the RVA catheter produces a fused QRS complex. The subsequent atrial activation is preceded (TCL now 322 ms) and suggests the presence of an accessory pathway. The increase in TCL to 364 ms in the following cycle is likely an expression of decremental anterograde AV node conduction. Note: The ventricular stimulus must be delivered His-synchronously for reliable assessment. However, a His signal is not visible here. An initial fusion of the QRS complex can be used as a surrogate, as shown here, in cases of difficult His catheter placement. CS = 10-pole catheter in the coronary sinus, HRA = 4-pole catheter in the RA, HIS = 8-pole His catheter, RVA = 4-pole catheter in the right ventricle

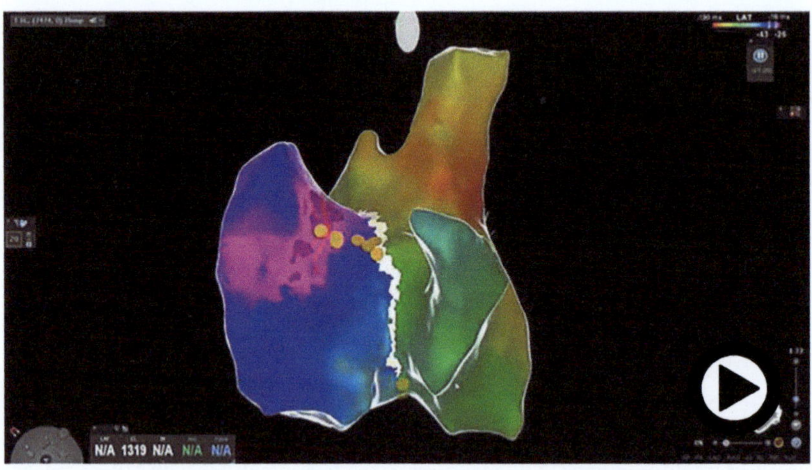

Fig. 10.8 Open Window Map of a right-sided posteroseptal accessory pathway with open preexcitation. The "window of interest" includes both the P wave and the QRS complex. The annotation is made on the steepest part of the unipolar signal. The *white line* marks the (non-conductive) AV valve annulus. The His bundle is marked in orange (https://doi.org/10.1007/000-d2q)

ongoing orthodromic AVRT. In addition to a fusion of the local atrial and ventricular potentials, an atrial signal in the ablation catheter as early as possible in relation to a reference catheter (e.g., in the coronary sinus) or an atrial action recognizable in the surface ECG is sought. Since an AVRT will terminate at the moment of successful ablation of the APB, ablation during tachycardia is associated with a certain risk of dislocation of the ablation catheter at that moment.

In the case of antegrade conducting AP, the earliest ventricular signal before the onset of ventricular depolarization in the surface ECG should be sought. For both strategies, consistent measurement based on a stable reference is important to achieve precise localization.

After stabilizing the catheter and starting the ablation, the AP should block within the first few seconds. An early block of the AP indicates a good catheter position. To avoid losing the localization of the AP during conventional fluoroscopic mapping, it can be advantageous to document the fluoroscopic position of the catheter at the moment of the block. The ablation pulse should be applied long enough to achieve a sustainable lesion.

After ablation, in the case of exclusively retrograde conducting pathways, renewed induction attempts should be made to conclusively confirm the diagnosis. In the case of antegrade conducting pathways, in addition to the block of antegrade conduction visible in the surface ECG, the retrograde conduction properties should be checked through ventricular stimulation. The use of adenosine can confirm the complete block of the AP in both directions. In the event of recovery after adenosine administration, a higher recurrence rate is to be expected. It is also advisable to observe a waiting period at the end of which the conduction properties are rechecked (Spotnitz et al. 2014).

10.5.2 T-Wave Inversions After Ablation of Antegrade Conducting AP

In patients with pre-excitation in the resting ECG, new T-wave inversions may occur after successful ablation of the AP. This is not the result of ischemia but rather the result of complex and not fully understood molecular mechanisms, including at the ion channel level. This phenomenon is summarized under the term "cardiac memory". It can also be observed in pacemaker or CRT-stimulated patients when stimulation is inhibited. The T-wave inversions usually regress within a few weeks after ablation (Shvilkin et al. 2015).

10.5.3 Success Rate and Complications in Ablation

The success rate of ablation is given as > 90%, but it is significantly dependent on the location of the AP and the experience of the person performing the ablation. Problems with catheter stabilization and the risk of AV block account for the lower success rate in ablation in the area of the superior TK annulus and near His AP (Brugada et al. 2020).

The same applies to complications during ablation, so figures here are also only generalizable to a limited extent. The overall complication rate is about 1.5%, and the mortality associated with ablation is 0.1% (Spector et al. 2009; Keegan et al. 2015). The risk of AV block requiring pacemaker implantation is reported to be about 0.5% (Garg et al. 2017).

10.6 Rare Forms of Accessory Pathways

There are rare variants of AP with decremental conduction properties, of which only the most well-known entities will be discussed here.

10.6.1 Permanent Junctional Reciprocating Tachycardia (PJRT; also: "Coumel Tachycardia")

These retrogradely decrementally conducting AP, usually located infero-septally in the area of the CS ostium, often lead to tachycardias with a long RP interval that occur already in early childhood. The stable reentry mechanism ensures that these tachycardias often persist for a long time and not infrequently lead to tachycardiomyopathy, which is usually reversible after ablation. Pre-excitation in the resting ECG is usually not found in these patients. PJRT is characterized by a long VA interval (usually > 200 ms) and must therefore be differentiated from an AT and atypical AVNRT by diagnostic maneuvers. The localization of the retrograde AP is achieved during ongoing tachycardia by mapping the earliest atrial excitation, based on a local potential significantly preceding the usually very distinct atrial actions in the surface ECG.

10.6.2 Atrio-fascicular and Long Atrio-ventricular Decremental Pathways

These AP, referred to as Mahaim fibers , connect the lateral or infero-lateral RA with the RV or parts of the right fascicle. Despite the anterograde conduction properties, these patients usually do not show obvious pre-excitation in the resting ECG. Since Mahaim fibers usually do not conduct retrogradely, antidromic reentry tachycardias occur. These present with a pronounced left bundle branch block due to their course. The mapping strategy targets a distinct, His-like, so-called M-potential, which is usually found in the area of the tricuspid valve vestibule.

For a further discussion of the aforementioned entities and other forms of decrementally conducting AP, refer to the detailed three-part publication "Unusual variants of pre-excitation: From anatomy to ablation" (Soares Correa et al. 2019a, b; Anderson et al. 2019).

References

AlMahameed ST, Buxton AE, Michaud GF (2010) New criteria during right ventricular pacing to determine the mechanism of supraventricular tachycardia. Circ Arrhythm Electrophysiol 3:578–584

Anderson RH, Sánchez-Quintana D, Mori S, Lokhandwala Y, Correa FS, Wellens HJ, Sternick EB (2019) Unusual variants of pre-excitation: from anatomy to ablation: part I-understanding the anatomy of the variants of ventricular pre-excitation. J Cardiovasc Electrophysiol 30(10):2170–2180. https://doi.org/10.1111/jce.14106

Arruda MS, McClelland JH, Wang X, Beckman KJ, Widman LE, Gonzalez MD, Nakagawa H, Lazzara R, Jackman WM (1998) Development and validation of an ECG algorithm for identifying accessory pathway ablation site in Wolff-Parkinson-White syndrome. J Cardiovasc Electrophysiol 9(1):2–12. https://doi.org/10.1111/j.1540-8167.1998.tb00861.x

Brugada J, Katritsis DG, Arbelo E, Arribas F, Bax JJ, Blomström-Lundqvist C, Calkins H, Corrado D, Deftereos SG, Diller GP, Gomez-Doblas JJ, Gorenek B, Grace A, Ho SY, Kaski JC, Kuck KH, Lambiase PD, Sacher F, Sarquella-Brugada G, Suwalski P, Zaza A, ESC Scientific Document Group (2020) 2019 ESC Guidelines for the management of patients with supraventricular tachycardia The Task Force for the management of patients with supraventricular tachycardia of the European Society of Cardiology (ESC). Eur Heart J 41(5):655–720. https://doi.org/10.1093/eurheartj/ehz467 (Erratum in: Eur Heart J. 2020 Nov 21;41(44):4258)

D'Avila A, Brugada J, Skeberis V, Andries E, Sosa E, Brugada P (1995) A fast and reliable algorithm to localize accessory pathways based on the polarity of the QRS complex on the surface ECG during sinus rhythm. Pacing Clin Electrophysiol 18(9 Pt 1):1615–1627. https://doi.org/10.1111/j.1540-8159.1995.tb06983.x

Garg J, Shah N, Krishnamoorthy P, Mehta K, Bozorgnia B, Boyle NG, Freudenberger R, Natale A (2017) Catheter ablation of accessory pathway: 14-year trends in utilization and complications in adults in the United States. Int J Cardiol 248:196–200. https://doi.org/10.1016/j.ijcard.2017.06.115

Gemma LW, Steinberg LA, Prystowsky EN, Padanilam BJ (2013) Development of rapid preexcited ventricular response to atrial fibrillation in a patient with intermittent preexcitation. J Cardiovasc Electrophysiol 24(3):347–350. https://doi.org/10.1111/j.1540-8167.2012.02398.x

González-Torrecilla E, Arenal A, Atienza F, Osca J, García-Fernández J, Puchol A, Sánchez A, Almendral J (2006) First postpacing interval after tachycardia entrainment with correction for atrioventricular node delay: a simple maneuver for differential diagnosis of atrioventricular nodal reentrant tachycardias versus orthodromic reciprocating tachycardias. Heart Rhythm 3(6):674–679. https://doi.org/10.1016/j.hrthm.2006.02.019

Ho RT, Frisch DR, Pavri BB, Levi SA, Greenspon AJ (2013) Electrophysiological features differentiating the atypical atrioventricular node-dependent long RP supraventricular tachycardias. Circ Arrhythm Electrophysiol 6(3):597–605. https://doi.org/10.1161/CIRCEP.113.000187

Katritsis DG, Boriani G, Cosio FG, Hindricks G, Jaïs P, Josephson ME, Keegan R, Kim YH, Knight BP, Kuck KH, Lane DA, Lip GY, Malmborg H, Oral H, Pappone C, Themistoclakis S, Wood KA, Blomström-Lundqvist C, Gorenek B, Dagres N, Dan GA, Vos MA, Kudaiberdieva G, Crijns H, Roberts-Thomson K, Lin YJ, Vanegas D, Caorsi WR, Cronin E, Rickard J (2017) European Heart Rhythm Association (EHRA) consensus document on the management of supraventricular arrhythmias, endorsed by Heart Rhythm Society (HRS), Asia-Pacific Heart Rhythm Society (APHRS), and Sociedad Latinoamericana de Estimulación Cardiaca y Electrofisiologia (SOLAECE). Europace 19(3):465–511. https://doi.org/10.1093/europace/euw301 (Erratum in: Europace. 2017 Apr 1;19(4):659)

Keegan R, Aguinaga L, Fenelon G, Uribe W, Rodriguez Diez G, Scanavacca M, Patete M, Carhuaz RZ, Labadet C, De Zuloaga C, Pozzer D, Scazzuso F, SOLAECE registry investigators (2015) The first latin American catheter ablation registry. Europace 17(5):794–800. https://doi.org/10.1093/europace/euu322

Knight BP, Ebinger M, Oral H, Kim MH, Sticherling C, Pelosi F, Michaud GF, Strickberger SA, Morady F (2000) Diagnostic value of tachycardia features and pacing maneuvers during paroxysmal supraventricular tachycardia. J Am Coll Cardiol 36(2):574–582. https://doi.org/10.1016/s0735-1097(00)00770-1

Michaud GF, Tada H, Chough S, Baker R, Wasmer K, Sticherling C, Oral H, Pelosi F, Knight BP, Strickberger SA, Morady F (2001) Differentiation of atypical atrioventricular node re-entrant tachycardia from orthodromic reciprocating tachycardia using a septal accessory pathway by the response to ventricular pacing. J Am Coll Cardiol 38:1163–1167

Nicolai P, Medvedowsky JL, Delaage M, Barnay C, Blache E, Pisapia A (1981) Wolff-Parkinson-White syndrome: T wave abnormalities during normal pathway conduction. J Electrocardiol 14:295–300

Pambrun T, El Bouazzaoui R, Combes N, Combes S, Sousa P, Le Bloa M, Massoullié G, Cheniti G, Martin R, Pillois X, Duchatea J, Sacher F, Hocini M, Jaïs P, Derval N, Bortone A, Boveda S, Denis A, Haïssaguerre M, Albenque J-P (2018) Maximal pre-excitation based algorithm for localization of manifest accessory pathways in adults. JACC: Clin Electrophysiol 4(8):1052–1061. https://doi.org/10.1016/j.jacep.2018.03.018

Pappone C, Vicedomini G, Manguso F, Saviano M, Baldi M, Pappone A, Ciaccio C, Giannelli L, Ionescu B, Petretta A, Vitale R, Cuko A, Calovic Z, Fundaliotis A, Moscatiello M, Tavazzi L, Santinelli V (2014) Wolff-Parkinson-White syndrome in the era of catheter ablation: insights from a registry study of 2169 patients. Circulation 130(10):811–819. https://doi.org/10.1161/CIRCULATIONAHA.114.011154

Shvilkin A, Huang HD, Josephson ME (2015) Cardiac memory: diagnostic tool in the making. Circ Arrhythm Electrophysiol 8(2):475–482. https://doi.org/10.1161/CIRCEP.115.002778

Skov MW, Rasmussen PV, Ghouse J, Hansen SM, Graff C, Olesen MS, Pietersen A, Torp-Pedersen C, Haunsø S, Køber L, Svendsen JH, Holst AG, Nielsen JB (2017) Electrocardiographic Preexcitation and risk of cardiovascular morbidity and mortality: results from the copenhagen ECG study. Circ Arrhythm Electrophysiol 10(6):e4778. https://doi.org/10.1161/CIRCEP.116.004778

Soares Correa F, Lokhandwala Y, Filho CF, Sánchez-Quintana D, Mori S, Anderson RH, Wellens HJJ, Back Sternick E (2019a) Part II – Clinical presentation, electrophysiologic characteristics, and when and how to ablate atriofascicular pathways and long and short decrementally conducting accessory pathways. J Cardiovasc Electrophysiol 30(12):3079–3096. https://doi.org/10.1111/jce.14203

Soares Correa F, Lokhandwala Y, Sánchez-Quintana D, Mori S, Anderson RH, Wellens HJJ, Back Sternick E (2019b) Unusual variants of pre-excitation: From anatomy to ablation: Part III – Clinical presentation, electrophysiologic characteristics, when and how to ablate nodoventricular, nodofascicular, fasciculoventricular pathways, along with considerations of permanent junctional reciprocating tachycardia. J Cardiovasc Electrophysiol 30(12):3097–3115. https://doi.org/10.1111/jce.14247

Spector P, Reynolds MR, Calkins H, Sondhi M, Xu Y, Martin A, Williams CJ, Sledge I (2009) Meta-analysis of ablation of atrial flutter and supraventricular tachycardia. Am J Cardiol 104(5):671–677. https://doi.org/10.1016/j.amjcard.2009.04.040

Spotnitz MD, Markowitz SM, Liu CF, Thomas G, Ip JE, Liez J, Lerman BB, Cheung JW (2014) Mechanisms and clinical significance of adenosine-induced dormant accessory pathway conduction after catheter ablation. Circ Arrhythm Electrophysiol 7(6):1136–1143. https://doi.org/10.1161/CIRCEP.114.002140

Veenhuyzen GD, Quinn FR, Wilton SB, Clegg R, Mitchell LB (2011) Diagnostic pacing maneuvers for supraventricular tachycardia: part 1. Pacing Clin Electrophysiol 34:767–782

Veenhuyzen GD, Quinn FR, Wilton SB, Clegg R, Mitchell LB (2012) Diagnostic pacing maneuvers for supraventricular tachycardias: part 2. Pacing Clin Electrophysiol 35:757–769

Xie B, Heald SC, Bashir Y, Katritsis D, Murgatroyd FD, Camm AJ, Rowland E, Ward DE (1994) Localization of accessory pathways from the 12-lead electrocardiogram using a new algorithm. Am J Cardiol 74(2):161–165. https://doi.org/10.1016/0002-9149(94)90090-6

Zhang Y, Li XM (2020) Pre-excitation cardiac problems in children: recognition and treatment. Eur J Pediatr 179(8):1197–1204. https://doi.org/10.1007/s00431-020-03701-9

Dierk Thomas and Hendrik Bonnemeier

11.1 Introduction: Mechanism of Typical Atrial Flutter

Typical atrial flutter is the most common atrial macroreentry tachycardia. The electrical excitation circuit takes its course in the right atrium in ~90% of cases (Saoudi et al. 2001; Bun et al. 2015) counterclockwise, i.e., ascending in the area of the atrial septum, then along the atrial roof, descending in the area of the free wall, and finally through the cavotricuspid area back to the interatrial septum (Fig. 11.1). The direction of excitation is assessed here considering the tricuspid valve annulus from the LAO ("left anterior oblique") perspective. Anatomically and functionally, the electrical excitation circuit is bounded anteriorly by the tricuspid valve and posteriorly by the

Supplementary Information The online version contains supplementary material available at https://doi.org/10.1007/978-3-662-65797-3_11. The videos can be accessed individually by clicking the DOI link in the accompanying figure caption or by scanning this link with the SN More Media App.

D. Thomas (✉)
Klinik für Kardiologie, Angiologie, Pneumologie, Zentrum für Innere Medizin, Universitätsklinikum Heidelberg, Heidelberg, Germany
e-mail: Dierk.thomas@med.uni-heidelberg.de

H. Bonnemeier
Klinik für Kardiologie, Helios Klinik Cuxhaven, Cuxhaven, Germany
e-mail: Hendrik.Bonnemeier@helios-gesundheit.de

openings of the superior and inferior vena cava, the crista terminalis, and the eustachian ridge. The so-called isthmus area between the inferior vena cava and the tricuspid valve ring provides the starting point for interventional ablation therapy. The course of the activation front counterclockwise with caudo-cranial septal excitation typically leads to "negative" flutter waves in the inferior leads II, III, and aVF with so-called "sawtooth waves" (Fig. 11.1). A clockwise excitation circuit ("clockwise") occurs in only ~10% of cases (Saoudi et al. 2001; Bun et al. 2015). The arrhythmia is then referred to as reverse or "reverse-typical" atrial flutter and is characterized by positive P-waves (sometimes notched) in the inferior leads (Fig. 11.2). The purely surface morphological distinction from atypical atrial flutter can be difficult here. Both forms usually have atrial rates between 240/min and 350/min, which can also be slower in the presence of structural changes in the atria or under antiarrhythmic treatment.

11.2 Cardioversion and Pharmacotherapy

In the case of an acute, symptomatic presentation of typical atrial flutter, electrical cardioversion is usually required. Instead of electrical cardioversion, pharmacological conversion attempts with amiodarone can also be undertaken, taking into account comorbidities and contraindications (Brugada et al. 2020).

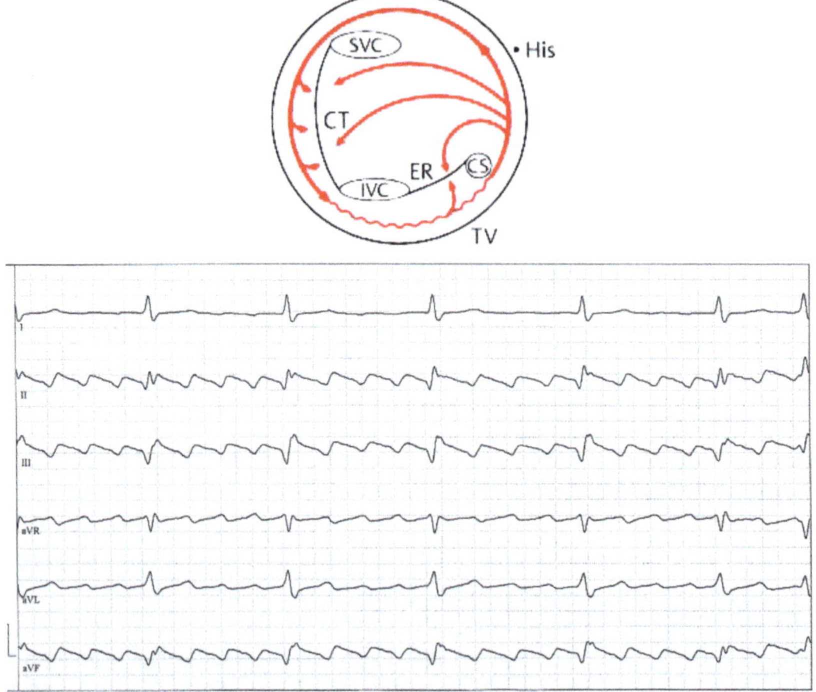

Fig. 11.1 The electrical excitation course in typical atrial flutter with ECG example (paper speed 50 mm/s). (Reproduced with permission from: Thomas et al. 2016)

Conversion with class Ic antiarrhythmics is contraindicated, as prolongation of the atrial cycle length can lead to 1:1 conduction of the tachycardia to the ventricle and thus to hemodynamic instability.

If catheter ablation is not desired or is delayed, medication-based rate or rhythm control must be considered. For rate control, beta-blockers or calcium antagonists (diltiazem, verapamil) can be used (Brugada et al. 2020). If rhythm control is the goal of treatment, amiodarone is used.

11.3 Electrophysiological Diagnostics and Catheter Ablation

11.3.1 Indication

In isthmus-dependent atrial flutter with a typical or "reverse-typical" right atrial excitation circuit, catheter ablation is the therapy of choice. Current European guidelines strongly recommend ablation of the arrhythmia in patients with symptomatic recurrent atrial flutter or with impaired left ventricular function due to tachyarrhythmic atrial flutter (Brugada et al. 2020). Catheter ablation can also be considered after the first occurrence of atrial flutter (Brugada et al. 2020).

▶ Typical, isthmus-dependent atrial flutter represents a common, clinically relevant supraventricular arrhythmia associated with significant symptoms and a risk of systemic embolism. Catheter ablation is an established, effective, and safe interventional treatment method.

11.3.2 Catheter Material and Electrophysiological Findings

For the electrophysiological diagnosis and ablation of typical atrial flutter, a multipolar electrode

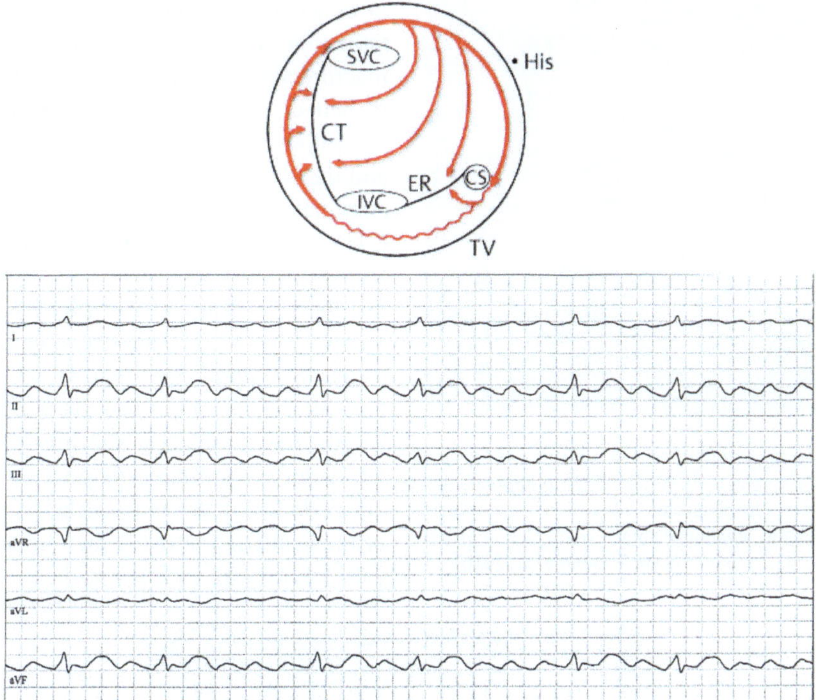

Fig. 11.2 Electrical excitation circuit in the right atrium in isthmus-dependent "clockwise" or "reverse typical" atrial flutter (detailed description see text) with exemplary ECG (paper speed 50 mm/s). (Reproduced with permission from: Thomas et al. 2016)

catheter ("Halo catheter"; Fig. 11.3) parallel to the tricuspid valve plane is very helpful. This catheter allows the simultaneous recording of electrical excitation from the atrial septum over the atrial roof, the lateral wall, and the cavotricuspid isthmus (CTI) to the coronary sinus (CS) ostium (Figs. 11.4 and 11.5). Additionally (or alternatively), another diagnostic catheter can be positioned in the CS (Fig. 11.3) to assess the prematurity of atrial excitation in the right versus left atrial side comparison, to increase the proportion of the captured cycle length in the total cycle of the tachycardia, and to perform stimulation in the CS. Finally, a standard diagnostic catheter can be positioned in the right ventricular (RV) apex to either bridge higher-grade AV blockages that may occur during the conversion of atrial flutter to sinus rhythm under ablation through ventricular stimulation or to unmask P-waves in the case of rapid AV conduction through premature ventricular extrastimuli. Furthermore, the RV-A catheter can mark the heart axis by marking the septal plane and serve as a landmark.

11.3.3 Diagnostic Maneuvers

In isthmus-dependent atrial flutter, the majority of the tachycardia cycle length is derived via the multi-electrode catheter. This already suggests the diagnosis of a right atrial macroreentrant tachycardia. To verify the isthmus dependency of the circuit activation, stimulation maneuvers are used, which can confirm the presence of "concealed entrainment" in the CTI area and thus the diagnosis of isthmus-dependent atrial flutter. For this purpose, fixed-frequency stimulation is performed in the CTI or lateral RA area with a cycle length 10–40 ms (by Bary et al. 2015) below the tachycardia cycle length. Concealed entrainment is present when, under stimulation, the intra-atrial excitation propagation is identical to the spontaneous tachycardia (albeit with a shortened cycle length corresponding to the stimulated frequency as an indication of effective stimulation = Capture) (Fig. 11.6). The presence

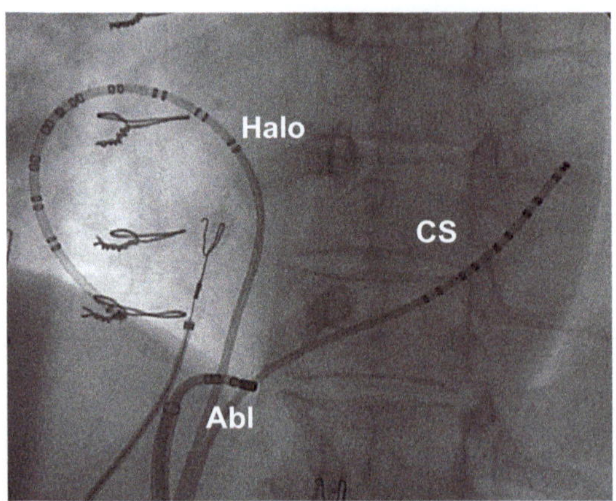

Fig. 11.3 Catheter positions during ablation of typical atrial flutter (LAO projection). A diagnostic multipolar catheter (Halo), a 10-pole diagnostic catheter in the coronary sinus (CS), and the ablation catheter (Abl) are depicted. (Reproduced with permission from: Thomas et al. 2016)

of concealed entrainment proves the active participation of the stimulated area in the electrical macroreentry. Additionally, in this diagnostic maneuver, the post-pacing interval (PPI) is determined, which lies between the stimulus and the subsequent spontaneous excitation at the stimulation site (e.g., catheter electrode on the CTI). If the PPI exceeds the spontaneous cycle length of the tachycardia by less than 20–30 ms, the stimulation site is very likely within the reentry (Fig. 11.6). This phenomenon is referred to as "resetting." However, if the PPI is more than 40–50 ms longer than the tachycardia cycle length, the stimulation site may not be part of the reentry. The time difference to the tachycardia cycle length arises from the propagation time of the excitation at the beginning and end of the

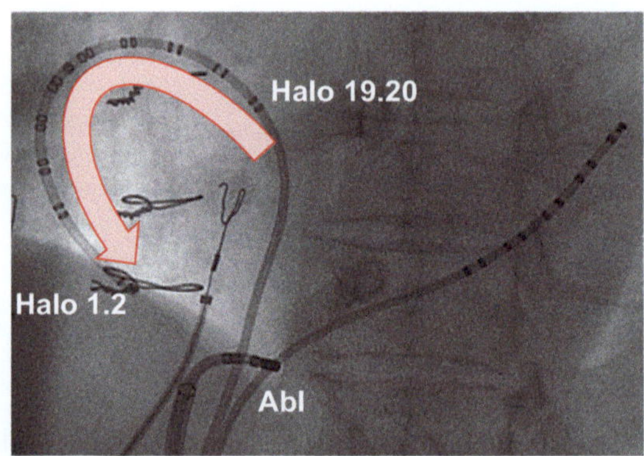

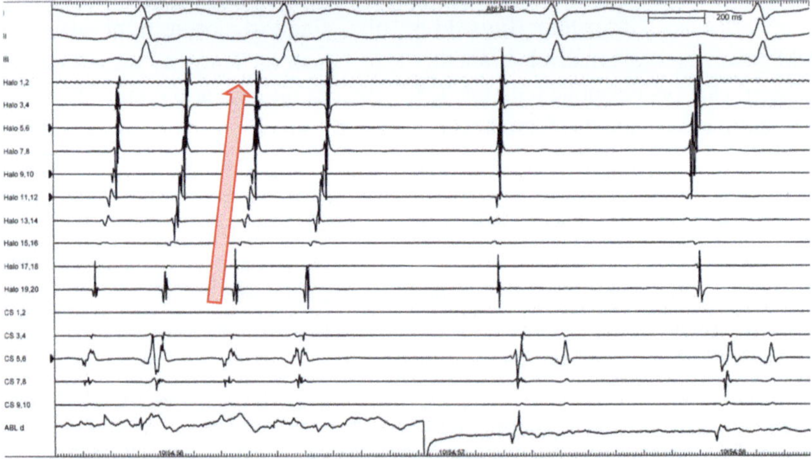

Fig. 11.4 Intracardiac activation sequence in typical atrial flutter. The *arrows* indicate the activation sequence in the LAO projection (*top*) and in the intracardiac signals (paper speed 100 mm/s). The excitation circuit runs from the Halo catheter electrodes 19 and 20 (Halo 19,20) counterclockwise (corresponding to a clock face in the LAO projection) to electrodes 1 and 2 (Halo 1,2) ("counterclockwise"). The arrhythmia running at the beginning of the recording is terminated in this example by the delivery of radiofrequency current via the ablation catheter (Abl). (Reproduced with permission from: Thomas et al. 2016)

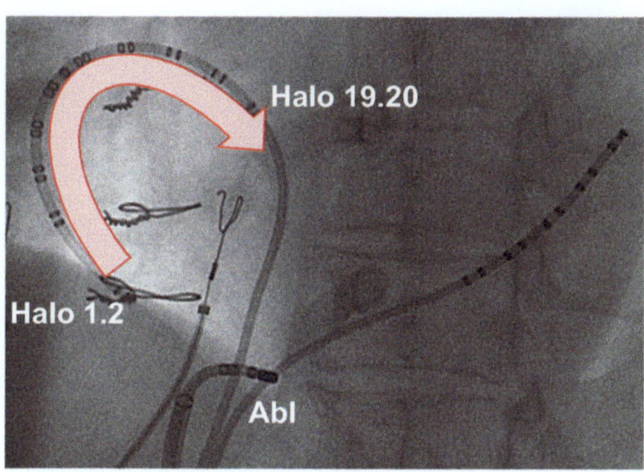

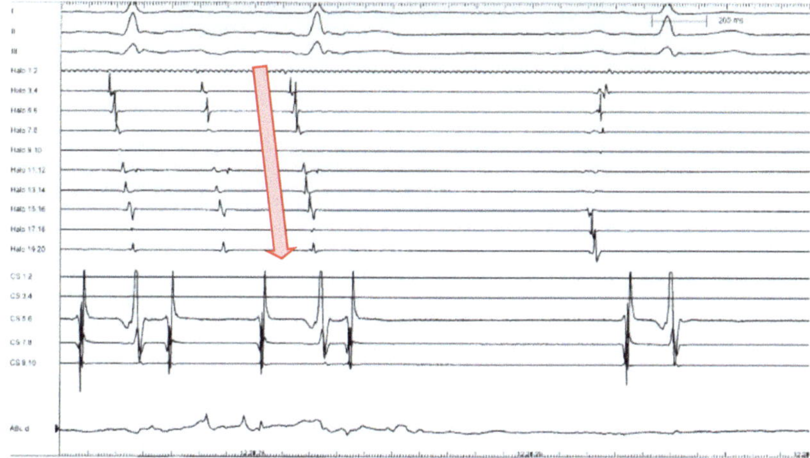

Fig. 11.5 Intracardiac activation sequence in reverse-typical-clockwise atrial flutter (paper speed 100 mm/s). The excitation circuit runs here in the LAO projection from the Halo catheter electrodes 1 and 2 (Halo 1,2) clockwise to electrodes 19 and 20 (Halo 19,20). In this example, the atrial flutter is terminated under ablation. (Reproduced with permission from: Thomas et al. 2016)

stimulation from the stimulation site to the reentry. If the listed criteria are met, the diagnosis of typical atrial flutter is made, and ablation is performed. In unclear cases, in addition to stimulation maneuvers, the use of a 3D mapping system can be useful to clarify the arrhythmia mechanism (Fig. 11.7 and 11.8).

11.3.4 Ablation and Success Control

The goal of catheter ablation is to interrupt the macroreentry in the area of the CTI between the tricuspid valve ring and the entry of the inferior vena cava. In most cases, radiofrequency current (rarely cryoenergy) is used to generate a continuous or point-by-point transmural linear ablation lesion. If atrial flutter is present at the beginning of the treatment, it must terminate during the ablation. The endpoint of the ablation is the demonstration of a bidirectional isthmus block. For this purpose, controllable ablation catheters with an 8-mm tip (temperature-controlled energy delivery max. 70°C/70W) or cooled ablation catheters (max. 40–45°C/40W) can be used. In cases of difficult completion of the CTI ablation line or more complicated anatomical situations, long intracardiac sheath systems are used in addition to cooled ablation catheters to increase accessibility. The correct position of the ablation catheter in the area of the CTI is checked in RAO and LAO projections; in LAO orientation, the catheter tip is located between 6 and 7 o'clock. At the beginning of the ablation,

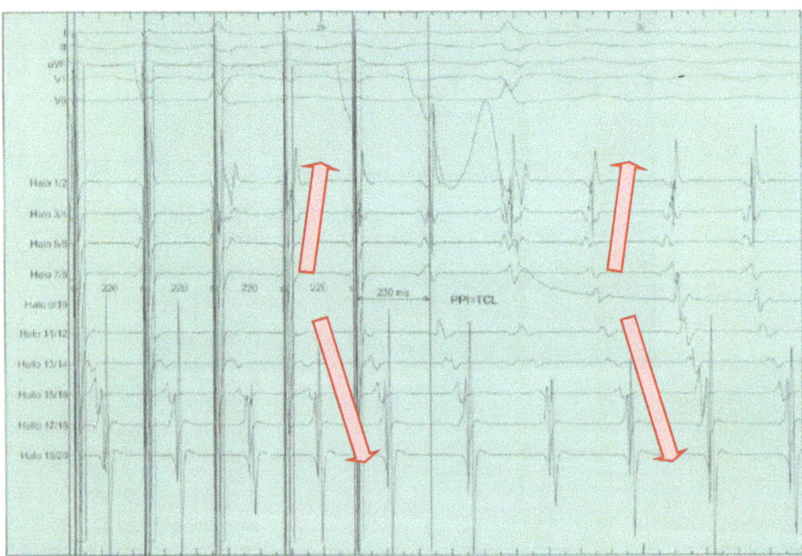

Fig. 11.6 Diagnostic criteria "Concealed Entrainment" and "Resetting". In this example, isthmus-dependent reverse-typical atrial flutter is present. During stimulation on the CTI with a base cycle length of 220 ms at a tachycardia cycle length (TCL) of 230 ms, concealed entrainment is present. Note that the sequence of excitation propagation (*arrows*) under stimulation is identical to the clinical tachycardia. There is also a resetting of the macroreentrant tachycardia: The length of the PPI corresponds to the TCL (explanations see text). (Reproduced with permission from: Thomas et al. 2016)

the ablation catheter is inserted into the right ventricle and withdrawn until the first atrial signals become visible in addition to the ventricular signal. Here, energy delivery begins, which is then continued under withdrawal and X-ray control of the catheter position up to the entry of the inferior vena cava.

After termination of the atrial flutter or during ablation in sinus rhythm, stimulation in the lower right atrium (block detection counterclockwise) and in the CS ostium (block detection clockwise) is performed to analyze the bidirectional isthmus block, and the sequential atrial activation is analyzed in the halo catheter (Fig. 11.9). In the case of a successful CTI block, the septum is activated last during inferolateral stimulation, whereas stimulation in the CS leads to the latest activation of the lower right atrium. During septal stimulation, wide double potentials with $\geq$ 110 ms latency should be found along the entire ablation line after isthmus block, which also confirms a successful CTI ablation. As long as the bidirectional isthmus block is not completely present (Figs. 11.10 and 11.11), gaps in the linear lesion are present, and further energy deliveries are required.

▶ **Troubleshooting in cavotricuspid isthmus ablation**

- To locate gaps, carefully check the isthmus area by probing with the ablation catheter
- Perform additional ablations where, despite previous ablation, atrial signals or closely coupled double potentials (< 90 ms) are still present
- Looping the ablation catheter in the right atrium with the catheter tip pressed against the cavotricuspid isthmus can be helpful
- Deviating the ablation line laterally or medially may be necessary

▶ Achieving bidirectional block in the cavotricuspid isthmus interrupts the right atrial reentry mechanism of typical atrial flutter and marks the endpoint of catheter ablation.

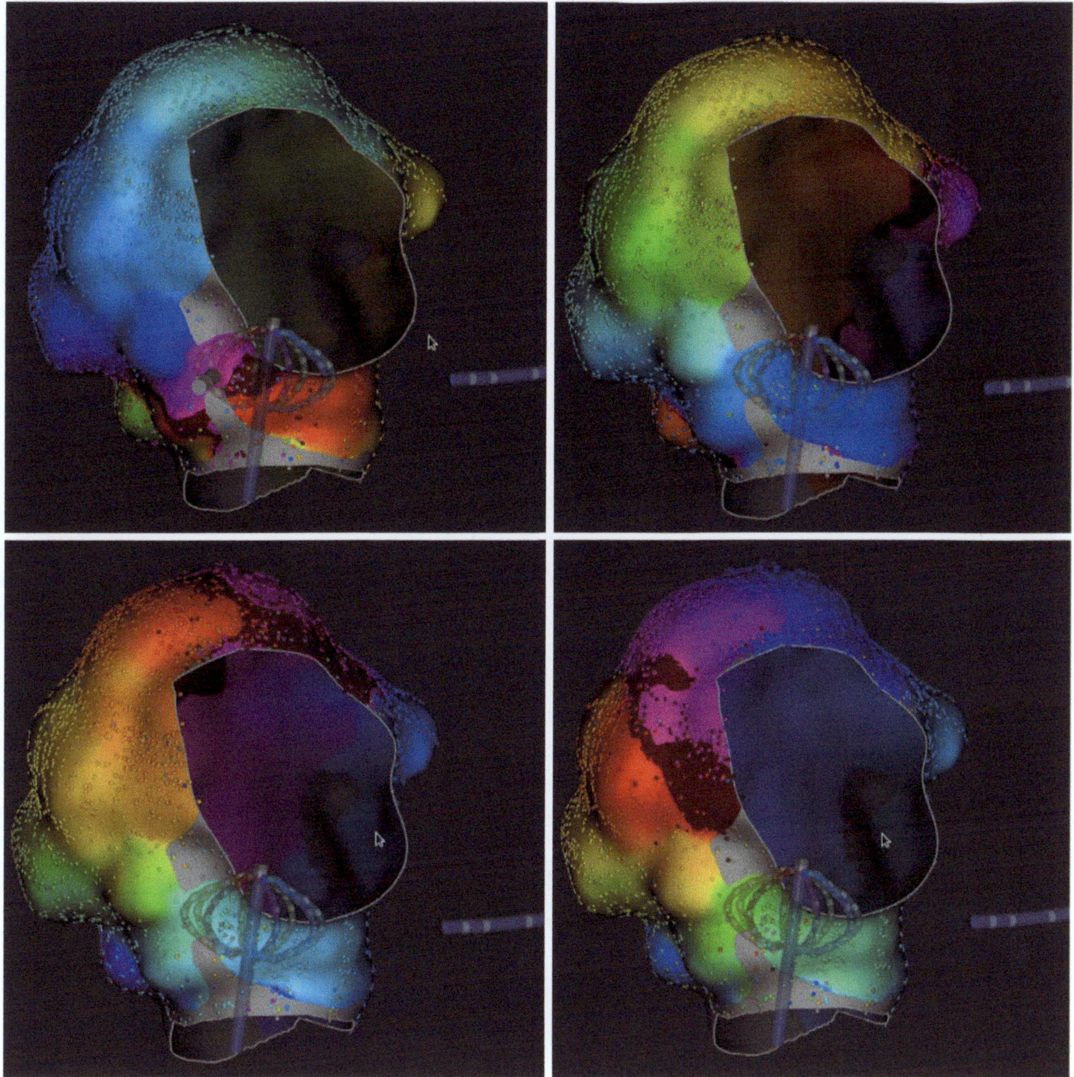

Fig. 11.7 Three-dimensional representation of the reentry in the right atrium during typical atrial flutter, created using Rhythmia HDx™. The excitation front is visualized in *red* and runs "counterclockwise" around the tricuspid valve ring

11.3.5 Success rates and possible complications

The acute procedural success rate of ablation of typical atrial flutter is very high, approximately 97% (Page et al. 2016). In contrast, the complication rate is pleasantly low (approximately 0.5%), with pericardial effusions (0.3%) and the need for pacemaker implantation (0.2%) being particularly relevant (Page et al. 2016). In the long term, the recurrence rate is up to approximately 11% (Page et al. 2016).

11.4 Embolism Prophylaxis and Anticoagulation

The data on the embolism risk in patients with typical atrial flutter is limited. It is assumed that typical atrial flutter carries a thromboembolic

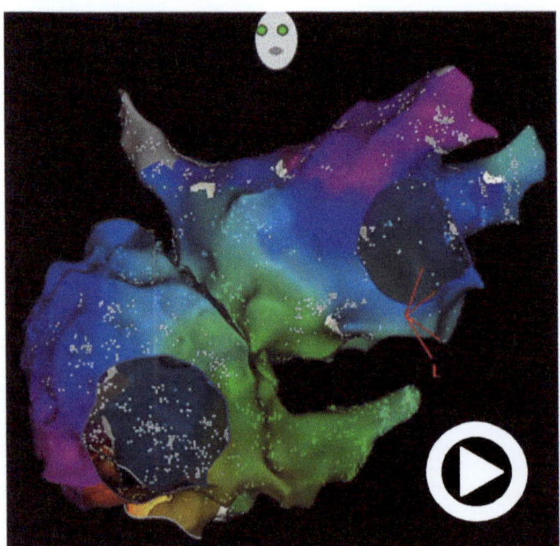

Fig. 11.8 Biatrial HD map of a typical atrial flutter ("counterclockwise"). Note the activation direction of the left atrium from inferior and septal as well as the *white* marked block line in the area of the crista terminalis (https://doi.org/10.1007/000-d2r)

risk comparable to atrial fibrillation. If catheter ablation of the arrhythmia is not performed, the indication for anticoagulation follows the current guidelines for the treatment of atrial fibrillation (Hindricks et al. 2021).

In patients who receive catheter ablation and exhibit atrial flutter at the time of treatment, a pre-procedural exclusion of thrombus via transesophageal echocardiography (if no adequate anticoagulation was performed for ≥ three weeks before the procedure) and post-procedural oral anticoagulation for at least four weeks are performed according to the recommendations for cardioversion (Hindricks et al. 2021). If adequate anticoagulation is not present at the time of ablation, a single dose of unfractionated heparin should be administered (e.g., 5000 IU heparin). Performing the ablation procedure under continued oral anticoagulation with vitamin K antagonists (INR > 2) or during continuous therapy with new (or non-vitamin K antagonist) anticoagulants (NOAC) is considered adequate and safe (Sticherling et al. 2015).

After an effective ablation of typical atrial flutter, the recurrence rate is low. However, there is a relevant coexistence of typical atrial flutter and atrial fibrillation. The majority of patients develop atrial fibrillation in the medium to long term after ablation of the cavotricuspid isthmus (Bun et al. 2015; Page et al. 2016). It is therefore recommended to perform oral anticoagulation in patients with a CHA2DS2-VASc score ≥ 2 even after recurrence-free ablation of atrial flutter (Sticherling et al. 2015).

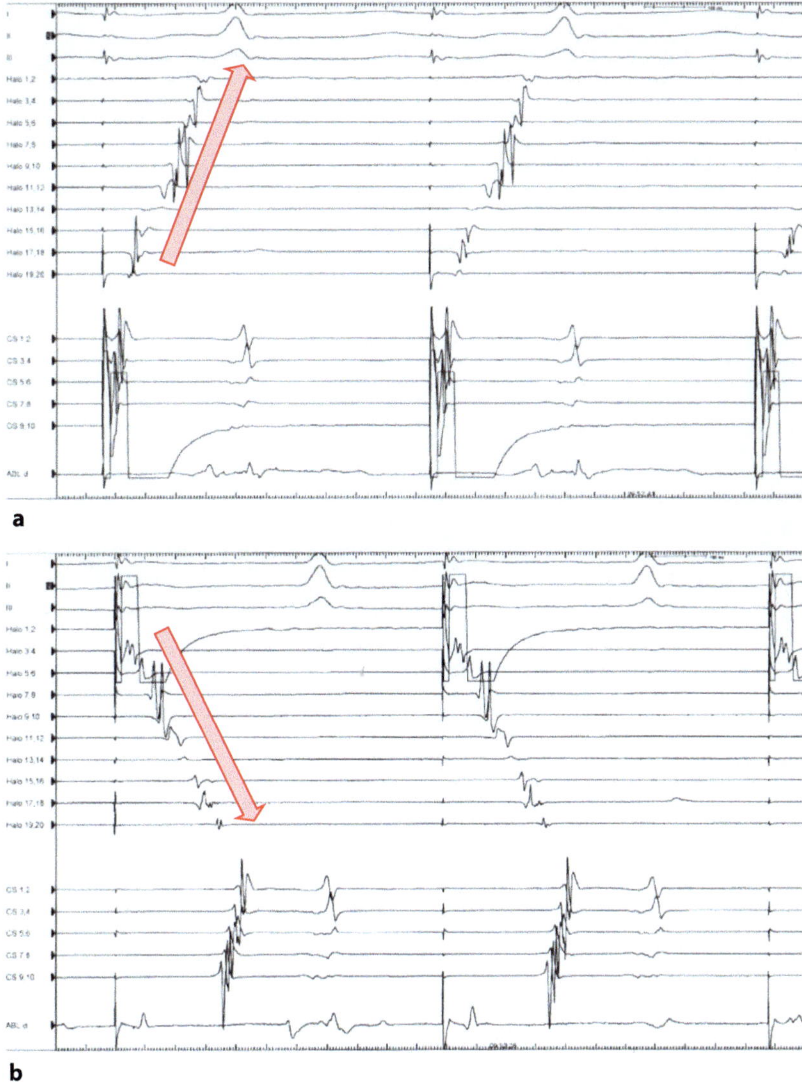

Fig. 11.9 Bidirectional conduction block, demonstrated by septal stimulation (**a**; stimulation site: proximal CS) and lateral stimulation (**b**; stimulation site: lower right atrium) of the ablation line on the CTI. During septal stimulation, the excitation front spreads counterclockwise (*arrow*), so that the inferolateral right atrium (Halo 1,2; see Figs. 11.3–11.5) is activated last. In contrast, the sequential activation of the right atrium during inferolateral stimulation (Halo 1,2) proceeds clockwise (*arrow*). At the very end of the sequence, the septum is electrically activated. (Reproduced with permission from: Thomas et al. 2016)

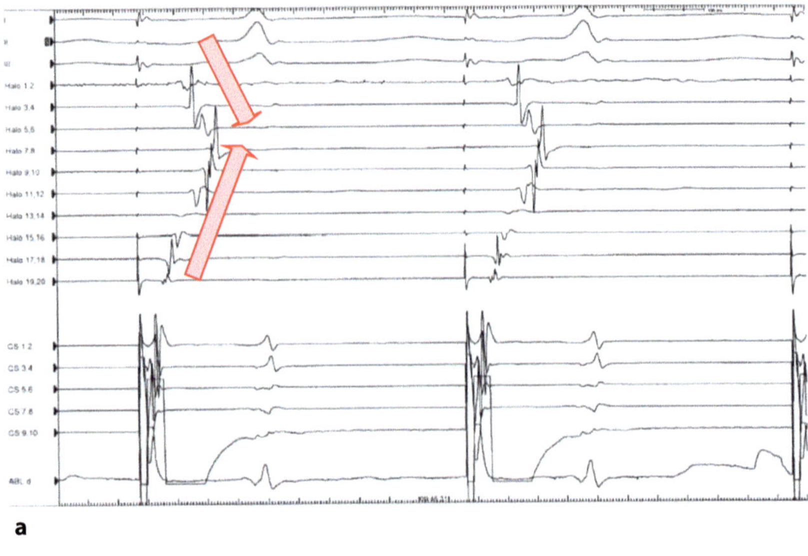

a

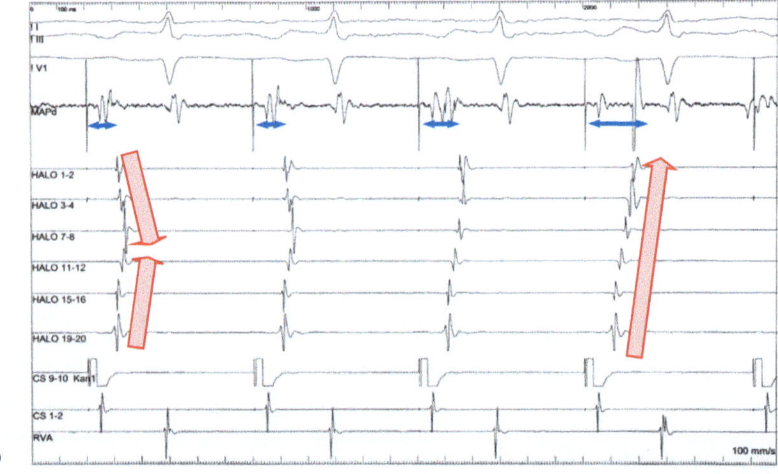

b

Fig. 11.10 Conduction delay without complete block in the area of the CTI, demonstrated during septal stimulation in the proximal CS. **a** The excitation spread occurs both clockwise (Halo 1,2 to Halo 5,6) and counterclockwise (Halo 19,20 to Halo 7,8). The clockwise conduction reflects conductivity with an incomplete ablation line between the proximal CS and the inferolateral RA. **b** In this example, there is also only a conduction delay without a complete CTI block at the beginning of the recording. During ablation, the complete interruption is shown in the further course. The ablation strategy here was based on the local electrical signal at the tip of the ablation catheter ("MAPd"): While a double potential with short coupling was present at the beginning, the latency increased during energy delivery, so that after complete ablation of the CTI, a widely split potential with latency > 110 ms is shown (*blue double arrows*). (Reproduced with permission from: Thomas et al. 2016)

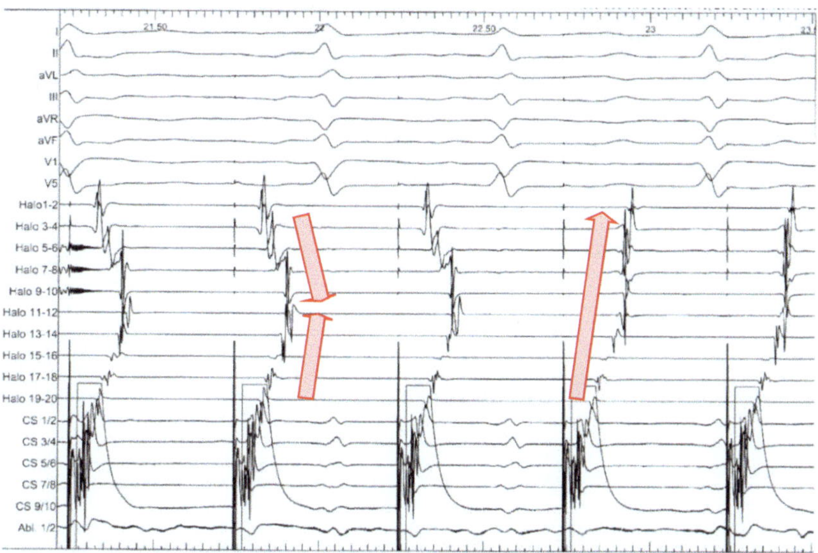

Fig. 11.11 Intracardiac activation pattern during stimulation via the basal coronary sinus. The desired CTI block occurs under energy delivery. (Reproduced with permission from: Thomas et al. 2016)

References

von Bary C, Eckardt L, Steven D, Neuberger HR, Tilz RR, Bonnemeier H, Thomas D, Deneke T, Estner HL, Kuniss M, Luik A, Sommer P, Voss F, Meyer C, Shin DI, Kriatselis C (2015) AV nodal reentrant tachycardia: Diagnosis and therapy. Herzschrittmacherther Elektrophysiol 26:351–358

Brugada J, Katritsis DG, Arbelo E, Arribas F, Bax JJ, Blomström-Lundqvist C, Calkins H, Corrado D, Deftereos SG, Diller GP, Gomez-Doblas JJ, Gorenek B, Grace A, Ho SY, Kaski JC, Kuck KH, Lambiase PD, Sacher F, Sarquella-Brugada G, Suwalski P, Zaza A, ESC Scientific Document Group (2020) 2019 ESC Guidelines for the management of patients with supraventricular tachycardia. Eur Heart J 41:655–720

Bun SS, Latcu DG, Marchlinski F, Saoudi N (2015) Atrial flutter: more than just one of a kind. Eur Heart J 36:2356–2363

Hindricks G, Potpara T, Dagres N, Arbelo E, Bax JJ, Blomström-Lundqvist C, Boriani G, Castella M, Dan GA, Dilaveris PE, Fauchier L, Filippatos G, Kalman JM, La Meir M, Lane DA, Lebeau JP, Lettino M, Lip GYH, Pinto FJ, Thomas GN, Valgimigli M, Van Gelder IC, Van Putte BP, Watkins CL, ESC Scientific Document Group (2021) 2020 ESC Guidelines for the diagnosis and management of atrial fibrillation developed in collaboration with the European Association for Cardio-Thoracic Surgery (EACTS). Eur Heart J 42:373–498

Page RL, Joglar JA, Caldwell MA, Calkins H, Conti JB, Deal BJ, Estes NA 3rd, Field ME, Goldberger ZD, Hammill SC, Indik JH, Lindsay BD, Olshansky B, Russo AM, Shen WK, Tracy CM, Al-Khatib SM (2016) 2015 ACC/AHA/HRS guideline for the management of adult patients with supraventricular tachycardia: a report of the American college of cardiology/American heart association task force on clinical practice guidelines and the heart rhythm society. J Am Coll Cardiol 67:1575–1623

Saoudi N, Cosío F, Waldo A, Chen SA, Iesaka Y, Lesh M, Saksena S, Salerno J, Schoels W, Working Group of Arrhythmias of the European of Cardiology and the North American Society of Pacing and Electrophysiology (2001) A classification of atrial flutter and regular atrial tachycardia according to electrophysiological mechanisms and anatomical bases; a Statement from a Joint Expert Group from The Working Group of Arrhythmias of the European Society of Cardiology and the North American Society of Pacing and Electrophysiology. Eur Heart J 22:1162–1182

Sticherling C, Marin F, Birnie D, Boriani G, Calkins H, Dan GA, Gulizia M, Halvorsen S, Hindricks G, Kuck KH, Moya A, Potpara T, Roldan V, Tilz R, Lip GY, Document reviewers (2015) Antithrombotic management in patients undergoing electrophysiological procedures: a European Heart Rhythm Association (EHRA) position document endorsed by the ESC Working Group Thrombosis, Heart Rhythm Society (HRS), and Asia Pacific Heart Rhythm Society (APHRS). Europace 17:1197–1214

Thomas D, Eckardt L, Estner HL, Kuniss M, Meyer C, Neuberger HR, Sommer P, Steven D, Voss F, Bonnemeier H (2016) Typisches Vorhofflattern: Diagnostik und Therapie [Typical atrial flutter: Diagnosis and therapy]. Herzschrittmacherther Elektrophysiol 27:46–56

Atypical Atrial Flutter

12

Marc Kottmaier and Tilko Reents

12.1 Introduction

Atypical atrial flutter is a cardiac arrhythmia characterized by rapid, repetitive, and regular depolarization of the atrial myocardium, which can lead to atrial rates of approximately 300/min (tachycardia cycle length 200 ms). Typically, there is regular conduction of the excitation to the ventricles, for example, three atrial excitations lead to one ventricular excitation, resulting in a 3:1 conduction. In rare cases, however, there may be variable conduction, where the ventricular rate is irregular, but the atrial rate is regular (Granada et al. 2000; January et al. 2019; Rodriguez Ziccardi et al. 2021). To differentiate from pseudo-regularized atrial fibrillation (e.g., in patients under antiarrhythmic medication), a

---

Supplementary Information The online version contains supplementary material available at https://doi.org/10.1007/978-3-662-65797-3_12. The videos can be accessed individually by clicking the DOI link in the accompanying figure caption or by scanning this link with the SN More Media App.

M. Kottmaier (✉)
Zentrum für Herzrhythmusstörungen Augsburg, Neusäß, Germany
e-mail: kottmaier@ep-augsburg.de

T. Reents
Klinik für Herz- und Kreislauferkrankungen, Deutsches Herzzentrum München, München, Germany
e-mail: reents@dhm.mhn.de

look at the surface ECG helps. Here, to distinguish from pseudo-regularized atrial fibrillation, the morphology (uniform) and the cycle length (regular, usually > 200 ms) of the atrial excitation should be considered (see Fig. 12.1). Any atrial macro-reentry tachycardia that does not mechanistically involve the cavotricuspid isthmus is referred to as atypical atrial flutter, both left and right atrial (Granada et al. 2000; January et al. 2019; Rodriguez Ziccardi et al. 2021).

The symptoms of patients are similar to those of atrial fibrillation, associated with palpitations, dyspnea, and reduced performance. Due to the usually tachycardic conduction, which responds less well to medication-based rate control compared to atrial fibrillation, patients with atypical atrial flutter often experience significant symptoms. As with atrial fibrillation, there is an increased risk of thromboembolic complications with atypical atrial flutter, so oral anticoagulation is indicated depending on comorbidities (CHA_2DS_2VASC score) (January et al. 2019).

Terminology and Mechanism
In the field of atrial tachycardias, there are significant overlaps in content and terminology between (atypical) atrial flutter and focal atrial tachycardias. For didactic reasons and clarity, the classification used here is named. In everyday language, the term atrial tachycardia and focal atrial tachycardia are often used synonymously. This is particularly the case in the context of SVT in structurally healthy atria. In

---

L. Iden et al. (eds.), *Invasive Electrophysiology for Beginners*, https://doi.org/10.1007/978-3-662-70158-4_12

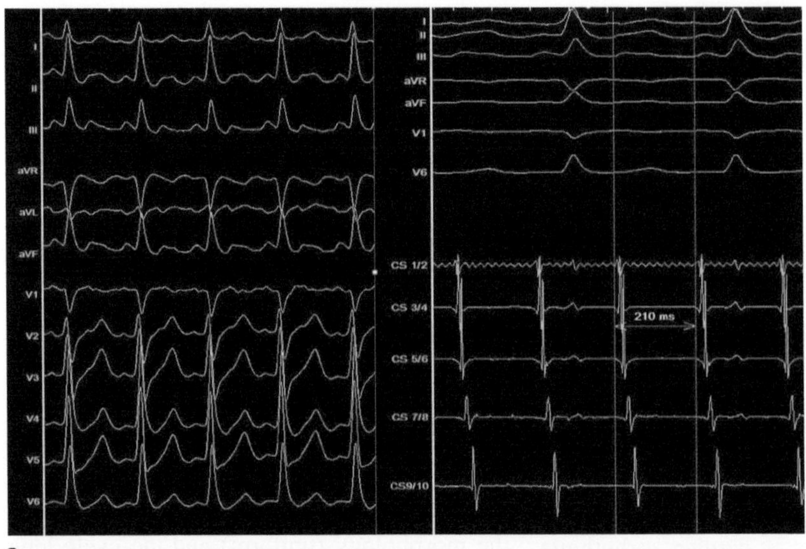

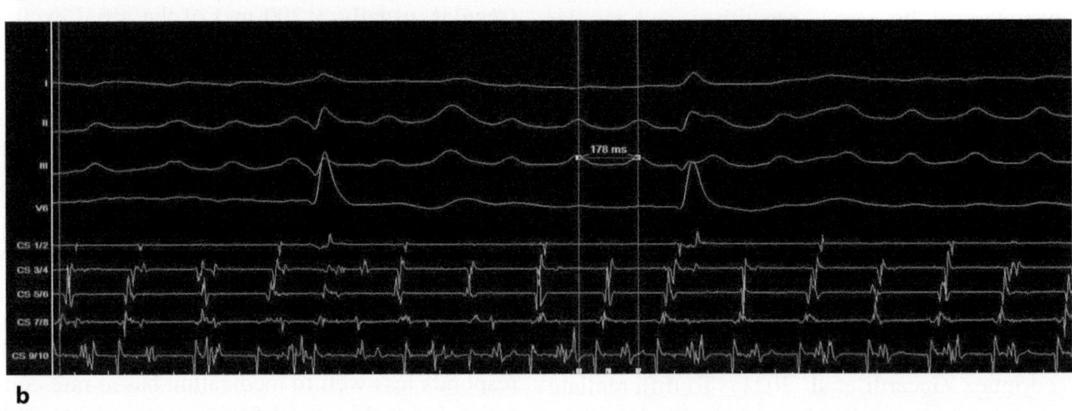

Fig. 12.1 **a** Atypical atrial flutter in the surface ECG with a cycle length of 210 ms. Corresponding intra-atrial leads of the regulated electrical activity in the coronary sinus with distal-proximal CS sequence. **b** Pseudo-regularized atrial fibrillation in the surface ECG with indicated "flutter waves". The intracardiac lead in the coronary sinus shows unregulated electrical activity in atrial fibrillation

contrast, the term atrial tachycardia in the context of a structurally altered atrium (previously ablated, previously operated, or dilated) represents a collective term for tachycardias of various mechanisms. It includes reentry tachycardias of various types, which are sometimes inconsistently named and handled in the nomenclature. The classification here and in the following is as follows:

then positive in at least two segments (e.g., the lateral and anterior left atrium). Good post-pacing intervals must therefore be shown in two different segments (see Sect. 12.2.1 "Entrainment Mapping"). In the context of mapping, almost the entire cycle length of the tachycardia can usually be recorded along the activation front in the affected atrium (Saoudi et al. 2001a) (see Fig. 12.2a).

Macro-Reentry Tachycardias (MR-ATs)
Mechanistically, MR-ATs involve multiple segments of the affected atrium. Entrainment is

Localized reentry tachycardias (LR-ATs)
LR-ATs are circulating excitations in a small area (typically about 2 cm^2), whose activation

front spreads centrifugally over the atrium. In the context of entrainment, a positive post-pacing interval (PPI) is shown only in one segment of the affected atrium. The PPI becomes shorter the closer one gets to the origin of the LR-AT and longer the further one moves away from it. Regarding mapping, more than 75% of the cycle length can usually be covered in the affected atrium (Jais et al. 2009). However, to accurately differentiate or identify the origin, high-resolution mapping catheters are usually necessary. MR-ATs are (mostly) easier to identify in activation mapping (see Fig. 12.2b).

Focal atrial tachycardia

Focal atrial tachycardias (FAT) are focal excitations of the atrium, originating from a point or cell cluster. In contrast to the aforementioned entities, the predominant mechanism is increased automaticity or triggered activity. The excitation of the atrium occurs centrifugally from the focus. The entire cycle length of the tachycardia is not necessarily mappable (Saoudi et al. 2001a).

This chapter focuses on macro-reentry tachycardias as well as localized reentry tachycardias; focal atrial tachycardias are covered in a separate chapter.

Etiology

Etiologically, atypical atrial flutter is a very heterogeneous condition and can be favored by various atrial preconditions, whereas it is rather rare in structurally healthy atria (Granada et al. 2000). In up to 15% of patients with atrial fibrillation and antiarrhythmic therapy with class Ic or class III antiarrhythmics (propafenone/flecainide or amiodarone), there can be a regularization of atrial activity, which can range up to a complete regularization to atypical atrial flutter (Granada et al. 2000; January et al. 2019; Rodriguez Ziccardi et al. 2021).

The pathophysiological correlate responsible for the development and maintenance of reentry tachycardias is summarized as "substrate".

Structural remodeling processes, caused by myocardial fibrosis or iatrogenically by ablation lesions and surgical incisions leading to scarring, together with anatomical structures such as the mitral or tricuspid valve, serve as "substrate" for reentry tachycardias.

These often arise in the border areas of scars, which usually exhibit very heterogeneous

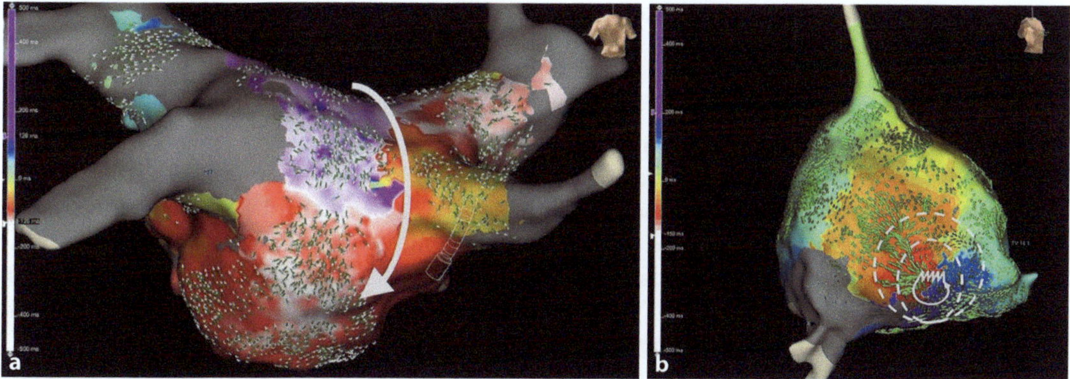

Fig. 12.2 a Macroreentry with activation front running over the roof of the left atrium. The cycle length is depicted 90% in the left atrium. Entrainment is positive at the roof as well as in the inferior left atrium (see subsection Entrainment). **b** Localized reentry in the area of the inferior crista terminalis in the right atrium. Almost the entire cycle length can be recorded at one spot with the multipolar mapping catheter. The activation appears centrifugal from one area. Unlike typical atrial flutter, the entrainment here is only positive in the area of the inferolateral wall of the RA (near the LR), while it would be negative in the proximal coronary sinus (positive in typical atrial flutter).

conduction properties regarding conduction velocities and refractory periods. Prerequisites for the development of a reentry tachycardia are:

1. **Unidirectional conduction block:** This can occur transiently, e.g., caused by an early premature beat, or permanently due to fibrosis or scarring processes that allow excitation propagation only in one direction.
2. **Zone of slow conduction:** Within areas of fibrosis/scars, vital myocytes with altered conduction properties are often found, which function as zones of slow conduction (so-called slow-conduction zones).
3. **Presence of an "excitable gap":** For the reentry circuit to form or be maintained, the circulating excitation must encounter non-refractory tissue.

Through a unidirectional conduction block, the electrical impulse excites the healthy myocardium via a zone of slow conduction (e.g., in the border area of a scar) and subsequently encounters a no longer refractory zone of slow conduction, allowing the reentry mechanism to form or be maintained (see Fig. 12.3).

In principle, although much less frequently, atrial flutter can also arise in "healthy" tissue on the basis of a reentry. A slow-conduction zone is not found here; the reentry then circles around an anatomical substrate (usually in dilated atria).

The following is a list of possible causes for the occurrence of atypical atrial flutter:

- **Iatrogenic substrate after ablation or incision**
  The substrate necessary for the development and maintenance of MR-AT can be caused by previous interventions (surgery or ablation) (Granada et al. 2000; January et al. 2019; Rodriguez Ziccardi et al. 2021). Atrial flutter often occurs after cardiac surgical procedures with atriotomy – for example, after closure of an atrial septal defect, a right atrial atriotomy as an access route for heart valve surgeries, or a MAZE procedure. Similarly, atypical atrial flutter can occur after previous ablations.

- **Idiopathic substrate due to fibrosis**
  In the context of extensive atrial fibrosis, either idiopathic or after, for example, mediastinal or thoracic irradiation, native atypical atrial flutter can occur. In a bipolar voltage mapping, these patients often show extensive areas with so-called "no" or "low-voltage".

- **Functional**
  Some potentially reversible factors that can lead to atrial fibrillation can also (although much less frequently) lead to atrial flutter. These include, for example, hyperthyroidism, intoxications, pericarditis, pulmonary embolisms, etc. The atria often do not show "low" or "no"-voltage areas, so after eliminating the trigger and rhythm control via cardioversion, there is a good prognosis regarding freedom from atypical atrial flutter (Granada et al. 2000; Saoudi et al. 2001b; January et al. 2019; Rodriguez Ziccardi et al. 2021).

12.2 Entrainment and Activation Mapping

12.2.1 Entrainment Mapping

Entrainment mapping enables the diagnosis and characterization of reentrant tachycardias. While activation mapping represents the temporal excitation sequence of a reentrant tachycardia, entrainment mapping checks whether the ablation catheter or diagnostic electrode catheter is located within the area of circulating excitation.

By stimulating with a cycle length of 20–30 ms below the tachycardia cycle length (TCL), the reentrant tachycardia is temporarily accelerated. It must be ensured that the reentrant tachycardia is actually accelerated ("captured") to the stimulation cycle length by measuring the atrial cycle length (for example, via leads of the CS catheter).

Whether the catheter is within the reentry circuit can be determined by the so-called post-pacing interval (PPI) or post-stimulation interval. The PPI is the interval between the last stimulated excitation and the first

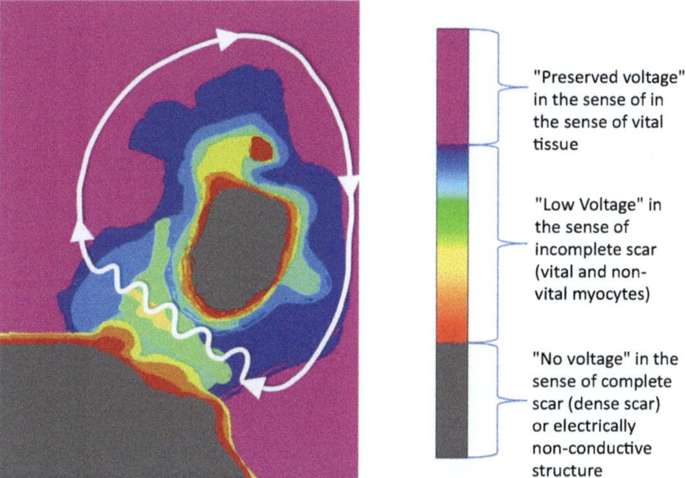

Fig. 12.3 Schematic representation of a reentry in the voltage map. Between two scar areas in gray (so-called no-voltage areas, as the tissue here exhibits no electrical activity) lies an area with partially fibrosed and vital myocytes. Due to the lower number of vital myocytes, the electrical amplitude is lower (low-voltage area, depicted with a color spectrum depending on the amplitude of the vital myocytes). The juxtaposition of vital and non-vital myocytes leads to a delay in the electrical conduction properties of a so-called slow-conduction zone (*curved line*). The reentry (*white arrow*) runs around the scar through vital tissue (preserved voltage, depicted in *violet*) and then encounters a no longer refractory slow-conduction zone, allowing the reentry to be maintained (*curved line*).

non-stimulated activation. If this interval is almost identical (< 30 ms above TCL) to the spontaneous cycle length of the tachycardia, then the catheter is within the reentry. Long PPIs (> 50 ms above TCL) indicate a catheter position outside the reentry circuit (see Fig. 12.4).

Furthermore, the presence of "concealed entrainment" is assessed. Here, under stimulation, both the intracardiac and surface morphology correspond to the clinical tachycardia.

The interpretation of entrainment can be complicated by acceleration or termination of the tachycardia. Additionally, there may be a change in the tachycardia mechanism or degeneration into atrial fibrillation. Therefore, it is advisable to stimulate or entrain only about 20–30 ms below the cycle length of the initial tachycardia. Another difficulty sometimes encountered is the lack of capture, meaning the tachycardia cannot be accelerated to the stimulated cycle length. Therefore, entrainment should always be performed from various stimulation sites. It should be noted that in atria with severe fibrosis and extensive "low-voltage" areas, entrainment or capture may be difficult.

12.2.2 Activation Mapping

The 3D mapping systems available since the late 1990s are capable of integrating electrophysiological data into a virtual three-dimensional geometry of the heart chamber. By scanning the atria with an ablation catheter or with multipolar mapping catheters, a three-dimensional geometry is generated and the recorded electrograms are simultaneously integrated into the 3D mapping system.

With activation mapping, the temporal sequence of a reentrant tachycardia can be displayed color-coded in a 3D mapping system. For the creation of an activation map, it is necessary to define a temporal reference, as there are no "early" or "late" signals in a macroreentry. For this purpose, the signals in the CS catheter are usually defined as the temporal reference. Based

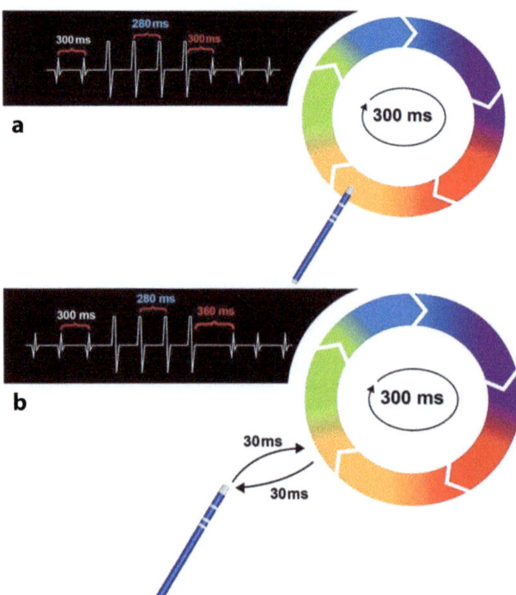

Fig. 12.4 Entrainment in atrial flutter with a cycle length of 300 ms. In the case of entrainment directly in the area of the reentry (macro- or localized reentry), the post-pacing interval approximately corresponds to the cycle length of the tachycardia (**a**). In the case of entrainment away from the reentry, the time required for electrical activation to the reentry and back to the catheter tip is added to the cycle length of the reentry.

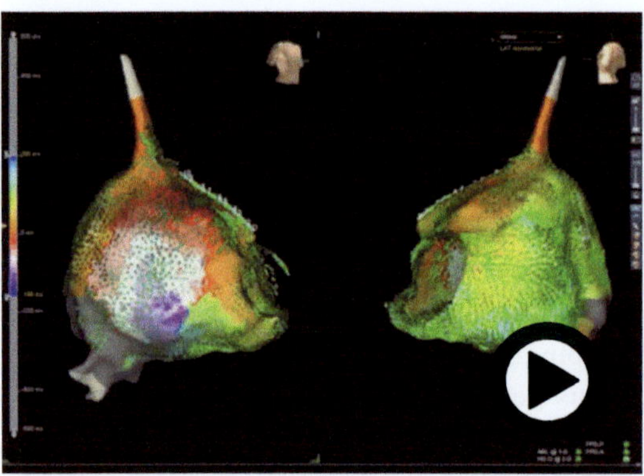

Fig. 12.5 LAT map of a right atrial localized reentry, created using HD mapping. The small extent of the reentry and the activation front are visible. The rest of the right atrium is activated centrifugally from the area of the reentry (https://doi.org/10.1007/000-d2t)

on this temporal reference, a so-called "Window of Interest" (WOI) is defined, which captures the signals that occur earlier or later in relation to the reference signal, color-coded in the 3D mapping system. The length of the WOI should generally correspond to 90% of the tachycardia cycle length and is limited by two intervals, an interval before the set reference in the CS catheter and an interval after the reference signal in the CS catheter. If the WOI is chosen correctly, a so-called "early-meets-late" zone typically appears in the color-coded 3D map for reentrant tachycardias. Furthermore, the critical zones of slow conduction (isthmus), which are necessary for the maintenance of the tachycardia, can be identified in the activation map.

For the creation of the activation map, both the ablation catheter and new multipolar mapping catheters can be used. The advantage of multipolar mapping catheters lies, in addition to the faster acquisition of activation points and the high spatial resolution due to the short distance between the individual electrodes, in the excellent signal quality. This allows even low-amplitude, fractionated signals to be visualized, which are often characteristic of zones of slow conduction (slow-conduction zone) (Markowitz et al. 2019b; see Figs. 12.5 and 12.6).

12.3 Most Common Forms of Atypical Atrial Flutter

Atypical atrial flutter is very heterogeneous. Regarding the nomenclature of atypical atrial flutter , an attempt is usually made to name the course of the activation front, for example, "peri-mitral." Here, the activation circles around the mitral valve. However, this nomenclature is only possible for MR-ATs. For LR-ATs, only the anatomical location is described, for example, an LR in the area of the anterior wall of the left atrium. With the advent of increasingly better mapping tools with high-resolution mapping catheters and optimized mapping algorithms, LR-ATs, but also MR-ATs, can be increasingly better differentiated. Thus, for example, after left atrial substrate modification or surgical MAZE procedure, an exact identification of the mechanism can be achieved.

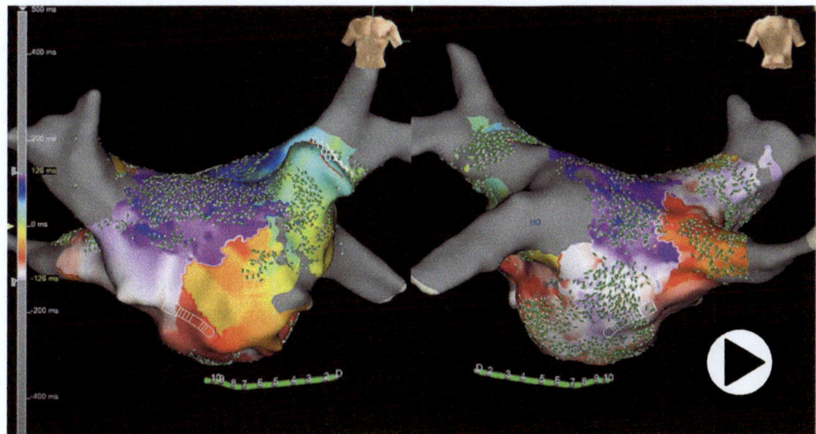

Fig. 12.6 LAT map of a roof-dependent macroreentry, created using HD mapping. A double-loop with a critical isthmus over the area of the atrial roof is visible. The two loops run around an anteroseptal block line and the (isolated) PV circles (https://doi.org/10.1007/000-d2s)

An example: In a patient with atypical atrial flutter after PVI, the entrainment at the roof of the left atrium and in the inferior LA is positive – one would assume roof-dependent atrial flutter. However, in the case of post-PVI, it could also be atrial flutter around the pulmonary veins with a slow-conduction zone in the area of the reconnected encircling (the circle around the pulmonary veins) and a simultaneous activation front over the roof of the LA. This could only be identified through detailed entrainment maneuvers. The creation of a roof line might lead to a change in the AT up to termination and conversion to SR, but the underlying substrate would not be addressed without re-pulmonary vein isolation, and the creation of the roof line might not have been necessary. The combination of entrainment and high-resolution activation mapping can therefore be very helpful.

The following provides an overview of the most common right and left atrial atypical atrial flutter forms (without claiming completeness).

Fig. 12.7 provides a schematic overview of the activation fronts or the activation course of the MR-ATs. In the subsection Ablation Strategy, a possible ablation line guidance or ablation strategy will be presented.

▶ For precise identification, the use of (ultra)-high-resolution mapping catheters in combination with entrainment mapping is recommended.

12.3.1 Right Atrial Atypical Atrial Flutter

Upper-Loop Reentry

Mechanism In an upper-loop reentry, a circulating excitation or activation front is observed around the superior vena cava, usually in a clockwise direction. A crucial component for maintaining this reentry is a slow-conduction zone in the area of the crista terminalis. The upper-loop reentry occurs in isolation or together with typical atrial flutter.

CS Sequence and Entrainment The upper-loop reentry usually shows a proximal-distal CS sequence, although this can be "steeper" than in typical atrial flutter. Positive entrainment is found in the area of the SVC junction as well as in the area of the superior crista terminalis.

Ablation Strategy The goal of ablation is to create a linear lesion in the area of the excitation passage in the crista terminalis. Due to the proximity to the phrenic nerve, it is highly recommended to mark the course of the nerve

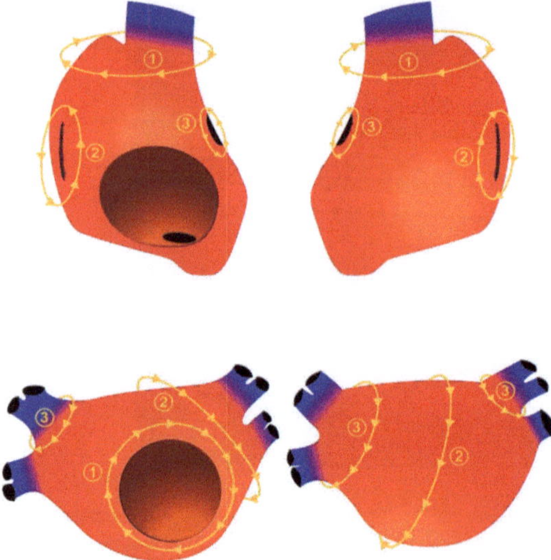

Fig. 12.7 Schematic representation of the activation front of selected macroreentry tachycardias **a** Right atrium in LAO and posterior view. *1* Upper-Loop-Reentry, *2* Reentry around a lateral atriotomy of the free right atrial wall, *3* Reentry around the fossa ovalis, this reentry actually belongs to the left atrial atypical atrial flutter forms, due to the representation, the septum is shown here from the right atrium. **b** Left atrium in AP and PA view. *1* Perimitral atrial flutter, *2* Roof-dependent atrial flutter, *3* Peri-pulmonary vein atrial flutter, the activation can run here over both ipsilateral or only one pulmonary vein

beforehand through "high-output pacing." In the case of too superior ablation, care must be taken to spare the sinus node (Tai et al. 2002).

Reentry at the Free Wall of the Right Atrium

Mechanism Atrial flutter, which includes the free wall of the right atrium, often occurs after cardiac surgical procedures where the lateral right atrium is opened. However, it is also found in patients without prior surgical intervention. A circulating excitation around a scar area in the lateral right atrium is observed. Typically, a line with double potentials (as a sign of a "local site of block") and singular fractionated areas at the lower or upper end of this scar area are found in this region (Saoudi et al. 2001b).

CS Sequence and Entrainment The CS sequence of this reentry usually runs from proximal to distal. Entrainment from both sides of the incision generally shows a post-pacing interval of < 30 ms. By extending the scar area to the inferior vena cava, this form of atrial flutter can be treated with a high success rate. In patients with typical atrial flutter who have a history of right atrial atriotomy, a voltage map and, if necessary, completion of the atriotomy scar is recommended. Here too, due to the proximity to the phrenic nerve, it is highly recommended to mark the course of the nerve beforehand through "high-output pacing."

Double-Loop Reentry

This form involves the simultaneous occurrence of different reentries. This can be a combination of an atriotomy-dependent atrial flutter and a typical atrial flutter or the simultaneous occurrence of an upper-loop reentry with a scar-associated atrial flutter. Often, the ablation of one mechanism leads to a transition of the atrial flutter, which often manifests through a change in cycle length and necessitates addressing the second mechanism through further ablations.

Scar-associated atrial flutter can also occur in other areas of the right atrium as an expression of a "diseased" right atrium, for example, in adults with congenital heart defects, but also after, for example, cannulation of a heart-lung machine. The ablation strategy for these forms of atrial flutter is always to connect the scar area with another anatomical barrier, for example, the inferior/superior vena cava, through a linear ablation strategy.

12.3.2 Left Atrial Atypical Atrial Flutter

Perimitral Atrial Flutter

Mechanism In perimitral atrial flutter, an activation front around the mitral valve is observed, either clockwise or counterclockwise. The slow conduction zone is often located in the area of the anterior wall. Perimitral atrial flutter can occur in combination with roof-dependent atrial flutter as double-loop reentry.

CS Sequence and Entrainment The CS sequence can appear proximal-distal (with a counterclockwise activation front) or distal-proximal (with a clockwise activation front) when the CS catheter is correctly positioned. Positive entrainment is observed both in the anterior LA and the lateral LA.

Ablation Strategy To interrupt the reentry, a line is usually created from the mitral annulus to an anatomical structure that does not conduct, such as the (isolated) pulmonary veins. The "line creation" is either an anterior line to the LSPV or RSPV or a lateral mitral isthmus line to the LIPV. The reconnection rates of the mitral isthmus line are significantly higher at about 70% compared to the anterior line at 40% due to the anatomical thickness of the tissue. Additionally, in about 60% of patients, an epicardial ablation via the coronary sinus is necessary to block the line. The slow conduction zone is usually located in the area of the anterior wall, and by combining activation mapping and voltage mapping, an intelligent line creation through no/low-voltage areas including the slow conduction zone can be achieved. During RF energy delivery, due to the higher tissue thickness in the area of the anterior wall and the mitral isthmus, longer energy delivery with medium power (40–50 W) is recommended. An ethanol injection into the Marshall vein network to achieve a mitral isthmus block appears to be superior to RF ablation of the mitral isthmus line alone (Sánchez-Quintana et al. 2014; Ammar et al. 2015; Kim et al. 2016).

Roof-Dependent Atrial Flutter

Mechanism In roof-dependent atrial flutter, an activation front is observed that runs "over" the roof of the left atrium. The slow conduction zone is often located in the area of the postero-superior left atrium. Especially with close anatomical relationships between the left and right pulmonary veins, roof-dependent atrial flutter can occur after PVI with wide antral ablation.

CS Sequence and Entrainment The CS sequence can appear steep, with nearly simultaneous activation of the distal and proximal CS poles, if the CS is perpendicular to the activation front, when the CS catheter is correctly positioned (not too far distal in the CS). Positive entrainment is found in the area of the roof of the left atrium as well as in the inferior LA.

Ablation Strategy In the ablation strategy, a line is created at the roof to connect the circles of the left and right pulmonary veins. This can be done either antero-superiorly or posteriorly. With an antero-superior line creation, the tissue to be ablated appears thicker, so a longer ablation duration per lesion with medium power seems reasonable. With posterior line creation, the tissue is thinner, and the anatomical proximity of the esophagus and the risk of atrio-esophageal fistula formation should not be underestimated. An ablation strategy with "High-Power-Short-Duration" (HPSD) can be useful here due to the less deep-reaching lesions. A common "reconnection site" of the posterior roof line is the transition to the ablation circle of the right superior pulmonary vein (RSPV).

Peri-PV Atrial Flutter

Mechanism The activation front in pulmonary vein-dependent atrial flutter runs around one or two ipsilateral pulmonary veins. This form of atypical atrial flutter often occurs after incomplete pulmonary vein isolation or reconnection, with the slow conduction zone often located in the area of the reconnected pulmonary vein circles. There is an overlap with roof-dependent atrial flutter.

CS Sequence and Entrainment Differentiating between roof-dependent or peri-PV atrial flutter can be particularly challenging in activation mapping, especially if the areas between the ipsilateral PVs have not been carefully mapped. Therefore, it is generally recommended to re-isolate reconnected pulmonary veins before ablating atypical atrial flutter. Not least because isolated pulmonary veins are essential as connection points for left atrial lines. The CS sequence can be distal-proximal, proximal-distal, or steep, depending on the affected pulmonary vein pair and the direction of the activation front.

Ablation Strategy As an ablation strategy, a circumferential, wide antral pulmonary vein isolation is recommended. It is often worth looking at signals "between" the pulmonary veins (carina region), as connections (including epicardial) can exist here.

Septal AT

Mechanism In septal atypical atrial flutter, the fossa ovalis represents the anatomical boundary around which the activation front circulates. This can occur either *"clockwise"* or *"counterclockwise"*. Here, the right pulmonary veins and the mitral valve annulus form the functional barriers of the reentry.

CS Sequence and Entrainment The CS sequence can be either distal-proximal or proximal-distal in this form of atrial flutter. Entrainment is positive in the entire septal area.

Ablation Strategy The tachycardia often terminates under ablation in the septal area; however, with an incomplete line, it can be relatively easily reinduced. Therefore, it is advisable to create an ablation line to connect the fossa ovalis, for example, to the right pulmonary veins or the mitral annulus. Due to the thickness of the septum, longer ablation times per lesion with medium to high energy are sensible; in some cases, ablation from the right atrium is also necessary.

12.4 Ablation of Atrial Flutter

In principle, the creation of ablation lines, especially in the left atrium, is associated with high reconnection rates and consequently with a high recurrence rate. Furthermore, "leaky" ablation lines are a substrate for further atrial arrhythmias. Therefore, optimal preparation is essential for the treatment of any type of atypical atrial flutter. The use of high-resolution mapping catheters to visualize the activation front, slow-conduction zones, and voltage to identify the best ablation strategy is advisable. Additionally, modern, cooled RF catheters, if possible with contact force measurement and optimized irrigation, should be used. For better stabilization, the use of (non-)steerable sheaths should be considered. After creating ablation lines, the bidirectional block of the line should be checked using "differential pacing" after an adequate waiting period (about 15–20 minutes). To increase the success rate of the ablation, it is also sensible to consider not only the voltage (regarding the line path) but also the (empirical) wall or tissue thickness. Newer ablation techniques such as high-power-short-duration can be particularly helpful in areas with thinner wall thickness (e.g., posterior wall of the LA) or critical adjacent structures (phrenic nerve; esophagus) (Ammar et al. 2015). Another point of contention is to what extent, in MR-ATs, merely ablating the slow-conduction zone (if identifiable) is sufficient compared to creating a complete line. After initial enthusiasm for a more limited ablation approach, several publications have shown higher recurrence rates compared to the "complete" line creation, so the limited procedure of ablating the slow-conduction zone should remain an individual decision (Markowitz et al. 2019a; Nakashima et al. 2020; Takigawa et al. 2018).

▶ **Summary**

- Atypical atrial flutter, like atrial fibrillation, is associated with a significantly increased risk of systemic embolism. Anticoagulation is recommended depending on the $CHADS_2VAS_2$ score.
- Atypical atrial flutter is an arrhythmia of the structurally altered or previously operated atrium. Furthermore, atypical atrial flutter can also occur functionally or under antiarrhythmic therapy.
- Radiofrequency ablation is an established, effective, and safe interventional treatment option for atypical atrial flutter.

- The success rate of ablation depends on the underlying disease or structural alteration of the atria as well as the underlying mechanism.
- Radiofrequency energy with cooled catheters is preferred; in the left atrium, the use of irrigated catheters is mandatory.
- The goal of ablation is to interrupt the reentry. Macro-reentry tachycardias are treated by creating a line between two non-electrically conductive structures. The endpoint should be a bidirectional conduction block within the framework of *differential pacing*.

References

Ammar S, Luik A, Hessling G, Bruhm A, Reents T, Semmler V, Buiatti A, Kathan S, Hofmann M, Kolb C, Schmitt C, Deisenhofer I (2015) Ablation of perimitral flutter: acute and long-term success of the modified anterior line. Europace 17(3):447–452. https://doi.org/10.1093/europace/euu297

Granada J, Uribe W, Chyou PH, Maassen K, Vierkant R, Smith PN, Hayes J, Eaker E, Vidaillet H (2000) Incidence and predictors of atrial flutter in the general population. J Am Coll Cardiol 36(7):2242

Jais P, Matsuo S, Knecht S, Weerasooriya R, Hocini M, Sacher F, Wright M, Nault I, Lellouche N, Klein G, Clementy J, Haissaguerre M (2009) A deductive mapping strategy for atrial tachycardia following atrial fibrillation ablation: importance of localized reentry. J Cardiovasc Electrophysiol 20:480–491. https://doi.org/10.1111/j.1540-8167.2008.01373.x

January CT, Wann LS, Calkins H, Chen LY, Cigarroa JE, Cleveland JC Jr, Ellinor PT, Ezekowitz MD, Field ME, Furie KL, Heidenreich PA, Murray KT, Shea JB, Tracy CM, Yancy CW (2019) 2019 AHA/ACC/HRS focused update of the 2014 AHA/ACC/HRS guideline for the management of patients with atrial fibrillation: A Report of the American College of Cardiology/American Heart Association Task Force on Clinical Practice Guidelines and the Heart Rhythm Society. Heart Rhythm 16(8):e66

Kim TH, Park J, Uhm JS et al (2016) Challenging achievement of bidirectional block after linear ablation affects the rhythm outcome in patients with persistent atrial fibrillation. J Am Heart Assoc 5(10):e3894. https://doi.org/10.1161/JAHA.116.003894

Markowitz SM, Thomas G, Liu CF et al (2019a) Atrial tachycardias and atypical atrial flutters: mechanisms and approaches to ablation. Arrhythm Electrophysiol Rev 8:131–137

Markowitz SM, Thomas G, Liu CF, Cheung JW, Ip JE, Lerman BB (2019b) Approach to catheter ablation of left atrial flutters. J Cardiovasc Electrophysiol 30(12):3057–3067. https://doi.org/10.1111/jce.14209

Nakashima T, Pambrun T, Vlachos K, Goujeau C, André C, Krisai P, Ramirez FD, Kamakura T, Takagi T, Nakatani Y et al (2020) Impact of Vein of Marshall ethanol infusion on mitral isthmus block: efficacy and durability. Circ Arrhythm Electrophysiol 13:e8884. https://doi.org/10.1161/CIRCEP.120.008884

Rodriguez Ziccardi M, Goyal A, Maani CV (2021) Atrial Flutter. In: StatPearls. StatPearls Publishing, Treasure Island

Sánchez-Quintana D, López-Mínguez JR, Macías Y, Cabrera JA, Farhood Saremi (2014) Left atrial anatomy relevant to catheter ablation. Cardiol Res Pract. https://doi.org/10.1155/2014/289720

Saoudi N, Cosio F, Waldo A et al (2001a) Classification of atrial flutter and regular atrial tachycardia according to electrophysiologic mechanism and anatomic bases: a statement from a joint expert group from the Working Group of Arrhythmias of the European Society of Cardiology and the North American Society of Pacing and Electrophysiology. J Cardiovasc Electrophysiol 12:852–866

Saoudi N, Cosio F, Waldo A, Chen SA, Iesaka Y, Lesh M, Saksena S, Salerno J, Schoels W (2001b) Classification of atrial flutter and regular atrial tachycardia according to electrophysiologic mechanism and anatomic bases: A statement from a joint expert group from the Working Group of Arrhythmias of the European Society of Cardiology and the North American Society of Pacing and Electrophysiology. J Cardiovasc Electrophysiol 12:852–866

Tai CT, Huang JL, Lin YK, Hsieh MH, Lee PC, Ding YA, Chang MS, Chen SA (2002) Noncontact three-dimensional mapping and ablation of upper loop re-entry originating in the right atrium. J Am Coll Cardiol 40(4):746–753

Takigawa M, Derval N, Frontera A, Martin R, Yamashita S, Cheniti G, Vlachos K, Thompson N, Kitamura T, Wolf M, Massoullie G, Martin CA, Al-Jefairi N, Amraoui S, Duchateau J, Klotz N, Pambrun T, Denis A, Sacher F, Cochet H, Hocini M, Haïssaguerre M, Jais P (2018) Revisiting anatomic macroreentrant tachycardia after atrial fibrillation ablation using ultrahigh-resolution mapping: Implications for ablation. Heart Rhythm 15(3):326–333. https://doi.org/10.1016/j.hrthm.2017.10.029

Atrial Fibrillation—Radiofrequency Ablation (Pulmonary Vein Isolation)

13

Sonia Busch and Till Althoff

13.1 Introduction

Spontaneous depolarizations from the pulmonary veins (PV) play a crucial role in the initiation and maintenance of atrial fibrillation (Haïssaguerre et al. 1998). Furthermore, specific electrophysiological properties of the pulmonary veins, particularly in the area of the transition to the left atrium, such as shortened refractory periods and reduced conduction velocities, have been demonstrated, which favor reentry mechanisms and thus constitute an arrhythmogenic substrate. Based on this, the concept of electrical isolation of the pulmonary veins was developed, which today represents the most effective

therapy for atrial fibrillation. Thus, pulmonary vein isolation (PVI) is the decisive endpoint of any interventional therapy for atrial fibrillation (Hindricks et al. 2020). PVI is predominantly performed catheter-based, using different energy sources and ablation techniques. One of the most well-established and widespread procedures remains sequential catheter ablation (point-by-point) using radiofrequency current application. Due to rapid technological advancements, this approach has continuously evolved since its introduction in 1998. The following will explain the technical implementation of this procedure using three-dimensional navigation systems. Special attention is also given to the importance of technological innovations and innovative ablation approaches for routine clinical procedures.

Supplementary Information The online version contains supplementary material available at https://doi.org/10.1007/978-3-662-65797-3_13. The videos can be accessed individually by clicking the DOI link in the accompanying figure caption or by scanning this link with the SN More Media App.

S. Busch
Medizinische Klinik II, Klinikum Coburg GmbH, Coburg, Germany
e-mail: Sonia.busch@klinikum-coburg.de

T. Althoff (✉)
Arrhythmia Section, Cardiovascular Institute, Hospital Clínic, University of Barcelona, Barcelona, Spanien
e-mail: ALTHOFF@clinic.cat

13.2 Accompanying Measures

13.2.1 Analgesia and Sedation

Due to the degree of invasiveness and the routinely applied deep sedation and analgesia, which are necessary to maintain stable examination conditions and adequate analgesia, guidelines from professional societies regarding structural prerequisites and sedation management have been developed (Tilz et al. 2017; Kuck et al. 2017).

These should be considered both from the perspective of patient safety and for forensic reasons.

13.2.2 Esophageal Temperature Monitoring

The question of whether esophageal temperature monitoring and corresponding titration of RF energy delivery reduce the risk of thermal esophageal lesions and thus particularly the life-threatening complication of an atrioesophageal fistula during RF ablation has not been conclusively clarified. Although a joint consensus paper of international professional societies on catheter-based and surgical ablation of atrial fibrillation considers temperature measurement to be useful (Calkins et al. 2018), no benefit of such an approach has been demonstrated in the randomized studies available to date. Additionally, the currently available temperature probes are hardly comparable, and none of the systems and corresponding temperature thresholds have been systematically validated regarding clinical endpoints. Due to this unclear evidence, the use of temperature probes is handled differently from center to center.

13.2.3 Periprocedural Imaging

Cross-sectional imaging techniques such as CT or MRI, as well as angiographic procedures, allow precise visualization of the left atrium along with the incoming PV and, if necessary, the detection of anatomical variants or anomalies. A combination of imaging and electroanatomical mapping can facilitate anatomical orientation. When visualizing the esophagus in the navigation system, the ablation line and energy delivery can be adjusted accordingly, potentially reducing the risk of esophageal lesions and associated complications.

Preprocedural MRI imaging with gadolinium contrast allows further characterization of the arrhythmogenic substrate in terms of atrial fibrosis through the detection of interstitial contrast agent accumulations ("late gadolinium enhancement"). Although there is not yet sufficient evidence for substrate-based ablation approaches, the individual substrate can be considered when deciding on PVI (Hindricks et al. 2020). Extensive fibrosis of the left atrium is associated with high recurrence rates (Marrouche et al. 2014). Due to the advancement of 3D mapping systems, periprocedural imaging currently plays only a minor role in routine PVI using RF ablation.

Another function of periprocedural imaging can be the preprocedural exclusion of intracavitary thrombi. For this purpose, transesophageal echocardiography is predominantly used, but computed tomography is also sufficiently validated in this regard. Under certain conditions, particularly continuous oral anticoagulation at an adequate dosage for at least three weeks before the procedure, preprocedural exclusion of intracavitary thrombi can be omitted (Hindricks et al. 2020).

13.3 Access

Regarding venous and left atrial access, please refer to Chap. 4. In addition, we recommend a dual transseptal access to avoid catheter exchanges over left atrial sheaths and thus minimize the risk of air embolisms. This dual access can be established either through a double transseptal puncture or, if a transseptal wire is already in the left atrium, by probing the puncture site with a second wire or the ablation catheter. In the latter approach, the independent steerability of the sheaths may be somewhat limited.

For the ablation catheter, a steerable sheath can be used to improve maneuverability and stability during RF applications. The latter is a critical determinant of lesion quality and thus crucial for procedural success. For the diagnostic mapping catheter, a non-steerable transseptal sheath is usually sufficient.

With the establishment of left atrial access, an *Activated Clotting Time*(ACT)-controlled heparinization (ACT $\geq$ 300 sec.) should be ensured to prevent thromboembolic complications (Calkins et al. 2018). Given the need for intensified anticoagulation throughout the left atrial procedure, the femoral vein should be punctured particularly gently, if necessary under ultrasound guidance. In the event of an arterial mispuncture, consistent compression for at least 3–4 minutes is advisable to avoid bleeding complications during the procedure.

13.4 Mapping

13.4.1 Mapping Catheter

For the visualization of PV signals, circular catheters were used almost exclusively for a long time, which can still be used today to create an electroanatomical geometry with the 3D mapping system (electroanatomical mapping). These differ in diameter as well as the number, size, and spacing of electrodes. In addition, there are both fixed and variably adjustable diameter variants. Meanwhile, in addition to these classic circular PV catheters, numerous non-circular multipolar mapping catheters are also available, which were primarily developed for high-resolution electroanatomical mapping of arrhythmias but are equally suitable for demonstrating PV isolation or locating gaps in an already established ablation line.

With regard to the highest possible sensitivity and spatial resolution in detecting local electrograms, catheters with microelectrodes (≤ 1 mm in size) and minimal electrode spacing ≤ 2 mm should be used if possible. This is given in most of the available multipolar mapping catheters, but not in the majority of currently available ablation catheters, which is why it is not advisable to forgo a diagnostic PV or mapping catheter.

13.4.2 3D Navigation System

For PVI, an anatomical representation of the left atrium and especially the pulmonary vein antra using a 3D navigation system is crucial. In principle, fluoroscopy can largely be dispensed with here; however, especially at the beginning of the learning curve, it should be used if in doubt. Multipolar mapping catheters in combination with automated annotation of individual mapping points have helped optimize and significantly streamline this process.

The higher the degree of interpolation set by the navigation system, the fewer annotated points are needed to create a three-dimensional geometry. However, increased interpolation comes at the expense of precision and should therefore not be set too tolerantly, especially for mapping particularly relevant structures.

To minimize motion artifacts due to respiratory excursions, the respiratory cycle should be taken into account if possible, and automatic respiratory compensation should be used. Annotation is performed exclusively within a defined range of the respiratory cycle, usually during expiration.

▶ The 3D navigation system is the main working tool for PVI in radiofrequency technology. Nowadays, in addition to pure anatomical representation, it offers a variety of other functions such as indices for lesion assessment and information about tissue contact of various catheters. Due to the complexity of modern systems, the investigator should have certain knowledge of the operation of the systems and algorithms used.

13.4.3 Anatomical Landmarks and Manual Annotation

Despite significant technological advances in the field of 3D mapping systems, a sufficiently precise representation of all structures relevant to ablation is not always possible, even with the use of additional imaging modalities. In particular, the anatomical transition between the left upper PV and the left atrial appendage ("left atrial appendage ridge") is often not correctly represented due to limited resolution, even with minimal interpolation. Here, manual marking of anatomical landmarks can be helpful. For example, the transition to the left atrial appendage can be defined by retracting the mapping catheter from the left upper PV while applying anterior pressure (rotation of the sheath and/or catheter counterclockwise). The catheter position is marked immediately before the "jump" towards the atrial appendage. Similarly, other relevant landmarks can also be marked in this way. Some investigators define their intended ablation line in this manner by "probing" the entire circumference of the pulmonary vein antrum with the catheter and marking accordingly. Alternatively, the ablation line can be pre-drawn in the 3D model.

13.4.4 Substrate Mapping

In addition to the anatomical geometry of the left atrium, electroanatomical mapping also provides the possibility of a color-coded representation of the bipolar electrograms in the form of a voltage map. Low voltage can be considered a surrogate for an arrhythmogenic substrate (possible threshold values for so-called low-voltage areas, e.g., < 0.1 mV or < 0.5 mV). Although there is currently no sufficient evidence for substrate-based ablation approaches, such a voltage map allows for the characterization of the individual substrate and phenotyping of the patient, which can be considered in further therapeutic decisions (Hindricks et al. 2020). Extensive left atrial low voltage is associated with high recurrence rates, which should be considered regarding a possible further escalation of rhythm control measures (Marrouche et al. 2014).

13.5 Ablation

13.5.1 Ablation Catheters

A variety of suitable ablation catheters from different manufacturers are available. These differ in terms of the controllable curve degree (curvature radius and arc length), the control mechanism, and the shaft construction, as well as electrode size and spacing. Regarding the safety and effectiveness of ablation, only externally cooled catheters are recommended, although the number and arrangement of the exit holes for the irrigation fluid can vary depending on the catheter. Many ablation catheters also offer the possibility of continuous measurement of tissue contact force, which allows for a certain standardization of ablation (see Sect. 13.5.4) and possibly an improvement in the safety profile.

13.5.2 Antral Ablation Guidance

While in the early days of PVI, a segmental ablation was pursued and each vein was electrically isolated individually, it is now assumed that the atrial myocardium in the area of the PV antra increasingly harbors arrhythmogenic foci and substrate. Therefore, today, during ablation using radiofrequency current, the isolation lines are guided to electrically isolate as much of the PV antra as possible. This ablation guidance also includes the carina, i.e., the area between the two ipsilateral PVs. The greater distance from the PV ostia also reduces the risk of ablation-induced PV stenosis.

▶ The wide antral circumferential ablation (WACA) is now standard in pulmonary vein isolation using radiofrequency technology for safety and effectiveness reasons.

13.5.3 Lesion Quality

Despite procedural success in terms of PVI, a significant proportion of patients experience recurrences, i.e., a reoccurrence of atrial fibrillation or atrial tachycardias after successful ablation. This is partly because the concept of PVI is not equally sufficient for all patients, especially in cases of advanced atrial myopathy or triggers outside the pulmonary veins. Additionally, PVI is not permanent in some cases. Thus, even with intraprocedural evidence of complete PVI, conduction recoveries and thereby electrical reconnection of the PV can occur over time, significantly promoting recurrences (Fig. 13.1). Numerous measures have now been established regarding lesion quality and the durability of the ablation line.

While until a few years ago, the catheter was predominantly moved during ablation in a so-called "dragging technique" under continuous RF application, modern ablation approaches guide the catheter point by point with sequential RF applications. This technique opens up the possibility of better controlling the quality of individual lesions.

13.5.4 Index-Guided Ablation and Lesion Distance

Traditionally, parameters such as reduction of the local signal amplitude and the drop in local impedance are used as surrogates for lesion quality or tissue heating. While these parameters still hold their value and can be used complementarily, many centers have now transitioned to primarily controlling the intensity of individual RF applications through indices that integrate various parameters such as contact force, power, and duration of the RF application into a weighted formula. These indices are capable of approximately predicting the extent of the lesions and thus the likelihood of transmurality .

In addition to the transmurality of the lesions, their continuity or overlap is also of crucial importance. This is determined, besides the extent of individual lesions, by the distance between adjacent ablation points ("interlesion distance"). The so-called CLOSE protocol is the first ablation protocol that considers both factors (Taghji et al. 2018). Validated target ranges for

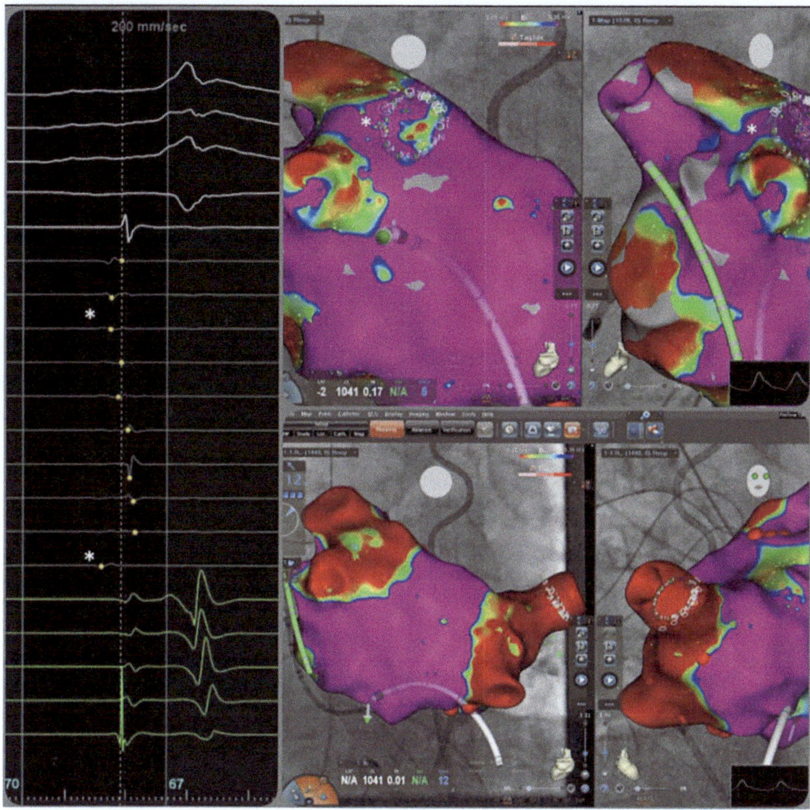

Fig. 13.1 Pulmonary vein reconnection in the voltage map. The voltage > 0.5 mV in the area of the left PV in combination with the derived PV signals indicate PV reconnection. The leading electrode pairs (*) indicate the location of the reconnection. Compare the voltage after re-isolation (*below*)

the respective indices and the desired distance between adjacent ablation points thus enable a standardized RF ablation for the first time. In Table 13.1 (Index-based ablation protocol), possible validated target criteria for index-guided ablation based on the CLOSE protocol are listed.

The criteria represent merely an example of a standardized protocol for index-guided PVI based on the CLOSE protocol.

In general, due to the anatomical peculiarities in the area of the posterior wall (proximity to the esophagus and thinner wall thickness), special caution is required; accordingly, lower index targets are recommended here. Some centers also reduce the applied power during ablation of the posterior wall. Regarding the recommended interlesion distance, it should be noted that the distance of 6 mm defined in the CLOSE protocol is a maximum tolerable distance and not a target value to be aimed for. While individual "outliers" with a distance of up to 6 mm may still be compatible with successful isolation, preclinical and clinical data suggest that significantly smaller distances around 4 mm should be aimed for to reliably generate gapless lesions (Hoffmann et al. 2020).

Index-guided ablation, taking into account the distances of adjacent RF applications, is enabled by 3D mapping systems, which on the one hand display the ablation index and the distance of the ablation catheter to the previous ablation point in real-time, and on the other hand automatically mark the individual ablation points. Optionally, a color coding according to the achieved index values as a surrogate for the intensity of the respective RF application is also possible (Fig. 13.2).

13.5.5 Catheter Stability

Since the stability of the catheter during ablation is also a crucial determinant of lesion quality, only those ablation points that meet predefined criteria of catheter stability are automatically annotated. The stability criteria defined in Table 13.1 represent a common setting. Measures such as general anesthesia with mechanical ventilation, especially special high-frequency ventilation procedures (high-frequency oscillatory ventilation) or the use of steerable sheaths can help improve catheter stability.

▶ Catheter stability is one of the most important determinants of lesion quality and can be improved by a number of measures in addition to the experience of the examiner. During ablation, special attention should be paid to catheter stability.

13.5.6 Ablation Sequence

In addition to the already mentioned variables of interlesion distance, ablation indices, and catheter stability, the local and temporal

Table 13.1 Standardized Index-guided PVI

Index Targets	Posterior target area	Ablation Index 300–400 Lesion Size Index 5.0–5.5
	Anterior target area	Ablation Index 450–550 Lesion Size Index 5.5–6.0
Interlesion Distance	Maximum tolerable point distance	6.0 mm
	Desired point distance	4.0 mm
Catheter Stability Criteria	Maximum movement radius	≤ 3 mm
	Stabilization duration	> 8 s
	Minimum contact force	5 g
	Time proportion with minimum contact force	> 50 %
Safety Criterion	Maximum contact force	40 g

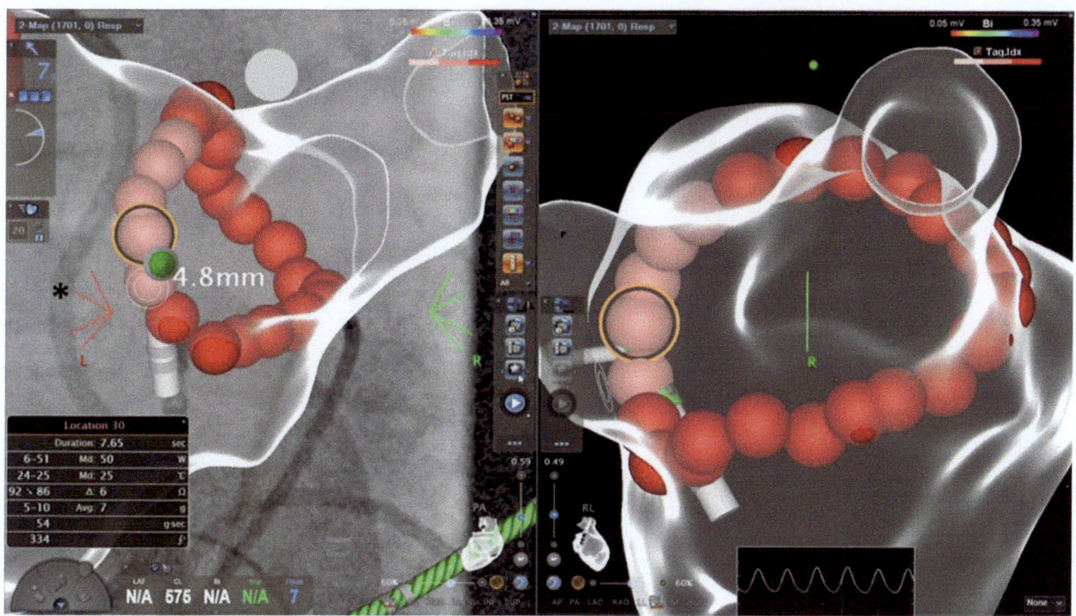

Fig. 13.2 Index-guided ablation. Example of an index-guided ablation with display of the distance to the last ablation point and color-coded visualization of the ablation index. Note the pale red coloration of the ablation points in anatomical proximity to the esophagus temperature probe (*)

sequence of lesion placement also influences lesion quality (Jankelson et al. 2021). Thus, a sequential, primarily gapless alignment of point lesions without time delay increases the effectiveness of the ablation. In addition to avoiding impairment of energy transfer by a developing local edema, a local heat accumulation effect ("heat stacking") probably also contributes to this (Barbhaiya et al. 2020). It should be noted that the effect of heat accumulation in the area of the posterior wall can promote heating of the esophagus and corresponding lesions and complications (Barbhaiya et al. 2020).

13.6 Power and Duration of RF Application

Traditional ablation approaches involve RF applications with a power of around 30–40 W over periods of about 20–40 s. With the aim of increasing the efficiency of ablation and minimizing collateral damage without sacrificing effectiveness, ablation approaches are increasingly being pursued in which RF energy is delivered at higher power (up to 90 W) over a shorter period ("high power-short duration ablation") (Althoff and Mont 2021). The relative predominance of direct (resistive) heat development over indirect heat development through conduction when applying high power over a short period results in a shallower or broader lesion geometry, which appears favorable given the thin atrial wall thicknesses and should allow for greater distances between adjacent ablation points (Fig. 13.3). Due to the shorter RF application times, the period over which the catheter must be stabilized is also reduced. Conversely, however, a brief loss of catheter position or wall contact during total application times of sometimes only 4 s can already result in significant losses in lesion quality, so catheter stability is likely to be of even greater importance with these approaches.

Numerous ablation protocols with target powers of 40–90 W have now been validated, including index-guided approaches with up to 50 W power (Althoff and Mont 2021). Due to the shorter duration of individual RF

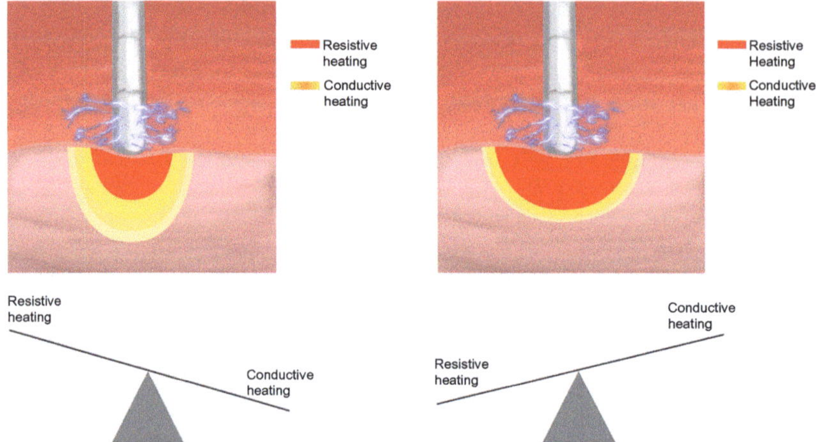

Fig. 13.3 High-Power-Short-Duration Ablation. Direct tissue heating via resistive heat development versus indirect heating via conduction

applications, these approaches are consistently associated with reduced ablation and procedure times. High-power ablation has proven to be safe and effective in principle. Despite convincing clinical data, however, certain concerns remain, particularly regarding the risk of localized tissue explosions, so-called "steam pops," as well as potential injuries to the esophagus. With regard to the latter, it seems advisable, based on the currently available data, to avoid both excessive energy deliveries and high contact pressures in the posterior wall area when applying high power (Althoff and Mont 2021; see Fig. 13.4).

13.7 Proof of Pulmonary Vein Isolation

13.7.1 Pulmonary Vein Signals

For the assessment of the endpoints of a pulmonary vein isolation and for the control of the procedure, understanding the electrical signals of the PV ostia is essential. Due to the myocardial fibers interwoven from the atrial myocardium and spirally extending into the PV, electrical potentials can be derived within the PV. Additionally, a far-field signal, caused by the

potentials of the atrial myocardium, can often be derived in the PV.

▶ Knowledge and correct interpretation of the electrical signals in the area of the PV antra are essential for performing a pulmonary vein isolation and are the basis of a safe and effective procedure.

Morphology, amplitude, and the relationship of these components to each other depend on the position of the mapping catheter at the PV ostium, the signal amplitude of the atrial myocardium, and the location in the atrium. Furthermore, the characteristics of the signals are influenced by the size and spacing of the electrodes of the chosen mapping catheter. For example, a high-amplitude far-field of the left atrial appendage can regularly be derived at the left upper PV, while a far-field from the superior vena cava can often be derived at the right upper PV. Typically, the far-field signals are derived before the PV signal in the temporal sequence due to the conduction from the atrium into the PV. At the beginning of the procedure, both components can also be fused (Fig. 13.5a).

In general, far-field signals have lower amplitude and rounded signal morphology, while near-field signals have higher amplitudes and sharper signal morphology. Particularly, far-field

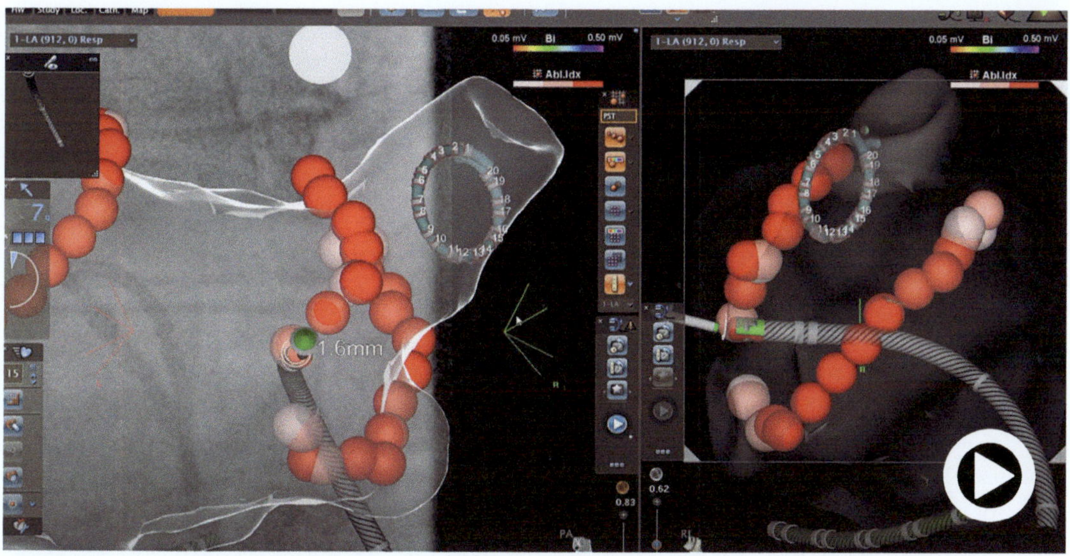

Fig. 13.4 Time-lapse recording of a PVI in radiofrequency technique using the ablation index. The creation of a voltage map is followed by ablation under visualization of the lesion distance (https://doi.org/10.1007/000-d2v)

signals from the atrial appendage are sometimes difficult to distinguish from the local PV signal. Sequential (temporally offset) excitation of the corresponding structures, for example, by stimulation in the left atrial appendage, can be used for differentiation. Through the temporally offset excitation (in this case, atrial appendage before PV), a temporal separation of the atrial appendage far-field and PV signal is achieved. While the atrial appendage far-field signal can be registered immediately after the stimulus, the local PV signal appears delayed depending on the local conduction velocity (Fig. 13.5b). This approach can also be applied analogously to differentiate other far-field signals, for example, to differentiate far-field signals from the superior vena cava and local signals of the right upper PV.

Signals registered and stored before the start of the PVI at the antral catheter position allow for later comparison between stimulated and spontaneous signal sequences and can thus facilitate the differentiation between near-field and far-field. Also, during ablation, the antral position of the circular catheter should be maintained as much as possible to notice any changes in the signals, such as a temporal separation of

atrial and PV signals. The separation of the signals is often particularly impressive when ablation is started at the roof of the ostium of the left upper PV (Fig. 13.5c).

In the antral position of the PV catheter, the temporal sequence of the PV signals can be helpful for locating a gap in the PV isolation line. Thus, the electrode pair with the earliest excitation at the PV ostium can approximately indicate the location (Fig. 13.5d). Important for this are a good apposition of the mapping catheter at the PV antrum and an adequate diameter of the mapping catheter concerning the PV ostium. In the case of relatively early excitation of an electrode pair in the area of the carina between the ipsilateral PVs, a gap in the area of the respective other vein should be considered, and a corresponding repositioning of the circular catheter should be considered.

After complete electrical isolation of the PV from the left atrium, dissociated activity can often be observed within the PV. Here, individual or regular signals, morphologically corresponding to the previously registered PV potentials, appear dissociated from the atrial excitation (Fig. 13.5f). Occasionally, it can also be observed that high-frequency electrical

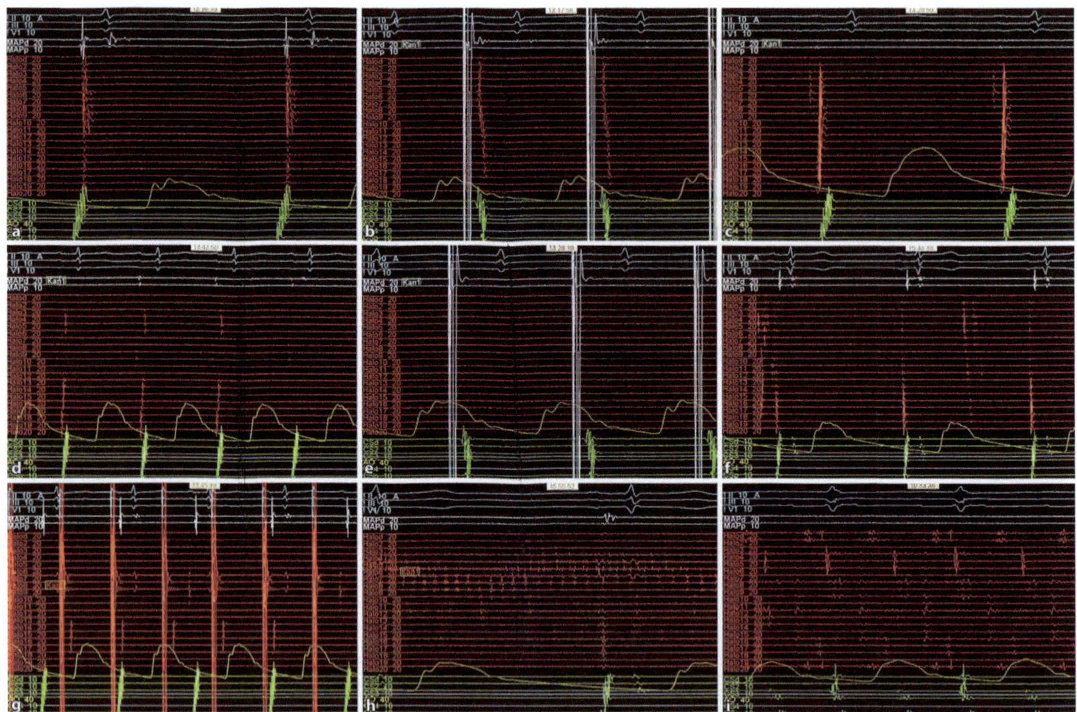

Fig. 13.5 Exemplary representation of pulmonary vein signals in various scenarios. **a** Fused components of the signal (LAA far-field and PV signal); **b** Stimulation via the ablation catheter from the LAA with separation of the components (LAA far-field fused with the stimulation spike, PV signal temporally offset); **c** Separation of the components during ablation; **d** Acute isolation of the PV, note the activation of the ablation catheter at the PV antrum clearly before the PV signal; **e** Stimulation from the LAA with evidence of an entrance block; **f** Dissociated activity in the PV with high-amplitude LAA far-field; **g** Evidence of an exit block during stimulation via the circular catheter in the PV, note the delayed signal (Halo 14-17) as a sign of local capture; **h** Derivation of high-frequency electrical activity within the pulmonary vein during dissociation, with sinus rhythm in the atrium; **i** Pulmonary vein-dependent reentry tachycardia with mapping of the entire cycle length of the tachycardia in the pulmonary vein during the isoelectric phase of the surface ECG

activity continues within an isolated PV while the atrium is excited in sinus rhythm (Fig. 13.5h).

13.8 Endpoints

In PVI, an immediate isolation with the first encirclement of the PV, without the need for subsequent RF applications, should be aimed for ("First-Pass Isolation"). To confirm complete PVI, in addition to an entrance block – that is, the absence of conduction of atrial impulses into the PV, characterized by the no longer or dissociated detectable PV signal – an exit block, that is, the absence of conduction during stimulation in the PV to the atrium, should be demonstrated in all PVs. To demonstrate an exit block, stimulation is usually performed sequentially from all bipoles of the circular PV catheter with 10 V and 2 ms pulse duration to test as much of the circumference of the respective PV as possible. Attention should be paid to the correct, antral catheter position and a local capture response in the stimulated PV (Fig. 13.5g).

A re-evaluation of entrance and exit block with a certain latency after ablation (usually 20 or 30 minutes waiting time), but also the application of adenosine, can be useful to unmask tissue that has not been effectively ablated and only temporarily does not conduct ("dormant conduction"). Furthermore, excitable tissue can also be unmasked by local stimulation along the ablation line (usually also 10 V over 2 ms) (Moser et al. 2017). These measures can help identify atrial myocardium that could contribute to conduction recovery and thus reconnection of the PV in the course after the procedure.

References

Althoff TF, Mont L (2021) Novel concepts in atrial fibrillation ablation-breaking the trade-off between efficacy and safety. J Arrhythm 37:904–911

Barbhaiya CR, Kogan EV, Jankelson L, Knotts RJ, Spinelli M, Bernstein S, Park D, Aizer A, Chinitz LA, Holmes D (2020) Esophageal temperature dynamics during high-power short-duration posterior wall ablation. Heart Rhythm 17:721–727

Calkins H, Hindricks G, Cappato R, Kim YH, Saad EB, Aguinaga L, Akar JG, Badhwar V, Brugada J, Camm J, Chen PS, Chen SA, Chung MK, Nielsen JC, Curtis AB, Davies DW, Day JD, d'Avila A, de Groot NMSN, Di Biase L, Duytschaever M, Edgerton JR, Ellenbogen KA, Ellinor PT, Ernst S, Fenelon G, Gerstenfeld EP, Haines DE, Haissaguerre M, Helm RH, Hylek E, Jackman WM, Jalife J, Kalman JM, Kautzner J, Kottkamp H, Kuck KH, Kumagai K, Lee R, Lewalter T, Lindsay BD, Macle L, Mansour M, Marchlinski FE, Michaud GF, Nakagawa H, Natale A, Nattel S, Okumura K, Packer D, Pokushalov E, Reynolds MR, Sanders P, Scanavacca M, Schilling R, Tondo C, Tsao HM, Verma A, Wilber DJ, Yamane T (2018) 2017 HRS/EHRA/ECAS/APHRS/SOLAECE expert consensus statement on catheter and surgical ablation of atrial fibrillation: executive summary. Europace 20:157–208

Haïssaguerre M, Jaïs P, Shah DC, Takahashi A, Hocini M, Quiniou G, Garrigue S, Le Mouroux A, Le Métayer P, Clémenty J (1998) Spontaneous initiation of atrial fibrillation by ectopic beats originating in the pulmonary veins. N Engl J Med 339:659–666

Hindricks G, Potpara T, Dagres N, Arbelo E, Bax JJ, Blomström-Lundqvist C, Boriani G, Castella M, Dan GA, Dilaveris PE, Fauchier L, Filippatos G, Kalman JM, La Meir M, Lane DA, Lebeau JP, Lettino M, Lip GYH, Pinto FJ, Thomas GN, Valgimigli M, Van Gelder IC, Van Putte BP, Watkins CL (2020) 2020 ESC Guidelines for the diagnosis and management of atrial fibrillation developed in collaboration with the European Association of Cardio-Thoracic Surgery (EACTS). Eur Heart J. https://doi.org/10.1093/eurheartj/ehaa612

Hoffmann P, Diaz Ramirez I, Baldenhofer G, Stangl K, Mont L, Althoff TF (2020) Randomized study defining the optimum target interlesion distance in ablation index-guided atrial fibrillation ablation. Europace 22:1480–1486

Jankelson L, Dai M, Aizer A, Bernstein S, Park DS, Holmes D, Chinitz LA, Barbhaiya C (2021) Lesion sequence and catheter spatial stability affect lesion quality markers in atrial fibrillation ablation. JACC Clin Electrophysiol 7:367–377

Kuck KH, Böcker D, Chun J, Deneke T, Hindricks G, Hoffmann E, Piorkowski C, Willems S (2017) Qualitätskriterien zur Durchführung der Katheterablation von Vorhofflimmern. Kardiologe 11:161–182

Marrouche NF, Wilber D, Hindricks G, Jais P, Akoum N, Marchlinski F, Kholmovski E, Burgon N, Hu N, Mont L, Deneke T, Duytschaever M, Neumann T, Mansour M, Mahnkopf C, Herweg B, Daoud E, Wissner E, Bansmann P, Brachmann J (2014) Association of atrial tissue fibrosis identified by delayed enhancement MRI and atrial fibrillation catheter ablation: the DECAAF study. JAMA 311:498–506

Moser J, Sultan A, Lüker J, Servatius H, Salzbrunn T, Altenburg M, Schäffer B, Schreiber D, Akbulak RÖ, Vogler J, Hoffmann BA, Willems S, Steven D (2017) 5-year outcome of pulmonary vein isolation by loss of pace capture on the ablation line versus electrical circumferential pulmonary vein isolation. JACC Clin Electrophysiol 3:1262–1271

Taghji P, El Haddad M, Phlips T, Wolf M, Knecht S, Vandekerckhove Y, Tavernier R, Nakagawa H, Duytschaever M (2018) Evaluation of a strategy aiming to enclose the pulmonary veins with contiguous and optimized radiofrequency lesions in paroxysmal atrial fibrillation: a pilot study. JACC Clin Electrophysiol 4:99–108

Tilz RR, Chun KRJ, Deneke T, Kelm C, Piorkowski C, Sommer P, Stellbrink CSD (2017) Positionspapier der Deutschen Gesellschaft für Kardiologie zur Kardioanalgosedierung. Kardiologe 11:369–382

Cryoballoon Ablation

Julian K. R. Chun and Andreas Metzner

14.1 Introduction

Catheter ablation is an established standard in the therapy of atrial fibrillation (AF) (Hindricks et al. 2021). The electrical isolation of the pulmonary veins (PV) as a procedural endpoint is the essential ablation strategy with demonstrable and reproducible benefits for both patients with paroxysmal and persistent AF (Verma et al. 2015). In addition to the established radiofrequency current (RFC)-based ablation using a 3D mapping system, new ablation systems have been developed, which particularly aim at simplifying this complex procedure as well as improving the safety and effectiveness profile. One of these systems is represented by the cryoballoon, which was first introduced in 2005 and has since developed into a standard tool for pulmonary vein isolation (PVI) alongside RFC therapy (Fig. 14.1).

The FIRE-and-ICE study (Kuck et al. 2016) could not show inferiority of the cryoballoon compared to RFC-based PVI in terms of safety and effectiveness in patients with paroxysmal AF. For patients with persistent AF, large multicenter, randomized studies are pending; however, the multicenter and prospective Freeze-AF cohort study showed comparable results of cryoballoon ablation compared to RFC ablation in patients with both paroxysmal and persistent AF. Furthermore, a short learning curve, high durability of lesions, and high reproducibility of long-term freedom from recurrence even outside high-volume centers are essential reasons for the now very widespread use of the cryoballoon for primary PVI (Providencia et al. 2016). Current randomized and multicenter studies have also demonstrated the superiority of cryoballoon PVI over antiarrhythmic drug therapy in the first-line strategy for patients with paroxysmal AF (Andrade et al. 2021; Wazni et al. 2021; Kuniss et al. 2021). These results not only show that early cryoballoon-based PVI is effective and safe in this patient group, but also that it can be primarily recommended to younger patients in the future, especially in light of the results of the EAST and ATTEST studies (Kirchhof et al. 2020; Kuck et al. 2021).

The following will present a practical and compact guide to the effective and safe application of the cryoballoon in the context of PVI,

Supplementary Information The online version contains supplementary material available at https://doi.org/10.1007/978-3-662-65797-3_14. The videos can be accessed individually by clicking the DOI link in the accompanying figure caption or by scanning this link with the SN More Media App.

J. K. R. Chun (✉)
Cardioangiologisches Centrum Bethanien – CCB, Frankfurt a. M., Germany
e-mail: j.chun@ccb.de

A. Metzner
Universitäres Herz- und Gefäßzentrum Hamburg-Eppendorf, Hamburg, Germany
e-mail: a.metzner@uke.de

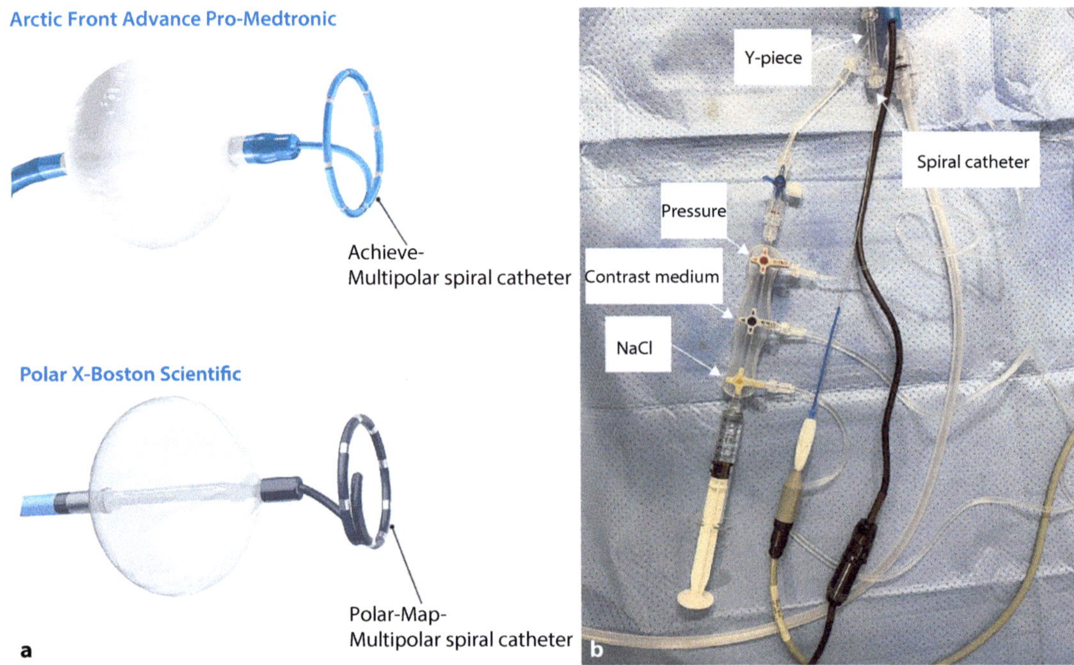

Fig. 14.1 Schematic representation of the two cryoballoon systems (**a**). Organization of the flushing system for contrast medium injection and the spiral catheter (**b**)

with special consideration of pre- and post-interventional aspects, safety algorithms, energy titration, and procedural tips and tricks.

14.2 Cryoballoon Systems

14.2.1 Arctic Front Advance Pro, Medtronic

This cryoballoon system essentially consists of three components:

1. the cryoballoon in its now fourth generation with a shortened distal tip (8 mm length), which is available in two different diameters (23 and 28 mm) and is combined with a modified spiral catheter with eight or ten electrodes as a guidewire and mapping catheter (Achieve, or Achieve Pro);
2. a unidirectional steerable 12-F sheath (Flexcath Advance; inner diameter 12F, outer diameter 15F); and,
3. the cryoconsole.

The cryoballoon, which has an inner and an outer balloon with a vacuum in between, is supplied with nitrous oxide (N_2O) via the console. This is injected into the balloon through a total of eight nozzles, transitions from the liquid to the gaseous state, and homogeneously cools the entire distal hemisphere of the balloon. The duration of the cooling cycle can be individually varied in 5-second steps via the console. During the application, the cycle duration and the current balloon temperature are displayed. At the end of a cooling cycle, the balloon automatically deflates as soon as a temperature of 20°C is reached. The modified spiral catheter (available in 15 mm, 20 mm, and 25 mm diameters) can record electrical signals from the respective PV during the cooling cycle when optimally positioned. This allows the registration of the individual isolation time point and, if necessary, integration into ablation protocols. Instead of the spiral catheter, a long wire can also be introduced through the central lumen of the cryoballoon to deliver improved mechanical balloon stability in the case of complex anatomy. Additionally, contrast medium is applied through the central lumen to verify PV occlusion. A lever on the handle of the cryoballoon can tilt the catheter downwards or upwards to improve the contact between the balloon and tissue by closing smaller occlusion gaps if necessary.

14.2.2 POLARx™, Boston Scientific

As the second cryoballoon-based ablation system, the POLARx™ (Boston Scientific) has been available since 2020. This system also consists of a console (SMARTFREEZE™, Boston Scientific), the cryoballoon (POLARx™) in combination with a modified spiral mapping catheter (POLARmap, 20 mm diameter), and a steerable sheath (POLARsheath, outer diameter 15.9F, inner diameter 12.7F). Similar to the Medtronic cryoballoon, the POLARx™, which has an outer diameter of 28 mm, also consists of an inner and an outer balloon with a vacuum in between. The spiral mapping catheter is introduced through the central lumen, and contrast medium is applied to verify PV occlusion. The cryoballoon tip is available in lengths of 5 and 12 mm.

▶ Both currently available cryoballoon systems consist of an inner and an outer balloon with a vacuum in between, as well as a spiral catheter for visualizing signals, and use nitrous oxide (N_2O) for cooling. There is the possibility to inject contrast medium through a central lumen and to visualize the achieved temperature.

14.3 Patient Selection

In Europe, the cryoballoon procedure is used both for the first ablation of paroxysmal and persistent AF. Particularly advantageous in the ablation of persistent AF is the size mismatch between the cryoballoon and normally dimensioned PV in favor of the balloon, as this not only isolates the PV but also ablates the antrum over a large area, thus providing additional substrate modulation.

Typical atrial flutter that can be present alongside atrial fibrillation does not constitute a contraindication for cryoballoon PVI. A cavotricuspid isthmus block can be easily performed before or after cryoablation under fluoroscopic navigation using a high-frequency current catheter. In contrast, the use of a 3D mapping system is recommended for more complex incidental findings, possibly left atrial or focal atrial tachycardias. Regarding anatomical variants, there is no general exclusion criterion for the use of the cryoballoon. In the case of a left common PV ostium with a long common "trunk" and an assumed distal isolation level, an RF/3D-map-based ablation can be considered instead of the cryoballoon.

14.4 Procedure Execution

In most centers, cryoballoon-based PVIs are performed under deep analgosedation. For this purpose, an initial bolus of a benzodiazepine (e.g., midazolam) and propofol can be administered, followed by a continuous propofol infusion. Before the start of the cryoapplications, a bolus of a morphine derivative (e.g., fentanyl or sufentanil) can be administered if necessary.

In addition to monitoring vital parameters such as oxygen saturation, body temperature, and pulse rate, non-invasive blood pressure measurement is usually performed at regular intervals (e.g., every 2 or 3 minutes). Depending on the respective clinic standard, blood pressure monitoring may also be performed invasively.

For a cryoballoon ablation, in addition to a left atrial access via a transseptal sheath, usually only one other vascular access is required for the insertion of a diagnostic catheter into the coronary sinus, which can later also be used for stimulation of the phrenic nerve.

14.4.1 Periprocedural Anticoagulation

According to current recommendations, procedures in patients on oral anticoagulation with vitamin K antagonists should be performed under continued anticoagulation with an INR value of 2–3. In the case of anticoagulation with non-vitamin K-dependent oral anticoagulants (NOACs), these can also be continued without interruption. However, in many centers, NOACs are currently paused on the morning of the intervention and resumed in a post-interventional safety interval (e.g., six hours after sheath removal). Overlapping therapy with heparin is therefore no longer necessary. During the procedure, an ACT of ≥ 300 s should be targeted. For this purpose, heparin (50–120 IU/kg BW) is administered immediately after the transseptal puncture. ACT measurements are predominantly performed at 15- or 30-minute intervals, and additional heparin is administered if necessary to achieve or maintain the target ACT.

14.4.2 Transseptal Puncture

For cryoballoon-based PVI, only a single transseptal access and thus a transseptal puncture is required. The transseptal puncture is usually performed with a non-steerable sheath (e.g., SL1, Abbott) in combination with a Brockenbrough transseptal needle. A diagnostic catheter positioned in the coronary sinus serves for better fluoroscopic and anatomical orientation during the transseptal puncture. Additionally, a wire or a pigtail catheter in the aortic root or a diagnostic catheter at the His bundle, which in this case indicates the caudal part of the aortic bulb, can be used for more precise orientation. The transseptal puncture is performed under pressure control in many centers.

The transseptal puncture should ideally be performed in a posterior-inferior position within the fossa ovalis. This position generally allows for the greatest possible manipulation and movement space within the left atrium and the best possible access to the right lower pulmonary vein, especially in the case of a very inferior takeoff.

Initially, the transseptal puncture is performed using a non-steerable sheath. Subsequently, a long wire is placed in the left upper PV. The non-steerable sheath is then exchanged for the steerable cryosheath over this wire. The distal end of the steerable cryosheath can ideally be "parked" in the proximal part of the left upper PV, which later ensures direct access to the PV using the spiral catheter and the cryoballoon without further sheath manipulation. Alternatively, the sheath can initially be curved and positioned in front of the mitral valve (Fig. 14.2).

If resistance is felt when inserting the cryosheath in the groin area or the interatrial septum, a clockwise rotation of the sheath is recommended to facilitate passage. If passage is still difficult, the introducer of the cryoballoon sheath can be used for pre-dilation. The cryosheath is continuously flushed during the procedure. Whenever a catheter is inserted through or removed from the sheath, aspiration should be performed to avoid potential air embolisms.

14.4.3 Pulmonary Vein Angiographies/Pre-interventional Imaging

Selective angiographies of the PV are helpful for visualizing the pulmonary venous and left atrial anatomy. For this purpose, the PV can be visualized using the non-steerable transseptal sheath and a multipurpose catheter (e.g., Cordis, 7F) through manual injection of contrast medium or using an injection pump. Various projections are possible, such as 30° right anterior oblique (RAO) for the septal PV and 40° left anterior oblique (LAO) for the left PV. The left upper PV is often visualized in both RAO and LAO to visualize both the entry into the left atrium and the course. As an alternative to the non-steerable transseptal sheath combined with a multipurpose catheter, the angiographies can also be performed directly via the non-steerable transseptal sheath or the Flexcath sheath, which can particularly facilitate access to the right lower PV. However, a potentially increased risk of air embolisms and atrial injuries due to the size and the rather rigid distal end of the sheath must be considered.

As an alternative to selective PV angiographies, some centers also perform pre-interventional CT or MRI imaging of the left atrium and the PV.

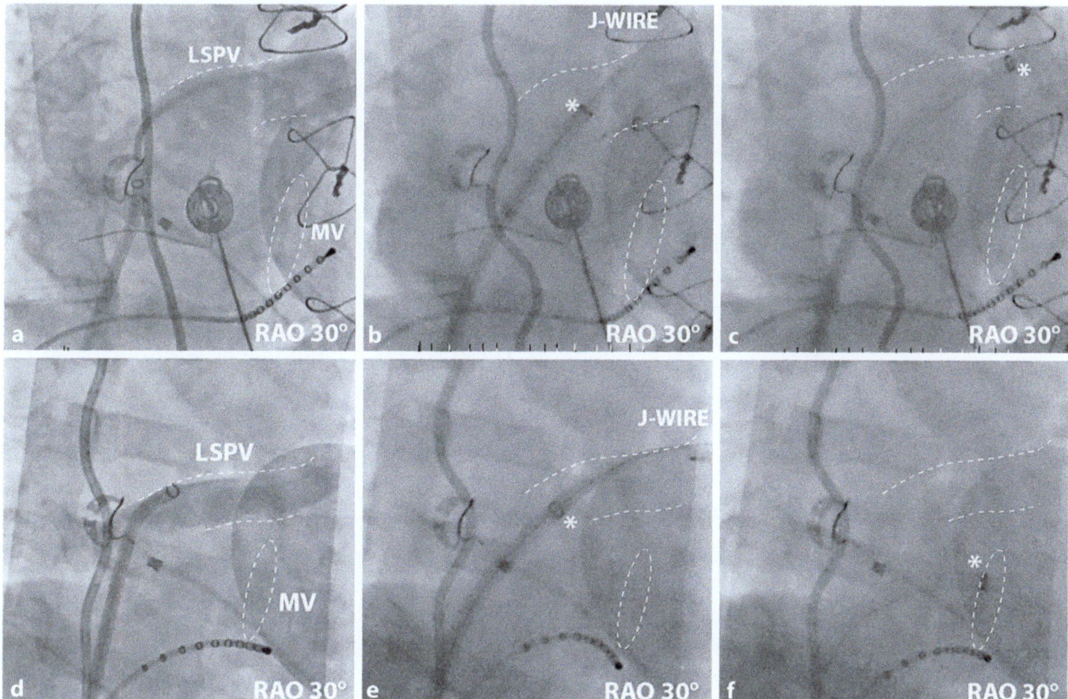

Fig. 14.2 Upper panel (**a,b,c**): Representation of the LSPV using selective angiography. Subsequently, secure positioning of the J-wire in the LSPV and exchange of the cryoballoon sheath in the LSPV. For further details, see text. Lower panel (**d,e,f**): Representation of the LSPV using selective angiography. Subsequently, insertion of the cryoballoon sheath into the left atrium while the J-wire remains in the LSPV. The cryoballoon sheath is curved and positioned in front of the mitral valve. For further details, see text. LSPV = left superior pulmonary vein, RAO = Right Anterior Oblique, MV—mitral valve

Both modalities are associated with increased procedural costs and, in the case of CT, also lead to increased radiation exposure for the patient. However, the acquired information of PV anatomy can potentially be used for patient selection.

14.4.4 Tips and Tricks, Energy Dosing, and Safety Algorithms

The electrical isolation of PV with a cryoballoon represents a simplified ablation procedure compared to RF ablation. Based on the primarily anatomically guided ablation principle, comparably good results with a low variance among different operators/centers can be achieved after a relatively short learning curve. Currently, two manufacturers offer their own version of the cryoballoon with similar properties: In both procedures, the key to successful ablation lies in the systematic implementation of three work steps.

1. Pulmonary vein occlusion with the cryoballoon.
2. Visualization of electrical pulmonary vein signals.
3. Dosing of the cryo energy

Step 1: Pulmonary Vein Occlusion with the Cryoballoon

With the "single big cryoballoon technique," techniques for optimizing cryoballoon positioning and pulmonary vein occlusion were introduced. Knowledge of the anatomy of the pulmonary veins is essential, both in absolute terms (the veins usually have a similar orientation in different patients) and in relative terms (the position of the pulmonary veins in relation to the transseptal puncture). The typical anatomies and orientations of the pulmonary veins (left field) and the occlusion techniques (right) are summarized in Fig. 14.3. The concept of coaxiality describes the principle that all cryoballoon components (balloon, sheath, spiral catheter) should be aligned in the same direction. If necessary, controlling the orientation of the catheter and sheath in a second fluoroscopic plane can be useful. It should be emphasized once again that an infero-posterior position of the transseptal puncture site is helpful for good cryoballoon PV occlusion (Figs. 14.3, 14.4 and 14.5).

Step 2: Visualization of electrical pulmonary vein signals

The real-time visualization of the time to isolation (TTI) is important to directly verify the effectiveness of the cryoablation (Fig. 14.6).

This way, ineffective applications can be terminated prematurely, or the total number of applications can be reduced in the case of short isolation times. An initial distal position of the spiral catheter (SC) improves the stability of the system. After inflating, the balloon is guided to the PV antrum with the SC positioned relatively deep in the vein. Once the balloon has taken a stable position at the PV (concept of coaxiality), the SC is pulled back proximally under rotating movements to capture PV signals. Once the visualization of the PV spike is verified, a contrast agent injection is performed to verify the degree of occlusion.

Step 3: Dosing the cold energy, applying safety algorithms

The freezing of cardiac tissue with the cryoballoon occurs radially, and animal experiments show that the depth of the lesion created is proportional to the application duration. The emergence of new and more potent generations of cryoballoons has raised the question of the ideal energy dosage/application duration to (1) enable a transmural lesion but (2) avoid damage to extracardiac structures. For this purpose, strategies have been investigated to avoid the empirical bonus-freeze and to shorten the application duration.

1—Omitting the "bonus-freeze" In the "FIRE-and-ICE" study, an ablation duration of 240 s with a subsequent empirical bonus application of the same duration was recommended in the study protocol. Subsequently, a randomized study showed that the bonus application can be omitted in the case of early PVI in real-time ("time to isolation"—TTI < 75 s) (Chun et al. 2017), while maintaining procedural efficacy and improving the safety of the procedure.

These results are consistent with other non-randomized studies that report high efficacy when using ablation protocols that empirically omit the "bonus" application. In line with these studies, it has often become established in clinical routine to forgo the empirical bonus application, although this is still recommended in the case of late PVI (TTI > 75 s).

2—Reducing the application duration Shortening the application duration is probably the best way to avoid deep-reaching, extracardiac lesions. While acute PVI is usually observed within the first 60 s, complications such as phrenic nerve palsy or deep temperatures in the esophagus predominantly occur only after 150 and 180 s.

The randomized and controlled "Circa-Dose" study was able to show that 2 × 120 s application time is similarly effective as 2 × 240 s. However, too short applications can actually lead to reduced effectiveness, as shown in the "PlusOne" study: In a group of patients treated with a TTI + 60-second protocol, an unexpectedly high rate of acute PV reconnections of 3.5% was observed. The use of TTI to shorten the application duration (TTI + 120 s) was tested with good clinical results. However, shortening the application is associated with a 48% probability of PV reconnections in the case of a re-procedure (29). In line with this observation, an empirical application of 240 s application duration was associated with a higher percentage of permanently isolated PV (87.5%) compared to patients treated with a fixed application duration of 180 s (69%) (Chen et al. 2019).

Considering this, the FALASA concept ("Freeze As Long As Safely Achievable") appears sensible. In this case, a single shot

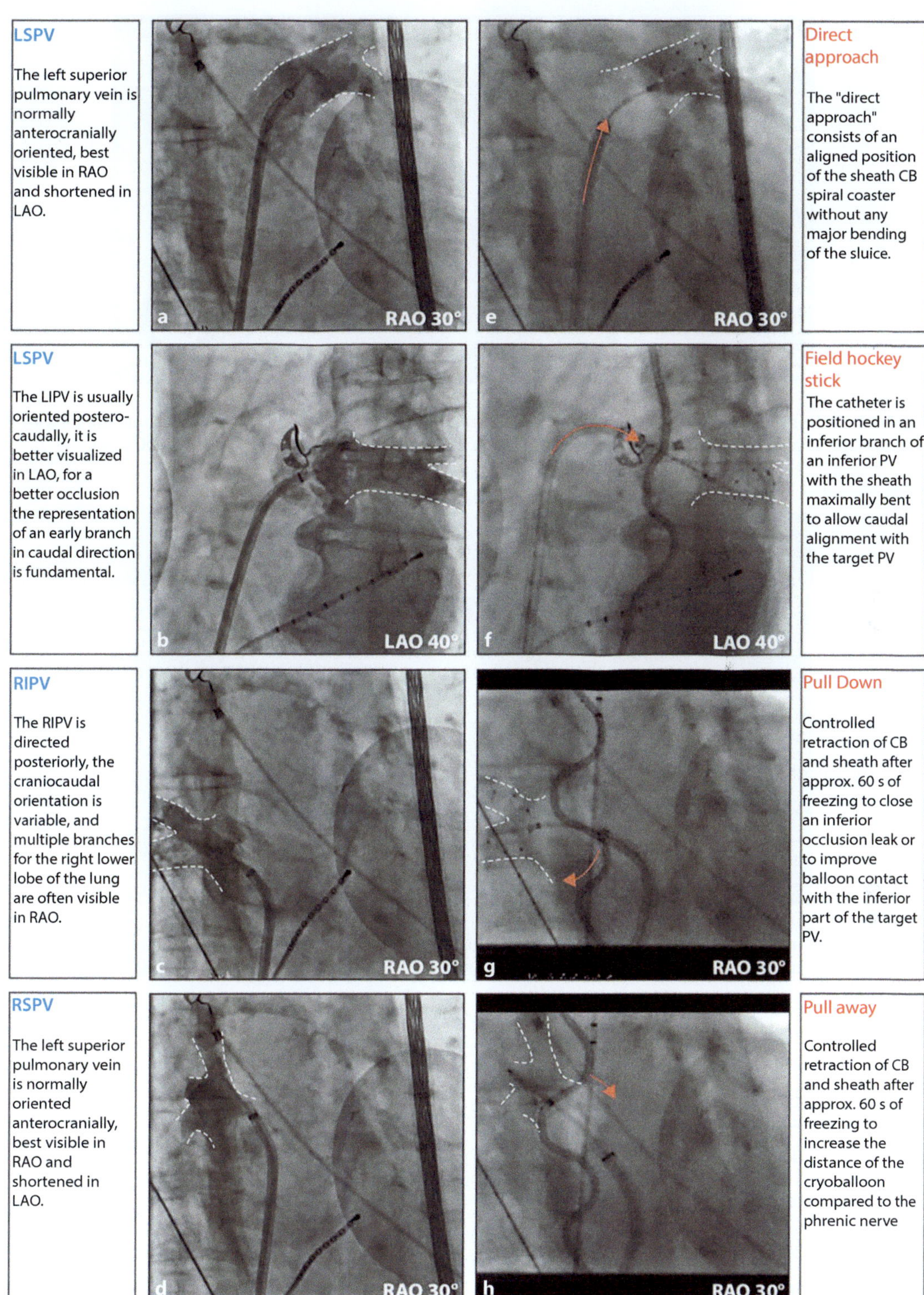

Fig. 14.3 Typical PV anatomies and orientations (left). Representation of successful PV occlusion techniques and cryoballoon maneuvers (right). PV = pulmonary vein, LAO = left anterior oblique, LSPV = left superior pulmonary vein, LIPV = left inferior pulmonary vein, RAO = right anterior oblique, RSPV = right superior pulmonary vein, RIPV = right inferior pulmonary vein

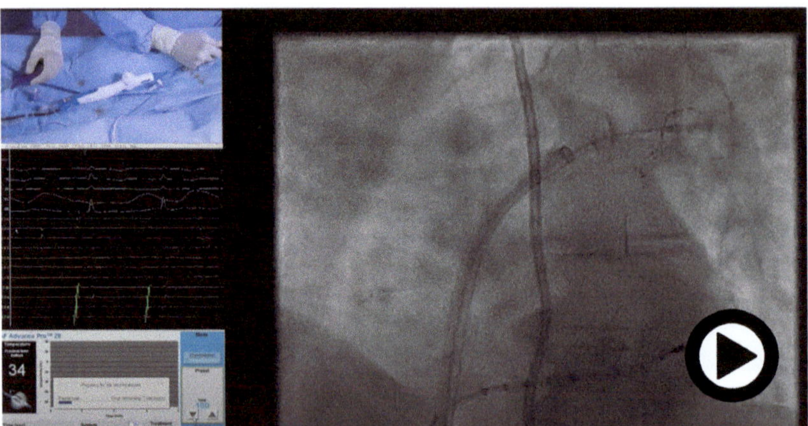

Fig. 14.4 Still image from Video 1. A practical guide to simplified navigation of the cryoballoon into the inferior PV is shown here (Part I shows the navigation for the ablation of the LIPV) (https://doi.org/10.1007/000-d2x)

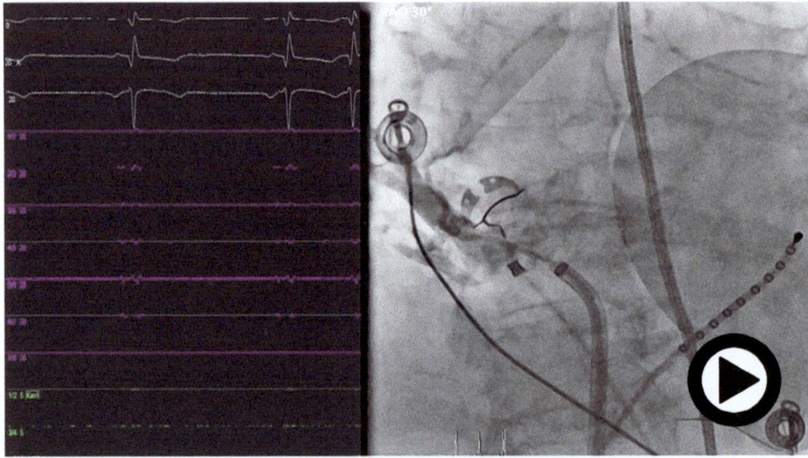

Fig. 14.5 Still image from Video 2. A practical guide to simplified navigation of the cryoballoon into the inferior PV is shown here (Part II shows the navigation for the ablation of the RIPV) (https://doi.org/10.1007/000-d2w)

application duration of 240 s is aimed for, which is only terminated prematurely in the event of extracardiac thermal damage or effects (N. phrenicus, esophageal temperature).

Course of temperature development during cryotherapy

The balloon temperature measured during a cryoapplication depends on the quality of the occlusion, the size of the pulmonary vein, and the duration of the application. A precise registration of the temperature urve provides valuable indications of the effectiveness of the energy delivery. A balloon temperature warmer than −35°C after 60s indicates suboptimal occlusion. At the end of an effective cold treatment, an average temperature between −45 and −50°C is to be expected. After the end of a cryotherapy, a longer thawing phase (e.g.: > 10 s until reaching 0°C) is associated with better long-term results. If the temperature drops to > −60 °C, the application should be terminated if necessary to avoid collateral damage. If the cryoballoon temperature drops unusually quickly, the balloon

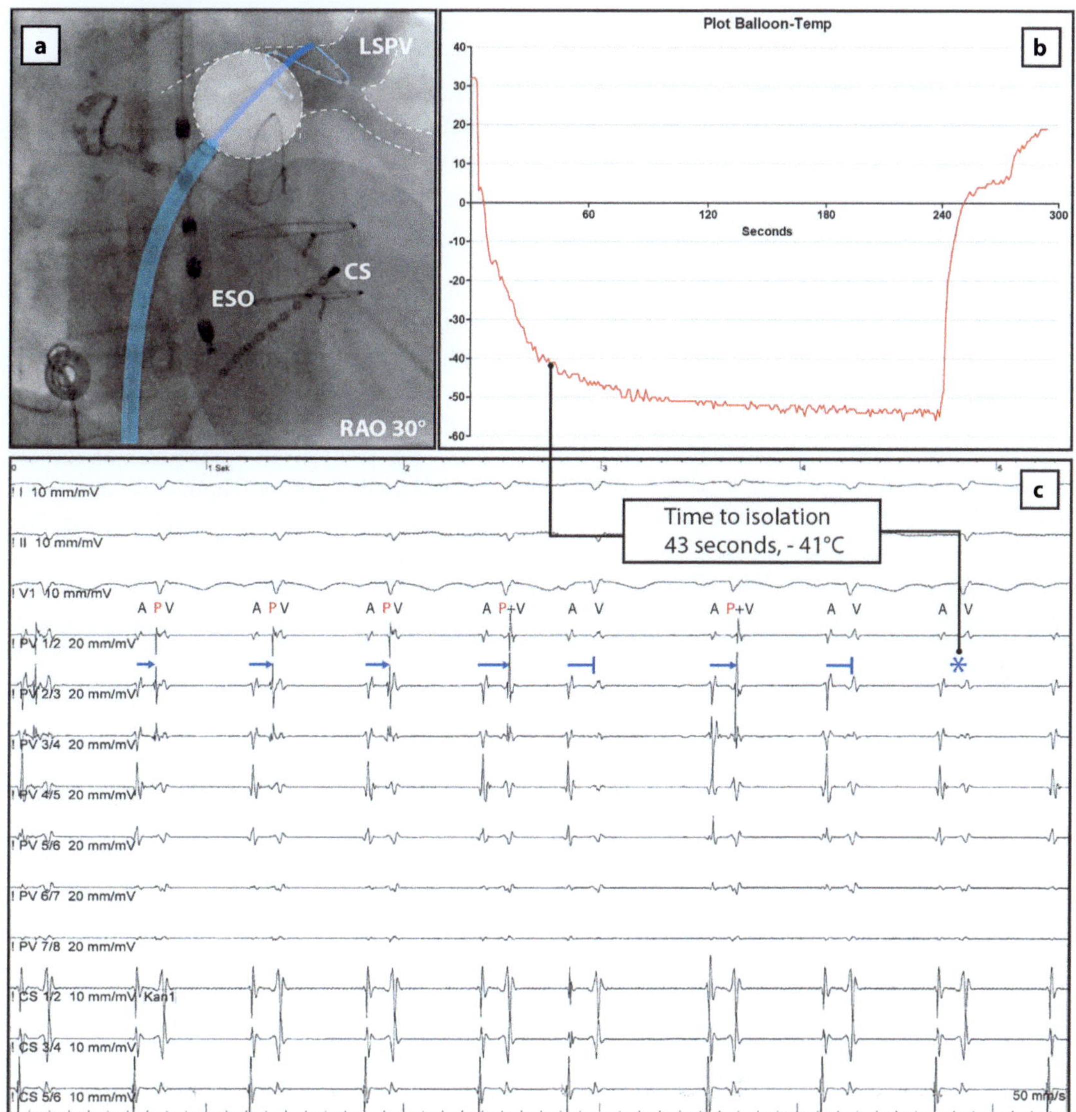

Fig. 14.6 **a** Complete occlusion of the left superior pulmonary vein using the "direct approach". Subsequently, a characteristic cryoballoon temperature curve with documentation of successful electrical isolation (*) after 43 s at a temperature of 41 °C. RAO = Right anterior oblique, LSPV = left superior pulmonary vein, ESO = temperature probe in the esophagus, CS = coronary sinus

position and balloon shape ("round" versus "compressed") should also be evaluated to avoid ablation within the pulmonary vein with corresponding complication potential.

The mentioned reference values refer to the treatment with the Artic-Front system. The first clinical experiences with the Polar-X platform show slightly colder measured balloon temperatures, which could be due to differences in material properties and the slightly changed positioning of the temperature sensor.

▶ The development of the temperature curve during ablation allows important conclusions to be drawn about the occlusion and a possible development to lower temperatures. It should therefore be observed throughout the entire ablation. The differences between the two currently available systems should be taken into account.

Safety

A crucial aspect for the widespread application of the cryoballoon procedure is its good safety profile (Table 14.1). In particular, the lower risk of potentially life-threatening cardiac tamponade is significant. However, there are specific safety-relevant parameters that should be continuously monitored to avoid thermal damage to extracardiac structures. This is especially true for the right-sided phrenic nerve (diaphragmatic paralysis) and the esophagus (atrio-esophageal fistula).

Monitoring the Function of the Phrenic Nerve
During ablation at the right PV, monitoring of diaphragmatic contraction and a systematic approach in case of phrenic nerve damage is required. This has been summarized in five basic rules (Bordignon et al. 2021):

1. Exclusive use of the 28-mm cryoballoon: Greater distance to the phrenic nerve and avoidance of a distal position of the balloon in the PV (Chun et al. 2008).
2. Achieving stable stimulation of the phrenic nerve: This is easier if a multipolar catheter is guided to the junction of the right subclavian vein, where the stimulation threshold for the phrenic nerve is lower. Additionally, a "far-field" stimulation with high voltage is recommended (electrodes 1–4, 12V@2.9 ms).

Table 14.1 Typical complications and frequencies in the context of cryoballoon AF ablation

Complication	Incidence (in %)
Phrenic nerve paralysis	2–7.3
Esophageal thermal lesions	1.5–22
Esophago-atrial fistula	< 0.01
Transient ischemic attack/stroke	0–1.4
Pericardial tamponade	0–0.9
High-grade pulmonary vein stenosis	0–1.3

3. Monitoring diaphragmatic contraction: In addition to abdominal palpation to detect diaphragmatic contraction, recording the compound motor action potential (CMAP) in the modified surface ECG helps to objectify a progressive loss of diaphragmatic function. A reduction in CMAP amplitude by > 30 % should lead to an interruption of the application. With the PolarX balloon, diaphragmatic contraction can additionally be monitored with the diaphragm movement sensor (DMS). The clinical benefit must be evaluated in further studies.
4. Use of a "pull-away" maneuver of the cryoballoon after 60 s of application duration to increase the distance between the cryoballoon and the phrenic nerve.
5. Active deflation of the cryoballoon ("double-stop" maneuver) in case of weakening of the phrenic nerve function to ensure rapid thawing and avoid sustained damage to the phrenic nerve (Ghosh et al. 2013).

▶ Phrenic nerve palsy represents a relevant but rare complication (< 3%) of cryoballoon ablation, which in most cases recovers within twelve months and whose incidence can be significantly reduced with various maneuvers and strategies.

Monitoring of Esophageal Temperature
During the ablation of atrial fibrillation, the benefit of monitoring the luminal temperature in the esophagus is controversial. For RF ablation, a randomized study recently showed that the use of intraesophageal temperature measurement has no impact on the likelihood of developing endoscopically diagnosed esophageal lesions. For cryoballoon PVI, however, it has been shown that the use of a temperature limit can reduce the incidence of thermal lesions in the esophagus from 19% to 1.7% (Fürnkranz et al. 2015). Due to a latency in the drop of esophageal temperature, a temperature of 15°C is recommended as the cut-off value for stopping cryoapplication.

In a series of > 1000 patients treated with cryoballoon PVI with esophageal temperature measurements (application duration: 240 s), the cut-off value of 15°C was reached in 19% of patients on average after 178 s. However, if for various reasons no temperature measurements are performed in the esophagus, the risk of thermal damage could potentially be reduced by empirically shortening the application duration to, for example, 180 s. However, a higher percentage of pulmonary vein reconnections must be accepted for this (Chen et al. 2019).

14.5 Post-procedural Management

14.5.1 Manual Compression or Suture Closure of the Puncture Site

Complications at the puncture site in the groin represent one of the most common adverse events in atrial fibrillation ablations, with around 2–4%. Therefore, sufficient closure of the puncture is crucial. Although cryoballoon PVI requires a relatively large-lumen vascular access of around 15F, interestingly, no significantly increased groin complications have been shown in large randomized studies compared to HFS ablations. Typically, the puncture site is manually compressed after sheath removal until hemostasis is achieved. A pressure bandage is then applied for at least six hours.

As an alternative to manual compression of the puncture site, temporary suture closure is increasingly being used (Fig. 14.7).

For this, a thread (for example, a monofilament non-absorbable 0-thread) is first placed subcutaneously from medial to lateral 5–10 mm distal to the puncture site with a widely curved needle. The thread is then guided across the puncture site and again subcutaneously from medial to lateral 5–10 mm proximal to the puncture site above the sheath running in depth with a second stitch. Thus, a Z-shaped suture is prepared over the puncture. The two free ends of the thread are grasped and brought together with a first surgical knot. After careful removal of the sheaths, the suture is tightened and fixed with

additional surgical knots until complete hemostasis is achieved. The thread can be removed the following morning. When placing the suture, care must be taken to guide the thread subcutaneously to avoid injury to large nerves and vessels. Studies on such closure using a "Z-suture" (or "figure-of-eight suture") show a good safety profile without significant differences in hematomas, rebleeding, vascular fistulas, or thromboses compared to conventional compression. This can reduce both the post-procedural stay in the EP lab and the duration of the pressure bandage application (Kumar et al. 2019).

14.5.2 "Same day discharge"

In recent years, in addition to questions of patient comfort, economic considerations have also led to the examination of discharging the patient on the same day as the treatment. Initial studies from North America and the UK have demonstrated a good safety profile with significant cost savings for selected patient groups. However, since very early discharge is significantly dependent on local care structures and individual follow-up, further data from the German-speaking area are necessary. It should also be critically considered that although severe complications such as pericardial tamponades are rare, they can still occur with more than a 24-hour delay and require rapid diagnosis and therapy. The current position paper on the quality criteria for atrial fibrillation ablation by the DGK calls for inpatient monitoring for 24–48 hours after the procedure.

14.5.3 Management of Atrial Fibrillation Recurrences after Cryopulmonary vein Isolation

In clinical and scientific practice, early recurrences (within three months after the index procedure) are distinguished from recurrences outside the so-called three-month "blanking"

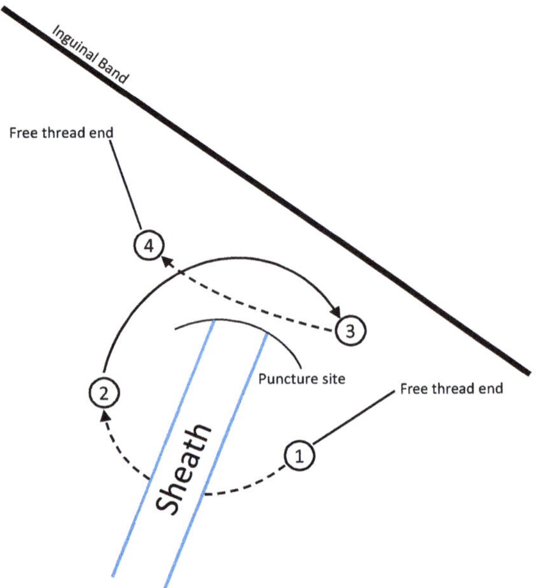

Fig. 14.7 Schematic representation of the placement of a Z-suture before sheath removal

period. This is based on the assumption that inflammation directly caused by ablation could be arrhythmogenic, while the effectiveness of catheter treatment, due to the delayed complete formation of a transmural ablation lesion, only fully manifests over the course of weeks. Although newer data suggest that early recurrences are often predictors of later recurrences, it remains common and justified from practical considerations to initially treat rhythm disturbances that recur after cryoablation with adjuvant antiarrhythmic medication and, if necessary, perform cardioversion.

Recurrences that occur in the medium to long term often necessitate a repeat ablation treatment. Since atrial fibrillation recurrences are usually associated with re-conducting PV even after an initially successful ablation, the focus remains on the established endpoint of PVI. Overall, based on the "FIRE-and-ICE-Redo-Study," there is a higher likelihood of durable isolation of the left-sided pulmonary veins after cryoballoon-based ablation compared to RF-g ablation (Kuck et al. 2019). Predilection sites for reconnections after cryoballoon-guided PVI are particularly the inferior part of the right lower PV and the superior aspect of the right upper PV. Regarding reablation in patients with AF recurrences after previous cryoballon or RF-based PVI and electrically reconnected PV, there is currently insufficient data for cryotreatment, so reablation with the cryoballoon can not be recommended routinely. Many factors speak for a switch to a 3D mapping procedure in combination with RF ablation. Typically, the site of reconnection can be pinpointed and then focally ablated. Additionally, RF strategies offer the option to analyze the underlying substrate more precisely using electroanatomical mapping and to target treatment in the case of existing atrial tachycardias. For the above reasons and the increasing frequency of durable isolation of all PV, the authors recommend the use of a 3D mapping system in the case of routine AF reablation.

▶ In the case of AF reablation, a 3D mapping system in combination with radiofrequency ablation should be used due to the greater flexibility and the possibility of very targeted ablation of gaps within the ipsilateral circular lesions and the ability to visualize the individual substrate.

14.6 Outlook

14.6.1 Ablation Strategies Beyond Pulmonary Vein Isolation

To date, PVI remains the only established endpoint in the treatment of atrial fibrillation, and both cryoballoon systems were explicitly developed for this purpose. The systematic extension of an ablation treatment to include modification of the left atrial substrate or electrical isolation of extrapulmonary vein atrial fibrillation triggers is controversially discussed and has predominantly not shown any advantage in randomized studies. Only for the supplementary electrical isolation of the left atrial appendage as the "fifth pulmonary vein" are there positive data available (Di Biase et al. 2016). In many cases, however, ablation treatment beyond PVI is associated with prolonged procedure times, increased radiation exposure, and a higher risk of complicating atrial tachycardias in the long term. Nevertheless, it may become necessary, for example, in cases of persistent atrial fibrillation despite electrically isolated pulmonary veins or intra-procedural atrial tachycardias, to consider an extension of the ablation treatment. It is interesting to note that strategies for the electrical isolation of the superior vena cava, the left atrial posterior wall (*"box lesion"*), or the left atrial appendage (Yorgun et al. 2019) have been described using a cryoballoon. Persistent superior vena cavas have also been successfully isolated primarily with a cryoballoon, and linear lesions such as a roofline have been bidirectionally blocked. However, all these extrapulmonary vein cryoballoon-based ablations must consider a specific risk profile, such as injuries to the epicardial coronary arteries and an increased post-procedural stroke risk with atrial appendage isolation, a lesion of the right phrenic nerve with superior vena cava isolation, or potential injury to the esophagus with ablation on the left atrial posterior wall. Moreover, no data from randomized studies are available so far, so these procedures should be reserved for the treatment of selected individual cases in experienced centers or should be performed within the framework of controlled studies.

▶ The ablation of structures outside the pulmonary veins is currently not recommended. In experienced centers and within controlled studies, ablation strategies beyond PVI are currently being evaluated.

Currently, additional isolation of the left atrial appendage using a cryoballoon for the treatment of persistent forms of atrial fibrillation (LALA-Land-AF; ClinicalTrials.gov identifier NCT04240366) or as an extended measure in electrically isolated pulmonary veins in the context of a reablation (ASTRO AF; NCT04056390) is being investigated in randomized controlled studies.

14.6.2 Intra-procedural Electroanatomical Mapping and Contrast-free Occlusion Testing

With the introduction of the novel imaging and electroanatomical mapping system KODEX (EPD-Solutions; Philips, Amsterdam, Netherlands), a direct integration of the Arctic Front cryoballoon system into a 3D imaging platform is now available. KODEX allows high-resolution electroanatomical representation of the heart anatomy by measuring dielectric coefficients between catheter electrodes as well as electrodes on the patient's body surface (Maurer et al. 2019). As it is an open platform, any appropriately validated electrode catheter can be calibrated for use. Thus, the Achieve catheter can also be used for left atrial imaging during a cryoballoon procedure. It has also been shown that KODEX is capable of quantifying the changes in the electric field around the catheter electrodes during the occlusion of a pulmonary vein by the cryoballoon. This can enable an assessment of adequate cryoballoon positioning—possibly even without the use of X-ray contrast medium.

14.7   Summary

The cryoballoon-based atrial fibrillation ablation is established as a standard procedure for index PVI in many centers and is recommended alongside RF ablation in the current guidelines as the gold standard for atrial fibrillation therapy. By applying systematic steps, a safe, simplified, and effective PVI can be achieved. The use of the cryoballoon for the ablation of extrapulmonary vein structures is the subject of ongoing scientific investigations and does not represent a routine procedure.

References

Andrade JG, Wells GA, Deyell MW, Bennett M, Essebag V, Champagne J, Roux J-F, Yung D, Skanes A, Khaykin Y, Morillo C, Jolly U, Novak P, Lockwood E, Amit G, Angaran P, Sapp J, Wardell S, Lauck S, Macle L, Verma A (2021) Cryoablation or drug therapy for initial treatment of atrial fibrillation. n Engl J Med 384:305–315

Di Biase L, Burkhardt JD, Mohanty P, Mohanty S, Sanchez JE, Trivedi C, Güneş M, Gökoğlan Y, Gianni C, Horton RP, Themistoclakis S, Gallinghouse GJ, Bailey S, Zagrodzky JD, Hongo RH, Beheiry S, Santangeli P, Casella M, Dello Russo A, Al-Ahmad A, Hranitzky P, Lakkireddy D, Tondo C, Natale A (2016) Left atrial appendage isolation in patients with longstanding persistent AF undergoing catheter ablation. J Am Coll Cardiol 68:1929–1940

Bordignon S, Chen S, Bologna F, Thohoku S, Urbanek L, Willems F, Zanchi S, Bianchini L, Trolese L, Konstantinou A, Fuernkranz A, Schmidt B, Chun JKR (2021) Optimizing cryoballoon pulmonary vein isolation: lessons from >1000 procedures – the Frankfurt approach. Europace 23:868–877

Chen S, Schmidt B, Bordignon S, Perrotta L, Bologna F, Chun KRJ (2019) Impact of cryoballoon freeze duration on long-term durability of pulmonary vein isolation. JACC Clin Electrophysiol 5:551–559

Chun K-RJ, Schmidt B, Metzner A, Tilz R, Zerm T, Koster I, Furnkranz A, Koektuerk B, Konstantinidou M, Antz M, Ouyang F, Kuck KH (2008) The "single big cryoballoon" technique for acute pulmonary vein isolation in patients with paroxysmal atrial fibrillation: a prospective observational single centre study. Eur Heart J 30:699–709

Chun KRJ, Stich M, Fürnkranz A, Bordignon S, Perrotta L, Dugo D, Bologna F, Schmidt B (2017) Individualized cryoballoon energy pulmonary vein isolation guided by real-time pulmonary vein recordings, the randomized ICE-T trial. Heart Rhythm 14:495–500

Fürnkranz A, Bordignon S, Böhmig M, Konstantinou A, Dugo D, Perrotta L, Klopffleisch T, Nowak B, Dignaß AU, Schmidt B, Chun JKR (2015) Reduced incidence of esophageal lesions by luminal esophageal temperature–guided second-generation cryoballoon ablation. Heart Rhythm 12:268–274

Ghosh J, Sepahpour A, Chan KH, Singarayar S, McGuire MA (2013) Immediate balloon deflation for prevention of persistent phrenic nerve palsy during pulmonary vein isolation by balloon cryoablation. Heart Rhythm 10:646–652

Hindricks G, Potpara T, Dagres N, Arbelo E, Bax JJ, Blomström-Lundqvist C, Boriani G, Castella M, Dan G-A, Dilaveris PE, Fauchier L, Filippatos G, Kalman JM, La Meir M, Lane DA, Lebeau J-P, Lettino M, Lip GYH, Pinto FJ, Thomas GN, Valgimigli M, Van Gelder IC, Van Putte BP, Watkins CL, ESC Scientific Document Group, Kirchhof P, Kühne M, Aboyans V, Ahlsson A, Balsam P, Bauersachs J, Benussi S, Brandes A, Braunschweig F, Camm AJ, Capodanno D, Casadei B, Conen D, Crijns HJGM, Delgado V, Dobrev D, Drexel H, Eckardt L, Fitzsimons D, Folliguet T, Gale CP, Gorenek B, Haeusler KG, Heidbuchel H, Iung B, Katus HA, Kotecha D, Landmesser U, Leclercq C, Lewis BS, Mascherbauer J, Merino JL, Merkely B, Mont L, Mueller C, Nagy KV, Oldgren J, Pavlović N, Pedretti RFE, Petersen SE, Piccini JP, Popescu BA, Pürerfellner H, Richter DJ, Roffi M, Rubboli A, Scherr D, Schnabel RB, Simpson IA, Shlyakhto E, Sinner MF, Steffel J, Sousa-Uva M, Suwalski P, Svetlosak M, Touyz RM, Dagres N, Arbelo E, Bax JJ, Blomström-Lundqvist C, Boriani G, Castella M, Dan G-A, Dilaveris PE, Fauchier L, Filippatos G, Kalman JM, La Meir M, Lane DA, Lebeau J-P, Lettino M, Lip GYH, Pinto FJ et al (2021) 2020 ESC Guidelines for the diagnosis and management of atrial fibrillation developed in collaboration with the European Association for Cardio-Thoracic Surgery (EACTS). Eur Heart J 42:373–498

Kirchhof P, Camm AJ, Goette A, Brandes A, Eckardt L, Elvan A, Fetsch T, van Gelder IC, Haase D, Haegeli LM, Hamann F, Heidbüchel H, Hindricks G, Kautzner J, Kuck K-H, Mont L, Ng GA, Rekosz J, Schoen N, Schotten U, Suling A, Taggeselle J, Themistoclakis S, Vettorazzi E, Vardas P, Wegscheider K, Willems S, Crijns HJGM, Breithardt G (2020) Early rhythm-control therapy in patients with atrial fibrillation. N Engl J Med 383:1305–1316

Kuck K-H, Brugada J, Fürnkranz A, Metzner A, Ouyang F, Chun KRJ, Elvan A, Arentz T, Bestehorn K, Pocock SJ, Albenque J-P, Tondo C (2016) Cryoballoon or radiofrequency ablation for paroxysmal atrial fibrillation. N Engl J Med 374:2235–2245

Kuck KH, Albenque JP, Chun KJ, Fürnkranz A, Busch M, Elvan A, Schlüter M, Braegelmann KM, Kueffer FJ, Hemingway L, Arentz T, Tondo C, Brugada J, FIRE AND ICE Investigators (2019) Repeat ablation for atrial fibrillation recurrence post cryoballoon or radiofrequency ablation in the FIRE AND ICE trial. Circ Arrhythm Electrophysiol 12(6):e7247

Kuck KH, Lebedev DS, Mikhaylov EN, Romanov A, Gellér L, Kalējs O, Neumann T, Davtyan K, On YK, Popov S, Bongiorni MG, Schlüter M, Willems S, Ouyang F (2021) Catheter ablation or medical therapy to delay progression of atrial fibrillation: the randomized controlled atrial fibrillation progression trial (ATTEST). Europace 23(3):362–369

Kumar V, Wish M, Venkataraman G, Bliden K, Jindal M, Strickberger A (2019) A randomized comparison of manual pressure versus figure-of-eight suture for hemostasis after cryoballoon ablation for atrial fibrillation. J Cardiovasc Electrophysiol 30:2806–2810

Kuniss M, Pavlovic N, Velagic V, Hermida JS, Healey S, Arena G, Badenco N, Meyer C, Chen J, Iacopino S, Anselme F, Packer DL, Pitschner HF, Asmundis C, Willems S, Di Piazza F, Becker D, Chierchia GB, Cryo-FIRST Investigators (2021) Cryoballoon ablation vs. antiarrhythmic drugs: first-line therapy for patients with paroxysmal atrial fibrillation. Europace 23(7):1033–1041

Maurer T, Mathew S, Schlüter M, Lemes C, Riedl J, Inaba O, Hashiguchi N, Reißmann B, Fink T, Rottner L, Rillig A, Metzner A, Ouyang F, Kuck K-H (2019) High-resolution imaging of LA anatomy using a novel wide-band dielectric mapping system. JACC Clin Electrophysiol 5:1344–1354

Providencia R, Defaye P, Lambiase PD, Pavin D, Cebron J-P, Halimi F, Anselme F, Srinivasan N, Albenque J-P, Boveda S (2016) Results from a multicentre comparison of cryoballoon vs. radiofrequency ablation for paroxysmal atrial fibrillation: is cryoablation more reproducible? Europace euw80

Verma A, Jiang C, Betts TR, Chen J, Deisenhofer I, Mantovan R, Macle L, Morillo CA, Haverkamp W, Weerasooriya R, Albenque J-P, Nardi S, Menardi E, Novak P, Sanders P (2015) Approaches to catheter ablation for persistent atrial fibrillation. N Engl J Med 372:1812–1822

Wazni OM, Dandamudi G, Sood N, Hoyt R, Tyler J, Durrani S, Niebauer M, Makati K, Halperin B, Gauri A, Morales G, Shao M, Cerkvenik J, Kaplon RE, Nissen SE, STOP AF First Trial Investigators (2021) Cryoballoon ablation as initial therapy for atrial fibrillation. N Engl J Med 384(4):316–324

Yorgun H, Canpolat U, Okşul M, Şener YZ, Ateş AH, Crijns HJGM, Aytemir K (2019) Long-term outcomes of cryoballoon-based left atrial appendage isolation in addition to pulmonary vein isolation in persistent atrial fibrillation. Europace 21:1653–1662

Localization of Ventricular Arrhythmias from the 12-Lead ECG

15

Leon Iden

15.1 Introduction

In the context of the ablation of ventricular arrhythmias, an approximate localization of the origin or the exit of the arrhythmia based on the 12-lead ECG is essential. This touches on aspects of indication, particularly the procedure planning regarding the access route, choice of materials, patient onsent, and possible escalation steps in case of procedural difficulties.

There are numerous published algorithms for localization that have not been validated against each other (Ito et al. 2003). Furthermore, many EPs develop an intuitive understanding of localization due to certain characteristic ECG patterns with increasing experience.

Here, a deliberately simple and practical representation is to be shown. It should be noted that due to the variability of the anatomical heart axis, thorax configuration, and the not always consistent placement of the chest leads, the precision of localization should generally not be overestimated.

The following basic principles should be considered for the localization of the arrhythmia (see Fig. 15.1):

L. Iden (✉)
Herz- und Gefäßzentrum, Segeberger Kliniken GmbH, Bad Segeberg, Germany
e-mail: leon.iden@segebergerkliniken.de

- An excitation front that approaches the tip of an ECG lead causes a positive deflection in the ECG. An excitation front that moves away from a lead causes a negative deflection in the ECG.
- If it is a focal arrhythmia, the origin of the arrhythmia can be estimated from the 12-lead ECG. If it is a (scar-associated) reentry, the systole of the tachycardia and thus the QRS complex begins at the exit of the tachycardia from the scar and is formed by the outer loop. The inner loop consists of a small number of simultaneously activated myocytes that are not visible on the surface ECG. This represents the diastole of the tachycardia, i.e., the period of the isoelectric or ST segment and T wave on the surface ECG.
- The right ventricle is significantly less involved in the formation of the vector due to the considerably lower myocardial mass compared to the LV. Furthermore, the RV is significantly less represented in the standard leads. Therefore, the localization of right ventricular arrhythmias is associated with greater uncertainty.

▶ In focal arrhythmias, the origin can be (approximately) determined from the 12-lead ECG, in scar-associated tachycardias the exit, i.e., the coupling of the excitation to the contractile myocardium at the border of the scar.

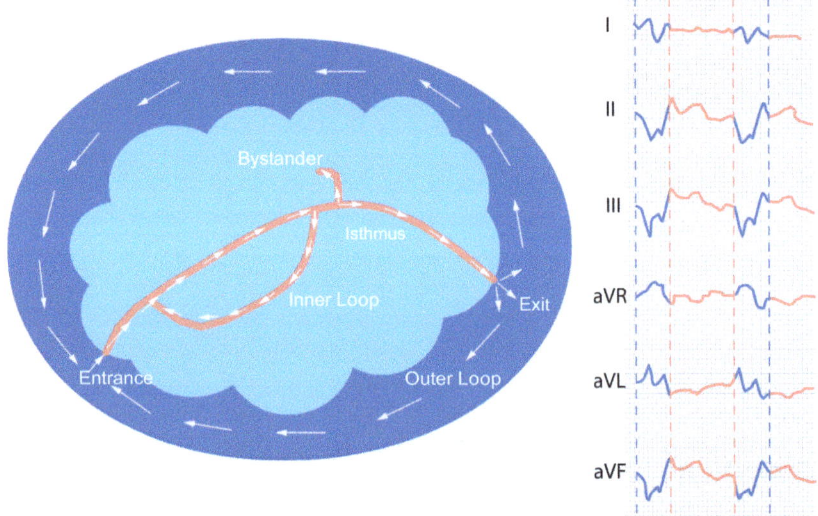

Fig. 15.1 Components of the reentry on the 12-lead ECG in scar-associated ventricular tachycardias: The systole of the tachycardia is caused by the contraction of the myocardium of the outer loop. The diastole of the tachycardia is due to the spread of excitation within the scar. The activated myocardial mass is too small to be visible on the surface ECG

15.2 An algorithm in four steps is suitable for localization

▶ The localization of an arrhythmia in the 12-lead ECG is carried out based on four steps, which correspond to individual spatial axes or dimensions, but are not completely perpendicular to each other.

1. Origin of the tachycardia superior or inferior?
   - Evaluation of the inferior leads II, III, aVF: A positive QRS complex indicates a cranial origin, a negative QRS complex indicates a caudal origin.
2. Origin in the right or left ventricle?
   - A left bundle branch block-like morphology of the chest leads indicates an origin in the right ventricle, a right bundle branch block-like morphology indicates an origin in the left ventricle.
3. Origin apical or basal?
   - An origin near the mitral or tricuspid valve is associated with a predominantly positive concordance of the chest leads, an apical origin is associated with a negative concordance.
4. Origin septal or lateral (here exemplified for the LV)
   - A septal origin is often characterized by a narrower QRS complex, while a lateral origin is often characterized by a wider QRS complex and pronounced RBBB or LBBB characteristics of the chest leads. In addition, the (approximately) horizontal leads I, aVL, and aVR provide information about the septal or lateral origin (see Fig. 15.2).

15.3 Localization in the outflow tract

PVCs or VT from the outflow tract are among the most common ventricular arrhythmias treated in the EP lab.

Due to some anatomical peculiarities of this region of the heart, a different algorithm must be used for localization here (Bala and Marchlinski 2007; Asirvatham 2009).

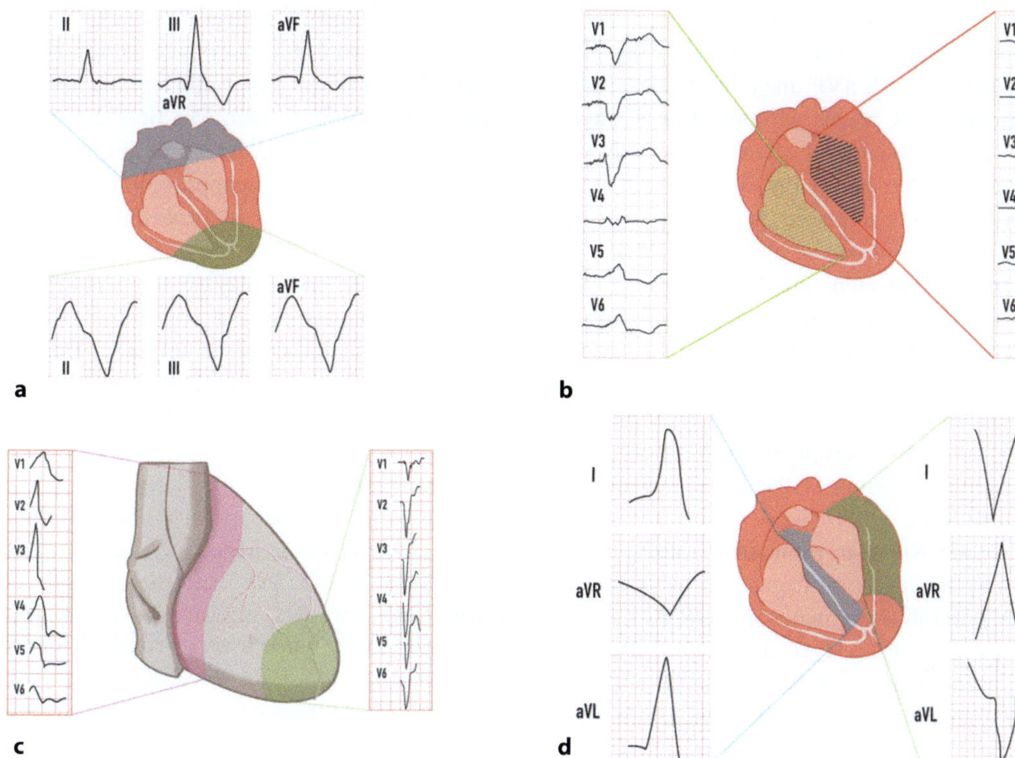

Fig. 15.2 Assignment of the characteristic morphologies and ECG features to the individual origins in the four different spatial axes or dimensions: **a** Positive QRS complexes in the inferior leads indicate a cranial origin, negative ones indicate a caudal origin. **b** A LBBB morphology indicates an origin in the right ventricle, a RBBB morphology indicates an origin in the left ventricle. **c** A positive concordance over the chest indicates a basal origin near the AV valves, a negative concordance over the chest indicates an apical origin. **d** Depending on the origin localized in step 2 in the left or right ventricle, the polarity of the leads I, aVR, and aVL in combination with the QRS width indicates a septal or lateral origin

- The outflow tract, i.e., the aortic root and pulmonary artery with their supra- and subvalvular portions, is among the most cranially located parts of the heart in the frontal plane.
- Both RVOT and LVOT couple to the septum in further propagation of excitation. From this and from the far cranial location, a positive excitation and LBBB-like morphology in V6 regularly result, without allowing differentiation between RVOT and LVOT.
- RVOT and LVOT are not adjacent in the frontal plane, but rather one behind the other. The base of the vector is therefore particularly different from leads V1–V3, while the sum vector almost always converges on V5 and V6, causing a positive QRS complex in these leads.

- Localization in the outflow tract follows different algorithms than in the ventricles: In the outflow tract, the R/S transition is crucial for differentiation between the right and left outflow tract, while in the ventricles, the RBBB or LBBB morphology is decisive.

- A source in the outflow tract is recognized by strictly positive QRS complexes in the inferior leads II, III, aVF, meaning the exclusive presence of R waves without Q or S waves. The axis of excitation often corresponds to a steep type: V6 is often positive. The distinction between a source in the outflow tract and adjacent regions can be blurred.
- In the second step, the R/S transition over the chest wall is considered to differentiate between RVOT and LVOT.
  - An early R/S transition means that the excitation vector is oriented towards leads V1–V3, thus originating posteriorly. The excitation origin is therefore attributed to the LVOT.
  - A late R/S transition analogously means that the vector propagates away from V1–V3 and thus originates in the RVOT.
- To assess an early or late R/S transition, the transition is often compared with the R/S transition of the QRS complex in sinus rhythm or during native ventricular excitation. There are further concepts for differentiating origins, especially in the area of the septal outflow tract. Practical considerations, such as the easier accessibility of the RVOT for primary mapping, often play a more important role in procedure planning (Betensky et al. 2011).
- Furthermore, lead I plays a role in differentiation. Thus, the presence of an S wave or a negative lead indicates an origin in the area of the anteroseptal RVOT or LVOT (Dixit et al. 2003; see Figs. 15.3 and 15.4).

Morphological Criteria

In addition to the pure polarity of individual leads, i.e., positive or negative, morphological criteria play a role. For example, a relatively narrow QRS complex suggests an endocardial and septal origin, while a very broad QRS complex with a pseudo-delta wave is suggestive of an epicardial origin (see Figs. 15.5 and 15.6).

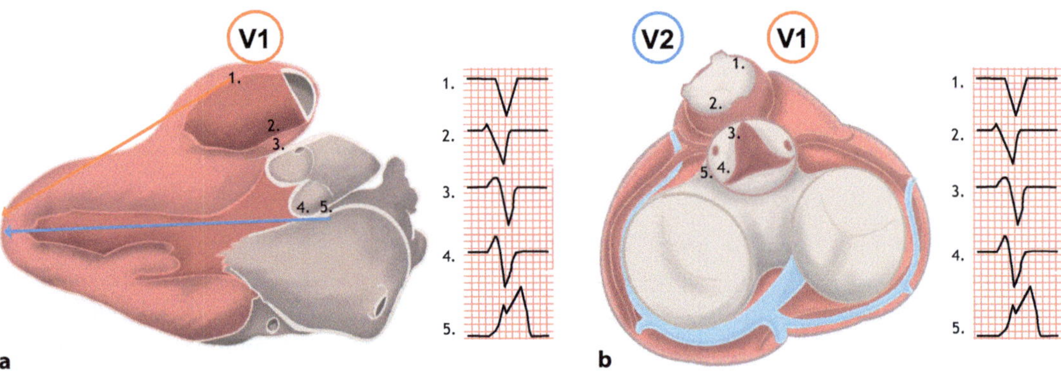

Fig. 15.3 a,b Anatomical positional relationship; the RVOT is ventral and close to leads V1 and V2; the LVOT is dorsal. Compare the different global vectors: Arrhythmias from the outflow tract differ in the base of the vector; the global propagation direction is similar, therefore the R/S transition over the chest leads is better suited as a differentiation criterion.

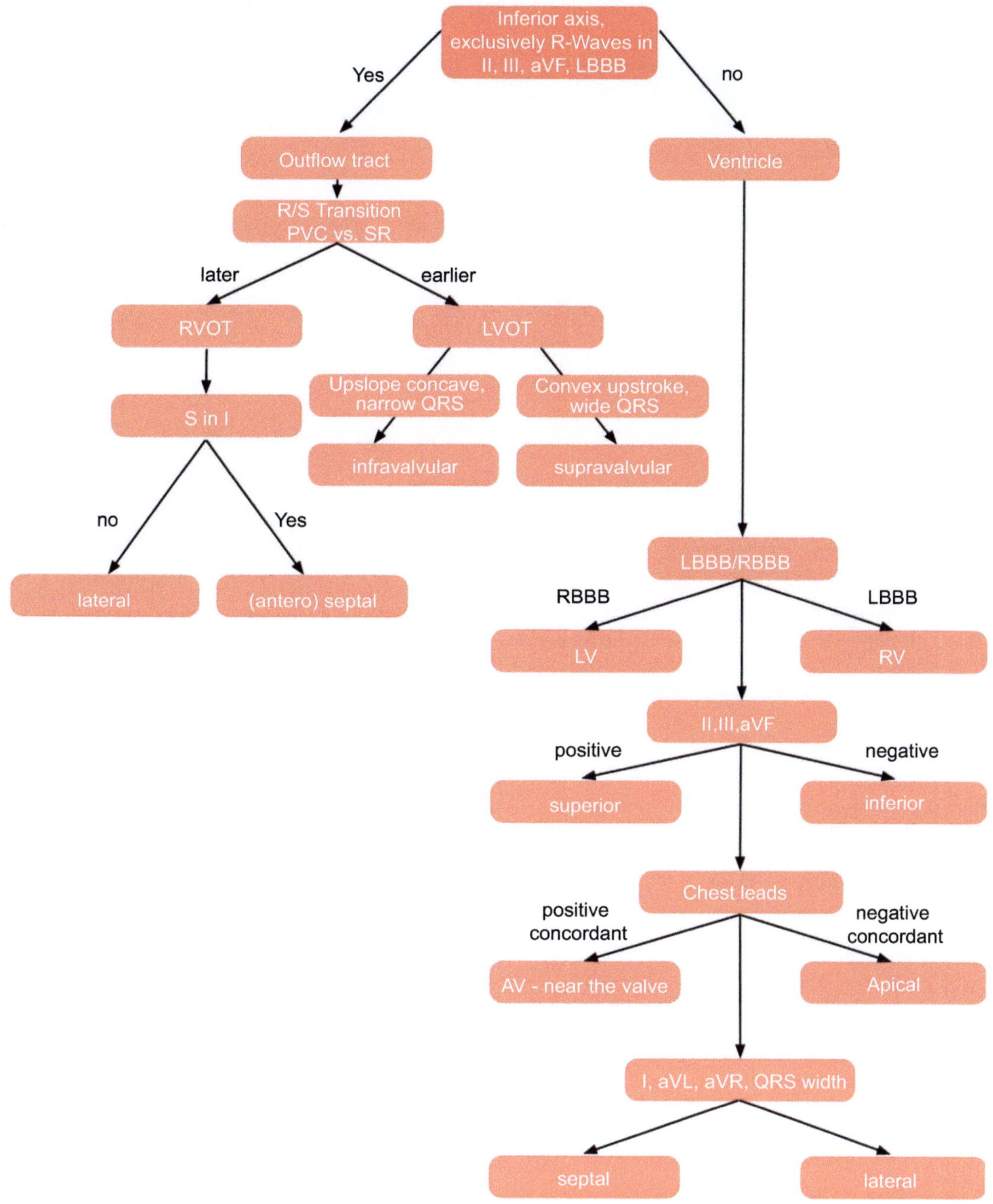

Fig. 15.4 Step algorithm for the localization of ventricular arrhythmias in different axes

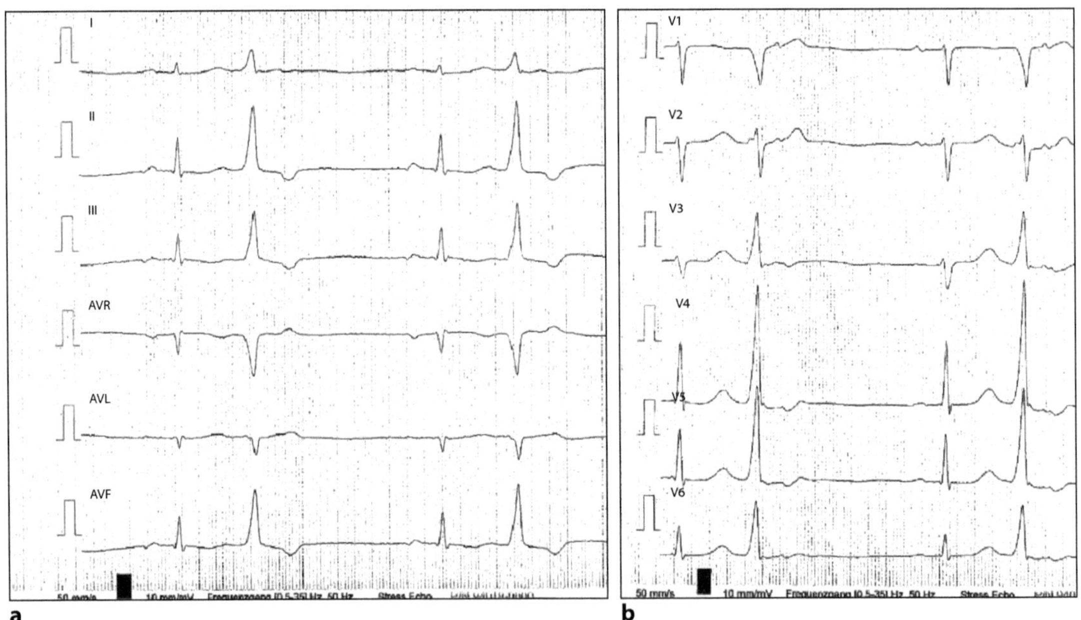

a   b

Fig. 15.5 Example of a septal, ventricular extrasystole originating close to the HIS-bundle: The retrograde P waves (best visible in V1) with compensatory pause identify the extra beats as clearly ventricular. The very narrow QRS complex with nearly identical vectors (11/12 leads) and very similar morphology compared to the intrinsic QRS complex suggest a septal, His-near origin.

Fig. 15.6 Example of a ventricular extrasystole from the area of the LV summit: The QRS duration of nearly 200 ms with the pronounced pseudo-delta wave suggests an epicardial origin. The pseudo-delta shows the propagation of excitation from epi- to endocardial, with the propagation speed increasing upon connection to the endocardial myocardium.

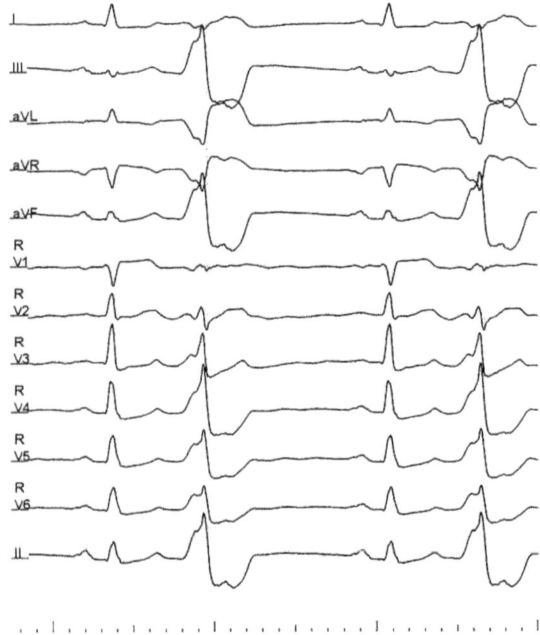

References

Asirvatham SJ (2009) Correlative anatomy for the invasive electrophysiologist: outflow tract and supravalvar arrhythmia. J Cardiovasc Electrophysiol 20(8):955–968

Bala R, Marchlinski FE (2007) Electrocardiographic recognition and ablation of outflow tract ventricular tachycardia. Heart Rhythm 4(3):366–370

Betensky BP, Park RE, Marchlinski FE, Hutchinson MD, Garcia FC, Dixit S et al (2011) The V(2) transition ratio: a new electrocardiographic criterion for distinguishing left from right ventricular outflow tract tachycardia origin. J Am Coll Cardiol 57(22):2255–2262

Dixit S, Gerstenfeld EP, Callans DJ, Marchlinski FE (2003) Electrocardiographic patterns of superior right ventricular outflow tract tachycardias: distinguishing septal and free-wall sites of origin. J Cardiovasc Electrophysiol 14(1):1–7

Ito S, Tada H, Naito S, Kurosaki K, Ueda M, Hoshizaki H et al (2003) Development and validation of an ECG algorithm for identifying the optimal ablation site for idiopathic ventricular outflow tract tachycardia. J Cardiovasc Electrophysiol 14(12):1280–1286

Idiopathic Ventricular Extrasystole

16

Sonia Busch and Heidi Estner

16.1 Definition and Epidemiology

Premature ventricular contractios (PVC) can frequently be found in people with healthy hearts. In epidemiological studies, PVC occur in approximately 5–10% of the population. The incidence increases with age and is particularly higher in women when originating from the right ventricular outflow tract (RVOT). Most often, these are monomorphic PVC, which can sometimes appear as bigeminy or as non-sustained to sustained ventricular tachycardias (VT) (Fig. 16.1).

By definition, non-sustained VTs have at least three consecutive beats and last a maximum of 30 seconds, with a heart rate of > 100/min.

Supplementary Information The online version contains supplementary material available at https://doi.org/10.1007/978-3-662-65797-3_16. The videos can be accessed individually by clicking the DOI link in the accompanying figure caption or by scanning this link with the SN More Media App.

S. Busch (✉)
Medizinische Klinik II, Klinikum Coburg GmbH, Coburg, Germany
e-mail: Sonia.busch@klinikum-coburg.de

H. Estner
Medizinische Klinik und Poliklinik I, LMU Klinikum der Universität München, München, Germany
e-mail: Heidi.estner@med.uni-muenchen.de

Accordingly, a VT is classified as sustained if it lasts longer than 30 seconds. About 70% of idiopathic PVC/VT originate from the right ventricular outflow tract (RVOT), followed by fascicular VTs, VTs from the aortic valve cusps, or from the basal left ventricle (LV), including epicardial or mitral valve region origins.

16.2 Clinical Presentation and Prognosis

The symptoms of isolated PVC do not always correlate with the frequency of occurrence and are very individual. The most common symptoms are palpitations, chest discomfort, or dizziness (e.g., due to a pulse deficit), while syncope is very rare in idiopathic PVC/VT. A large portion of patients are asymptomatic despite numerous PVC. In contrast to PVC in the presence of structural heart disease, the prognosis of idiopathic PVC is usually very good (Al-Khatib et al. 2018; Hasdemir et al. 2011). Only smaller observational studies indicate that frequent PVC, even in structurally normal hearts, are associated with an increased risk of sudden cardiac death (Ataklte et al. 2013; Massing et al. 2006). In clinical practice, distinguishing PVC on the basis of rare but serious cardiomyopathies, such as arrhythmogenic right ventricular cardiomyopathy (ARVC), can be challenging in individual cases.

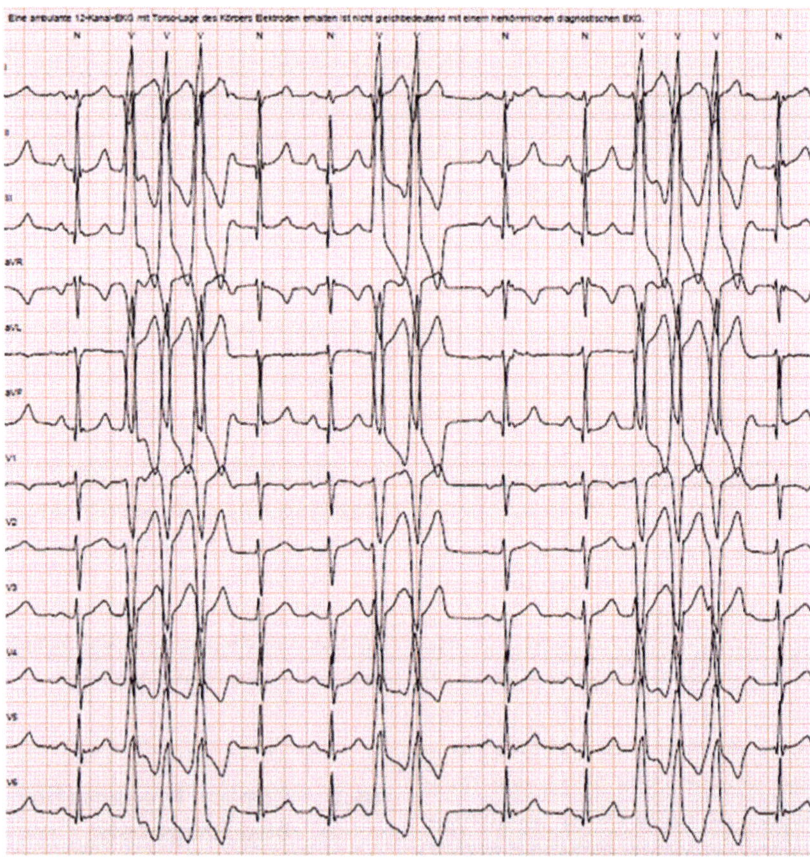

Fig. 16.1 Excerpt from a 24-hour 12-lead ECG. Frequent monomorphic PVC from the RVOT are shown as couplets and as non-sustained VTs

The following factors can be helpful for risk stratification:

- **PVC with short coupling** (≤ 350 ms). An association with idiopathic ventricular fibrillation has been described here (Viskin et al. 2005).
- **Polymorphic PVC.** These are often indicative of structural heart disease, which should be excluded invasively and/or through advanced imaging (e.g., cardiac CT, magnetic resonance imaging).
- Distinguishing PVC on the basis of CPVT and ARVC can be particularly challenging. In CPVT, as an ion channel disease, there is typically exercise-dependent polymorphic, and in rare cases bidirectional, (non-)sustained VTs. In ARVC, there are usually right precordial T-wave inversions (beyond V2) and different PVC morphologies. Therefore, the clinical exclusion of a serious but less obvious cardiomyopathy should not be made imprudently, as otherwise an increased mortality risk might not be recognized and treated.

16.3 Cardiological Evaluation

A 12-lead ECG, a transthoracic echocardiography (TTE), and an exercise ECG should be performed for risk stratification and evaluation of structural heart disease. A positive family history of sudden cardiac death can be an indication of ARVC. In the case of abnormal findings, further diagnostics using (stress) MRI and/or invasive coronary diagnostics should be performed. For classic idiopathic PVCs such as

RVOT-PVCs or fascicular left ventricular PVCs (RBBB/overturned left axis type), further diagnostics are generally not required. In the case of atypical PVC morphology or other abnormalities, an MRI examination should be performed early, as myocarditis or arrhythmogenic right ventricular cardiomyopathy can be detected better and/or at an earlier stage than with conventional echocardiography. Both diagnoses may influence the prognosis and should be considered in the therapeutic decision. Frequent PVCs can trigger a usually reversible tachycardiomyopathy. It is important to emphasize that not all patients with frequent PVCs develop tachycardiomyopathy. The most studied predictors are the PVC burden and the QRS duration: The wider the QRS complex, the higher the risk of tachycardiomyopathy (Table 16.1).

The minimal frequency of PVC/24 h, which is associated with a restriction of pump function, seems to be around 15–25 % (Baman et al. 2010; Hasdemir et al. 2011). Through successful treatment, e.g., the ablation of PVC, the reduction of LV- function can generally be reversed (Hachiya et al. 2000). Since PVC can be not only a cause but also a consequence of cardiomyopathy, it is difficult to differentiate between cause and effect (Simantikaris et al. 2012). Therefore, the diagnosis can often only be made retrospectively after the disappearance of PVC and subsequent recovery of LV function (Hasdemir et al. 2011). Some studies have investigated predictors for tachycardiomyopathy. A left ventricular end-diastolic diameter (LVEDD) > 66 mm is predictive of irreversible cardiomyopathy. In 2017, Penela et al. presented an algorithm to predict underlying structural heart disease: A QRS duration > 130 ms, a PVC burden < 17 % and an LVEDD > 63 mm were predictive that patients would not recover even after successful elimination of PVC (positive predictive value of 97 %). A cardiac MRI examination also has a high value here. The exclusion of scars seems to be predictive of the recovery of LV function.

16.4 Therapy

16.4.1 Indication and Therapy Options

The decision to treat PVC is based on the symptomatology and/or a reduced LV function, as it is possible here to improve LV function again with a significant reduction in PVC burden (Priori et al. 2015; Bogun et al. 2007). Even in patients with CRT due to severely reduced LV function, successful treatment of frequent PVC may be necessary to increase the proportion of biventricular stimulation (Lakkireddy et al. 2012).

Pharmacologically, PVC can initially be treated with β-blockers or calcium antagonists

Table 16.1 Predictors for the development of tachycardiomyopathy

Predictor	Result	Reference
Male gender	–	Hasdemir et al. 2011
Symptoms	Asymptomatic symptoms duration	Hasdemir et al. 2011 Yokokawa et al. 2012
PVC burden	> 16% > 17% > 24%	Hasdemir et al. 2011 Penela et al. 2017 Baman et al. 2010
Circadian rhythm	PVC burden constantly high	Hasdemir et al. 2011
Recurrent monomorphic VT	–	Hasdemir et al. 2011
QRS duration	> 150 ms	Yokokawa et al. 2012
PVC interpolation	–	Olgun et al. 2011
PVC morphology	Non-fascicular, right ventricular epicardial	Munoz et al. 2011 Yokokawa et al. 2012

of the non-dihydropyridine type. However, both substance groups are often hardly more effective than a placebo (10–15 %). Antiarrhythmics of classes Ic or III, on the other hand, are often effective in the treatment of PVC but have a higher rate of side effects, including a proarrhythmic effect.

An indication for catheter ablation arises in individual Cases:

- If there is symptomatology and the frequency of PVC allows successful systematic mapping (e.g., > 10 % monomorphic PVC, in at least one holter ECG)
- In asymptomatic patients, if a decrease in LV function or LV dilation is detectable over time.
- In CRT patients, to achieve an adequate proportion of biventricular stimulation.

16.4.2 Basis of Electrophysiological Examination of Idiopathic PVC

Idiopathic PVC are classified based on their clinical presentation (e.g., exercise-induced) or the underlying mechanism (adenosine-sensitive, triggered, β-blocker dependent, automaticity, etc.).

The following parameters indicate triggered activity:

- Clinical presentation: spontaneous PVC (especially with a fixed coupling interval) or repetitive non-sustained monomorphic VT
- Response to pharmacological therapy: spontaneous onset influenced by sympathetic or vagal tone
- Inducibility by isoproterenol, psychological stress, or physical activity
- Termination by adenosine, verapamil, or β -blockers
- Inducibility by "burst pacing" (atrial and ventricular)
- Overstimulation and entrainment are not possible
- Normal local electrograms with absence of fractionated potentials

- The activation map shows a very small area with early activation and centrifugal spread of excitation

Since PVC can be the first hallmark in the early stages of structural heart disease, abnormal signals ("low-voltage," late and fractionated electrograms) should be looked for during mapping. Ablation at the site of origin is often associated with an acceleration ("heating up") of the PVC, followed by termination.

16.4.3 Mapping and Ablation— Activation Mapping

The focal mechanism of idiopathic PVC allows for activation mapping to identify the earliest site of ventricular activation. Activation mapping or prematurity mapping or LAT (local activation time mapping) is the preferred and most precise mapping strategy, especially in combination with the unipolar electrogram with QS morphology (Fig. 16.2).

It can be used in combination with pace mapping (see below). Activation mapping of the PVC requires inducibility. Too deep sedation should be avoided; isoproterenol infusions or (less commonly) various stimulation maneuvers can induce PVC. In activation mapping, it is very helpful to analyze both the bipolar and unipolar electrogram. Detailed mapping with a high point density is necessary to detect the earliest site, as the area excited within 10 ms can already be up to 3 cm^2 in size (Fig. 16.3).

Three-dimensional mapping systems and multi-electrode mapping can be helpful, as well as "non-contact" mapping in infrequent PVC. Electrograms at successful ablation sites show a prematurity of 10–50 ms before the onset of the QRS complex. In the unipolar electrogram, a QS configuration is found at the successful ablation site as an expression of the propagation of the wavefront awaa from this point. It should be emphasized that each heart chamber has a point/ area of earliest excitation somewhere, but this does not necessarily have to be the origin if the non-causal ventricle was mapped or the ectopy is

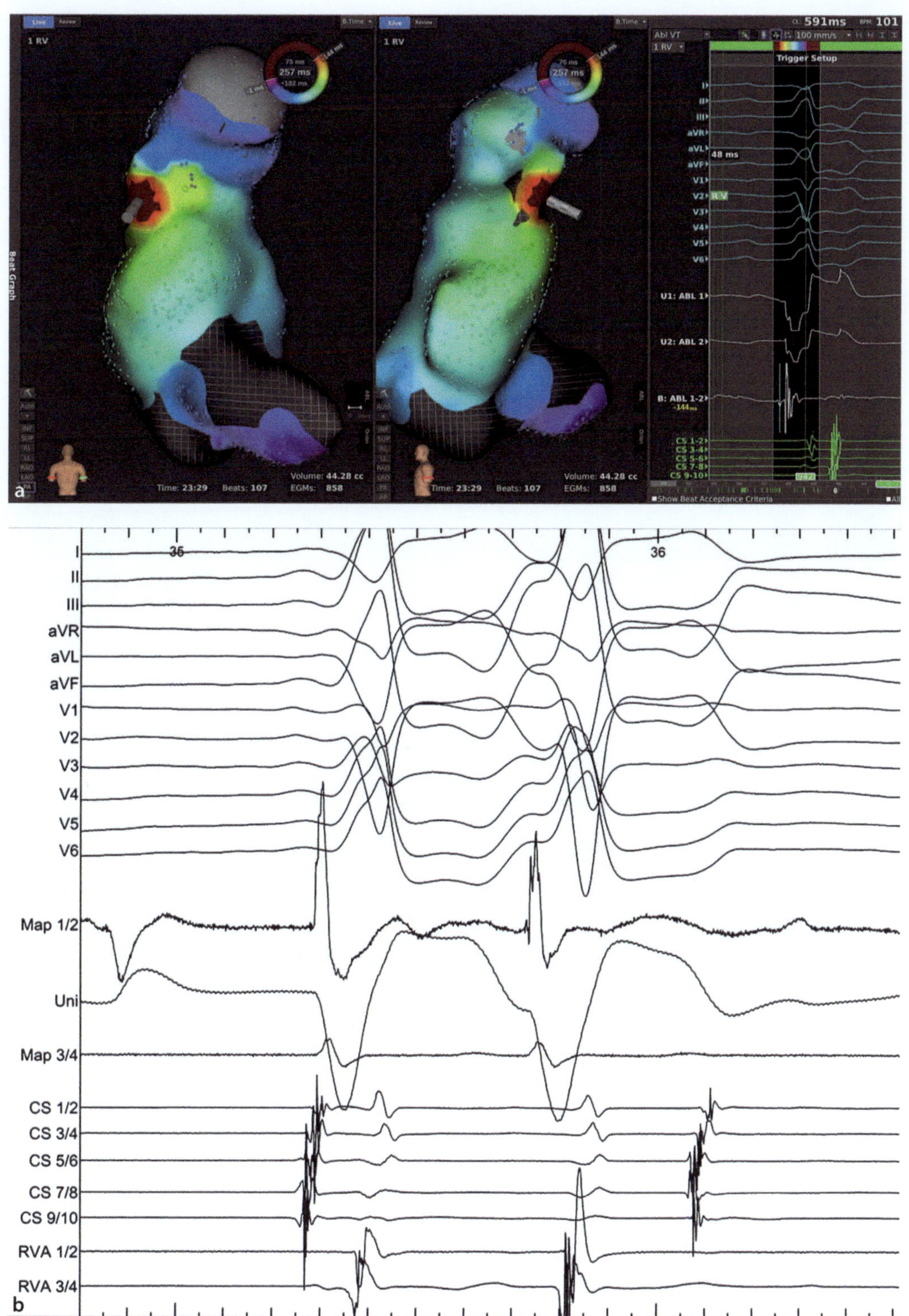

Fig. 16.2 **a** High-resolution three-dimensional map of the RVOT (in PA and left lateral) with earliest focal activity in the septal RVOT (*dark red*) and corresponding electrogram. **b** 12-channel ECG and electrophysiological study of the PVC: "Map 1/2" and "Uni" show the bipolar and unipolar electrograms at the successful ablation site. The prematurity is 46 ms before the onset of the QRS complex

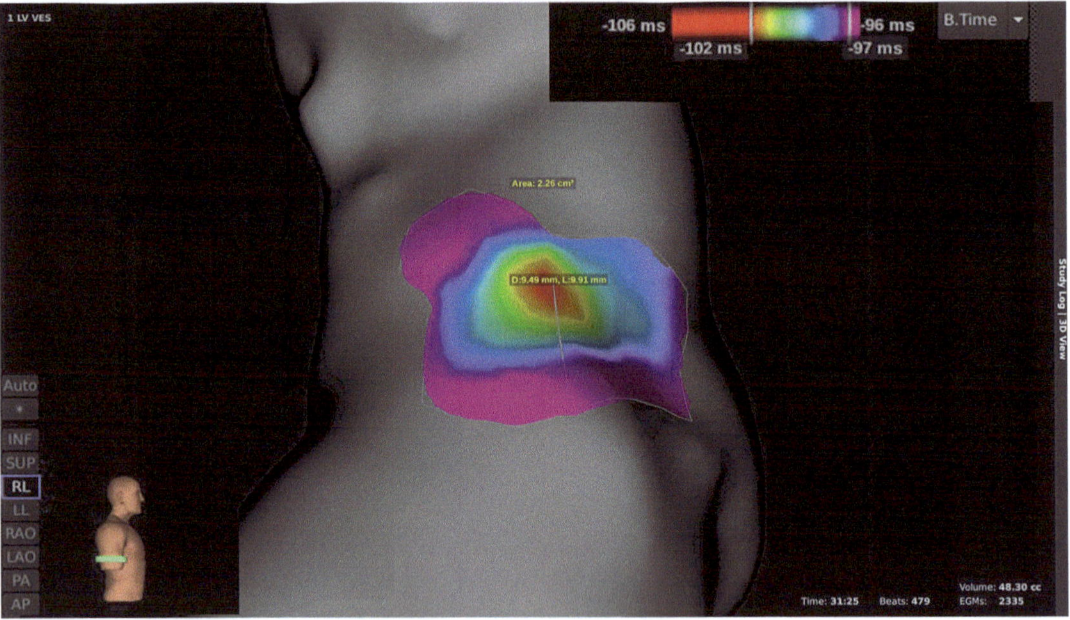

Fig. 16.3 Representation of the area (2.2 cm²) or the radius (9.9 mm) at onset (*red point*) and the following 10 ms after onset (*in color*). The figure illustrates how precise the mapping must be to map the exit of the PVC. An inaccuracy of 10 ms already means a distance of 1 cm from the site of origin, and the area excited within 10 ms is already > 2 cm² in size

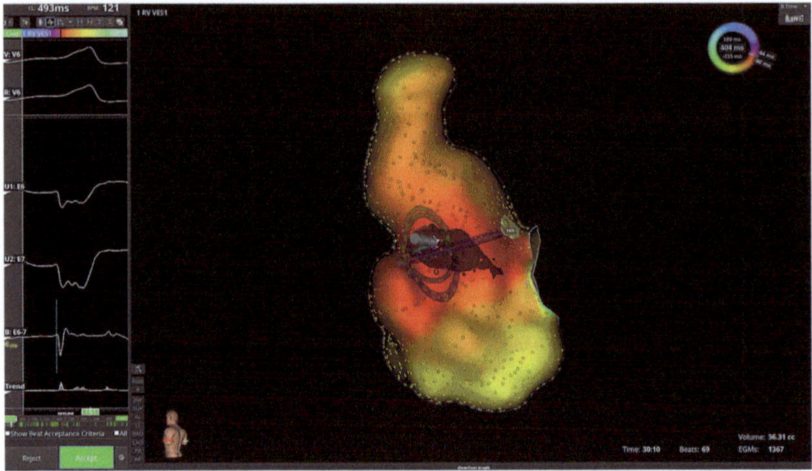

Fig. 16.4 Rounded multi-electrode catheter (Intellamap Orion) in the area of the earliest activation of a right ventricular, His-near PVC with marking of the catheter position and the point with the earliest activation. Note also the uni- and bipolar local electrograms with QS configuration of the unipolar electrogram and the significant prematurity before the onset of the QRS complex. Created with the RHYTHMIA-HDx mapping system

epicardial or located in the aortic root. Therefore, it must be critically reviewed whether the unipolar and bipolar electrogram in the mapped area show corresponding prematurities, especially if the maximum prematurity is detected in an entire area rather than at a single point (Figs. 16.4 and 16.5).

16.4.4 Mapping and Ablation—Pacemapping

In cases of rare ectopy, creating a pacemap is a good alternative (Jadonath et al. 1995). The principle is based on comparing a stimulated QRS morphology with the clinical QRS complex (and typically providing a percentage for correspondance). Pacemapping based on the PVC morphology in the clinically documented 12-lead ECG is not recommended, as the chest leads for the electrophysiological study often cannot be placed identically to the clinical documentation. In individual cases, it may be useful to mark the position of the ECG electrodes after recording the PVC, e.g., during an exercise ECG, or to leave the electrodes in place to enable pacemapping when PVC are not inducible. However, possible vector changes due to different positions (sitting vs. lying) should be considered. Ideally, stimulation from the origin area shows a perfect QRS match between ectopy and stimulated QRS complex (Fig. 16.6).

The higher the stimulation amplitude, the less specific the pacemapping maneuver becomes, as a larger area is directly excited. Therefore, stimulation should be performed with an energy just above the pacing threshold.

Modern workstations or mapping systems offer automated ECG morphology analysis. Here, the match should be $\geq 95\%$. The automatic analysis seems to be more accurate than the visual one. Depending on the algorithm used, all twelve leads are weighted equally, or there is a weighting according to the amplitude of the lead. Therefore, there can be significant differences between the algorithms, especially in low-amplitude leads. Nevertheless, it must be emphasized that the spatial resolution of pacemapping is low, and the arrhythmia origin can be up to 2 cm away from the site of the perfect pacemap. Therefore, pacemapping is inferior to activation mapping in terms of spatial resolution but represents an important complement.

16.4.5 Special Features in the Ablation of Outflow Tract PVC

Outflow tract PVC represent a subgroup of idiopathic PVC, which are mainly located in the right or left ventricular outflow tract. Since induction is possible through atrial or ventricular stimulations, isoproterenol facilitates induction, and adenosine or propranolol hinders it, a catecholamine-sensitive cAMP-mediated triggered

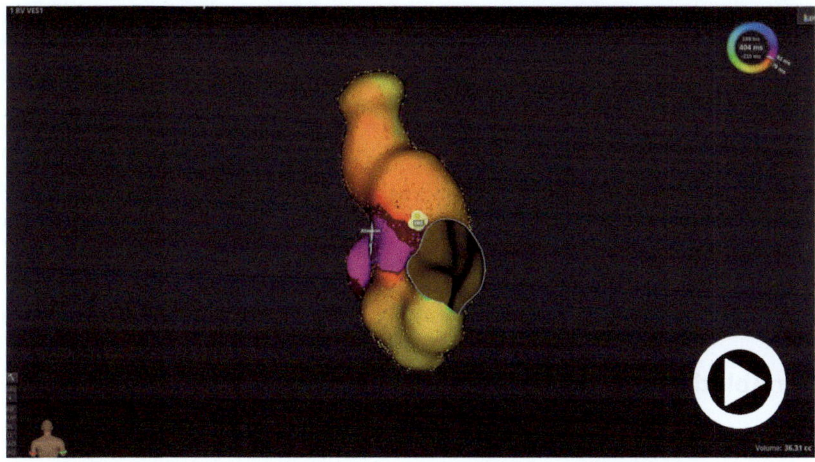

Fig. 16.5 Activation map of a right ventricular, His-near ventricular extrabeat (initial left lateral view). The tricuspid valve annulus is cut out as an anatomical structure, the His bundle is marked. Created with the RHYTHMIA-HDx mapping system (https://doi.org/10.1007/000-d2y)

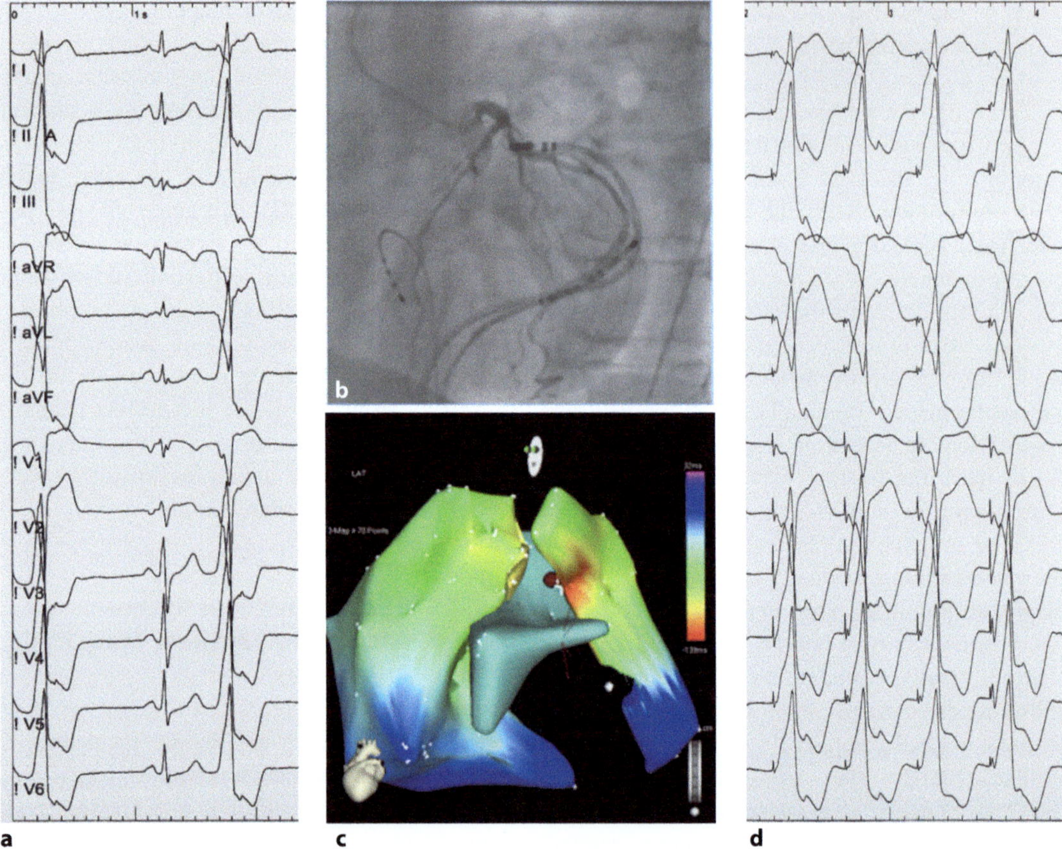

Fig. 16.6 **a** 12-lead ECG of the clinical PVC. **b** Position of the ablation catheter in the coronary sinus (CS) with LAD (Left anterior descending) depiction (LAO [Left anterior oblique] projection). **c** 3D activation map showing the earliest activation (*in red*) in the CS. Additionally, depiction of the right ventricle and the aorta. **d** Pacemapping in the CS at the site of the earliest activation in the area of the LV summit (cooled ablation in the CS with 25 W)

activity is assumed. β receptor agonists activate adenylate cyclase, which in turn promotes the conversion of ATP to cAMP and causes intracellular calcium overload. This increased calcium overload induces late afterdepolarizations. The release of calcium is negatively influenced by adenosine, which is why these PVC are usually "adenosine sensitive" (Lerman et al. 1986).

Indication for Ablation in Outflow Tract PVC/VT

The catheter ablation of idiopathic PVC and VT, especially from the RVOT, is very successful (> 90%). The complication rates are low, with a perforation rate of now < 1%. The greatest limitation is usually the poor inducibility of VT during the electrophysiological study. Patients with frequent symptomatic idiopathic PVC or VT from the outflow tract have an indication for catheter ablation, whereby in the international recommendations, due to the different success rates and the more complex anatomy, RVOT arrhythmias (Class I, also as first-line therapy) are differentiated from left ventricular outflow tract (LVOT) arrhythmias (Class IIa, usually after previous ineffective drug therapy) (Priori et al. 2015).

Anatomy

The majority of the RVOT is normally located anterior and to the left of the aortic root (see also Chap. 15 "Localization of Ventricular Arrhythmias"). The interventricular septum defines the medial boundary, and the free wall defines the lateral boundary of the RVOT. Superiorly, the RVOT is bounded by the pulmonary valve and inferiorly by the tricuspid valve. Coming from the tricuspid valve, the RVOT is located above and to the left (Fig. 16.7; Ho 2009).

The pulmonary valve, in turn, is located 1–2 cm above the aortic valve. Autopsy data have shown that in about 50–70% of cases, myocardial muscle strands extend from the RVOT to above the pulmonary valve. These muscle fibers may represent the substrate for ectopy, as they can exhibit abnormally triggered activity. About 1/3 of all idiopathic PVCs originate from the LVOT. The LVOT consists of the aortic root, the area below the aortic valve, the aortomitral continuity, and basal portions of the LV ("LV

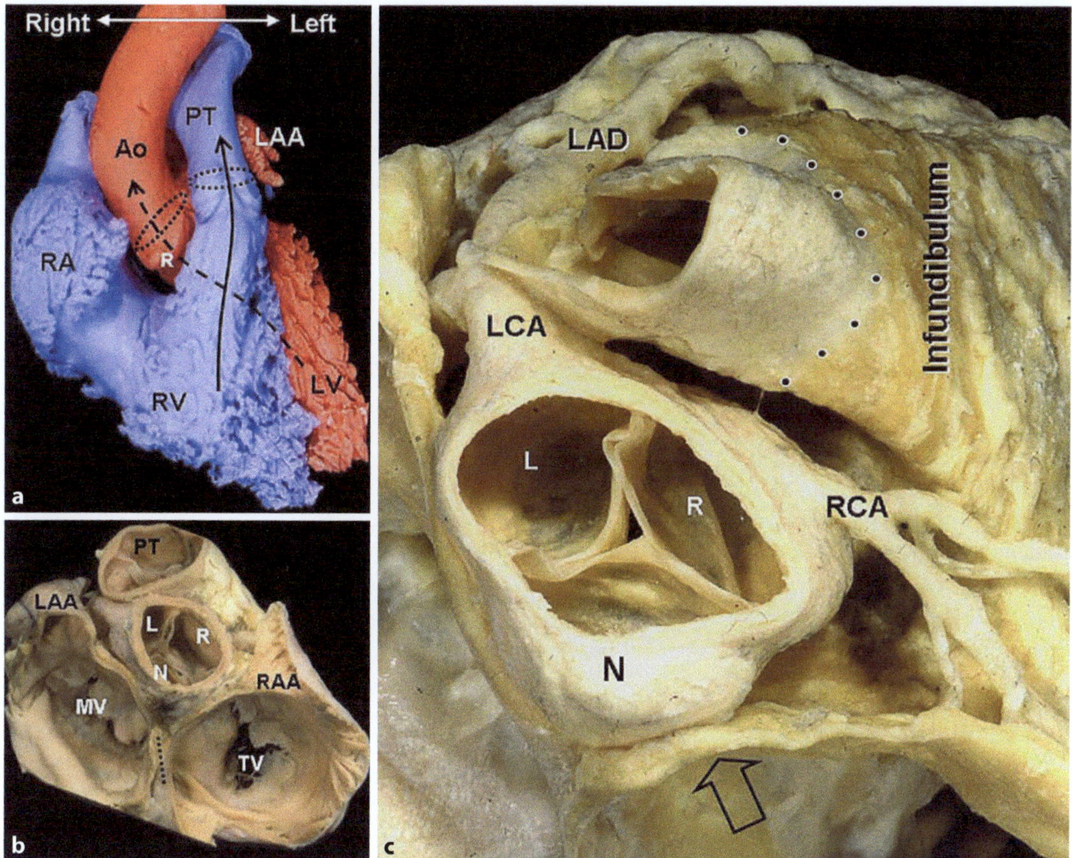

Fig. 16.7 **a** The outflow of a normal heart shows the overlap of the RVOT and LVOT in the frontal view (*arrows*). The dotted ovals represent the pulmonary and aortic valves. **b** Transection of the atria as well as the pulmonary and aortic valves at the level of the sinotubular junction opened. The view from the right rear shows the central location of the aortic valve. The *dotted line* shows the interatrial septum. **c** After removal of the epicardial fat, the ventriculoarterial junction is clearly visible (*dotted line*). *Open arrow* shows the positional relationship of the aortic root to the right atrium. Ao = aorta; L = left coronary aortic sinus; LAA = left atrial appendage; LCA = left coronary artery; LAD = left anterior descending artery; LV = left ventricle; MV = mitral valve; N = noncoronary aortic sinus; PT = pulmonary trunk; R = right coronary aortic sinus; RA = right atrium; RAA = right atrial appendage; RCA = right coronary artery; RV = right ventricle; TV = tricuspid valve. (Courtesy of Ho 2009)

summit"). The aortic root is centrally located in the heart. Depending on the size of the atrial appendages, the right or left atrial appendage extends to the right or left coronary aortic sinus. The LVOT consists of muscular and fibrous components. Only the anterior and lateral LVOT contain myocardium. The posterior portion consists of fibrous tissue that extends from the cardiac skeleton to the anterior leaflet of the mitral valve (aortomitral continuity). The septal portion consists of a mixture of muscular and fibrous components from the interventricular septum. The non-coronary aortic leaflet is located inferiorly and posteriorly, the left coronary superiorly, and the right coronary aortic leaflet anteriorly.

ECG Characteristics RVOT vs. LVOT

Various algorithms have been published that enable differentiation between RVOT and LVOT origin based on surface ECG in different cohorts. A comprehensive algorithm was published by Ito et al. (2003). Typically, the ECG shows a left bundle branch block pattern with an inferior axis. The following criteria are helpful for further discrimination of the location (Table 16.2):

- **Precordial QRS transition** septal: early transition; free wall: late transition (after V4); very early transition (V2 or V3) can indicate LVOT or aortic valve, and a late transition can indicate an origin in the RVOT. If the QRS transition is earlier than in sinus rhythm, it indicates an LVOT origin (Betensky et al. 2011).
- **QRS vector in I:** positive in septal and posterior RVOT origin, negative in anteroseptal ectopy; S in lead I indicates LVOT (Dixit et al. 2003).
- **QRS width**: septal RVOT narrow QRS complex, free wall with wide QRS
- **"Notching" in the inferior leads:** RVOT from free wall
- **S in V5–V6:** ectopy from aortic valve or below (Hachiya et al. 2000).

Table 16.2 ECG characteristics of outflow tract tachycardias

	RVOT		LVOT	Aortic cusps	Epicardial
	Septal	Free wall			
ECG Feature	–	–	–	–	–
Precordial QRS Transition	Early transition ≤ V3	Late transition ≥ V4	Very early transition (V2 or V3) or transition earlier than in sinus rhythm	Very early transition (V2 or V3) or transition earlier than in sinus rhythm	–
QRS Vector in I	Positive in septal and posterior ectopy	Negative in anteroseptal ectopy	Negative	–	–
QRS Morphology in V5–V6	–	–	–	S	–
QRS Complex	Narrow	Notching in the inferior leads	–	–	Wide
QRS Morphology in V1	–	–	–	"M" or "W": left coronary pouch QS or QR: right coronary pouch	–
Others	–	–	–	–	aVL/aVR Q-wave ratio > 1.740 maximum deflection index > 0.55

- **QRS morphology in V1:** "M" or "W": from the left coronary cusp, QS or QR: from the right coronary cusp (Ouyang et al. 2002).
- **aVL/aVR Q-wave ratio:**> 1.740 indicates an epicardial focus, as does the maximum deflection index > 0.55 (Daniels et al. 2006).

The ECG analysis helps to plan the access route and procedure to save examination time. Nevertheless, in individual cases, intensive mapping of the RVOT, LVOT, and aortic valve or even the epicardial myocardium (e.g., via coronary sinus) must be performed (Fig. 16.6). This is particularly true if the maximum prematurity is less than 20 ms, especially in the septal RVOT. Then, the LVOT or other adjacent structures should be thoroughly mapped to avoid missing the ectopic origin. A common reason for unsuccessful ablation attempts is incomplete mapping. The bipolar electrograms can show high-frequency low-amplitude activity preceding the main electrogram. A so-called "reversed polarity," i.e., the reversal of electrogram components between sinus rhythm and PVC, is often associated with successful ablation.

In the aortic valve, the unipolar electrograms can appear later than the bipolar signals, and a pacemap is often negative or cannot be performed due to the lack of local capture. An irrigated ablation catheter is necessary, and coronary angiography is recommended to estimate the proximity to the coronary arteries.

16.4.6 Special features in the ablation of fascicular PVCs

In patients with healthy hearts, these PVCs often arise from triggered activity, whereas in patients with structural heart disease, reentry mechanisms are also significant (Baman et al. 2010). The surface ECG is characterized by a right bundle branch block-like configuration with an left or right axis deviation, regardless of the underlying mechanism. These VTs are often induced by physical activity or catecholamines.

Frequently, localized presystolic or mid-diastolic potentials are found in the area of the distal fascicles, indicating localized reentry mechanisms. The goal in mapping fascicular VT is the earliest Purkinje potential before the QRS complex during VT. If the VT is not inducible, pacemapping is an alternative. Pacemapping at the Purkinje potential not only provokes an identical QRS complex, but the S-QRS interval also corresponds to the Purkinje-QRS interval. Unfortunately, QRS deviation often occurs because pacemapping excites not only the Purkinje potential but also the surrounding ventricular myocardium directly. Fascicular PVCs can be distinguished from papillary muscle PVCs. Papillary muscle PVCs have a wider QRS complex and monophasic R or qR in V1 without Q in the limb leads. Often, a Purkinje potential can also be detected at the successful ablation site, but it is late in sinus rhythm. Ablation can be difficult because the focus may lie deep in the papillary muscle, and anatomical peculiarities can make adequate catheter stabilization challenging. Intracardiac ultrasound can be helpful here, as 3D systems may not adequately represent the anatomy of the papillary muscle.

16.4.7 PVC from the Area of the AV Valves

Up to 5% of idiopathic PVC originate from the area of the mitral or tricuspid valve annulus. Pacemapping and mapping of small presystolic potentials along the valve apparatus are often helpful. In contrast to outflow tract PVC, pacemapping is an important maneuver here, as even small localization changes can cause significant QRS changes. Technically, catheter ablation along the valves is similar to the ablation of accessory pathways: good wall contact is essential, and the ablation catheter is positioned below the mitral valve (in the case of retrograde access) or navigated using steerable sheaths (in the case of anterograde access).

16.5 Summary

Idiopathic PVC are predominantly found in patients with structurally normal hearts. They almost always have a good prognosis. Diagnostics should primarily exclude (incipient) cardiomyopathy. There is an indication for treatment in cases of severe symptoms, high PVC burden, or deterioration of left ventricular function. Catheter ablation represents the most successful therapy, which is often curative. Idiopathic PVC usually have a focal origin. The localization of the origin is based on the creation of an activation map with the best prematurity, with or without the combination of pacemapping. A precise ECG analysis should always be performed beforehand to plan the ablation. The most common anatomical sites of origin for idiopathic PVC are the right and left ventricular outflow tracts, the posterior (and anterior) fascicle of the left bundle branch of the conduction system, and the mitral valve annulus.

References

Al-Khatib SM, Stevenson WG, Ackerman MJ (2018) 2017 AHA/ACC/HRS guideline for management of patients with ventricular arrhythmias and the prevention of sudden cardiac death: a report of the American college of cardiology/American heart association task force on clinical practice guidelines and the heart rhythm society. J Am Coll Cardiol 72:e91–e220

Ataklte F, Erqou S, Laukkanen J, Kaptoge S (2013) Meta-analysis of ventricular premature complexes and their relation to cardiac mortality in general populations. Am J Cardiol 112:1263–1270

Baman TS, Lange DC, Ilg KJ et al (2010) Relationship between burden of premature ventricular complexes and left ventricular function. Heart Rhythm 7:865–869

Betensky BP, Park RE, Marchlinski FE et al (2011) The V(2) transition ratio: a new electrocardiographic criterion for distinguishing left from right ventricular outflow tract tachycardia origin. J Am Coll Cardiol 57:2255–2262

Bogun F, Crawford T, Reich S et al (2007) Radiofrequency ablation of frequent, idiopathic premature ventricular complexes: comparison with a control group without intervention. Heart Rhythm 4:863–867

Daniels DV, Lu YY, Morton JB et al (2006) Idiopathic epicardial left ventricular tachycardia originating remote from the sinus of Valsalva: electrophysiological characteristics, catheter ablation, and identification from the 12-lead electrocardiogram. Circulation 113:1659–1666

Dixit S, Gerstenfeld EP, Callans DJ, Marchlinski FE (2003) Electrocardiographic patterns of superior right ventricular outflow tract tachycardias: distinguishing septal and free-wall sites of origin. J Cardiovasc Electrophysiol 14:1–7

Hachiya H, Aonuma K, Yamauchi Y et al (2000) Electrocardiographic characteristics of left ventricular outflow tract tachycardia. Pacing Clin Electrophysiol 23:1930–1934

Hasdemir C, Ulucan C, Yavuzgil O et al (2011) Tachycardia-induced cardiomyopathy in patients with idiopathic ventricular arrhythmias: the incidence, clinical and electrophysiologic characteristics, and the predictors. J Cardiovasc Electrophysiol 22:663–668

Ho SY (2009) Anatomic insights for catheter ablation of ventricular tachycardia. Heart Rhythm 6:S77–S80

Ito S, Tada H, Naito S et al (2003) Development and validation of an ECG algorithm for identifying the optimal ablation site for idiopathic ventricular outflow tract tachycardia. J Cardiovasc Electrophysiol 14:1280–1286

Jadonath RL, Schwartzman DS, Preminger MW, Gottlieb CD, Marchlinski FE (1995) Utility of the 12-lead electrocardiogram in localizing the origin of right ventricular outflow tract tachycardia. Am Heart J 130:1107–1113

Lakkireddy D, Di Biase L, Ryschon K et al (2012) Radiofrequency ablation of premature ventricular ectopy improves the efficacy of cardiac resynchronization therapy in nonresponders. J Am Coll Cardiol 60:1531–1539

Lerman BB, Belardinelli L, West GA, Berne RM, DiMarco JP (1986) Adenosine-sensitive ventricular tachycardia: evidence suggesting cyclic AMP-mediated triggered activity. Circulation 74:270–280

Massing MW, Simpson RJ Jr., Rautaharju PM, Schreiner PJ, Crow R, Heiss G (2006) Usefulness of ventricular premature complexes to predict coronary heart disease events and mortality (from the Atherosclerosis Risk In Communities cohort). Am J Cardiol 98:1609–1612

Munoz FDC, Syed FF, Noheria A et al (2011) Characteristics of premature ventricular complexes as correlates of reduced left ventricular systolic function: study of the burden, duration, coupling interval, morphology and site of origin of PVCs. J Cardiovasc Electrophysiol 22:791–798

Olgun H, Yokokawa M, Baman T et al (2011) The role of interpolation in PVC-induced cardiomyopathy. Heart Rhythm 8:1046–1049

Ouyang F, Fotuhi P, Ho SY et al (2002) Repetitive monomorphic ventricular tachycardia originating from the aortic sinus cusp: electrocardiographic characterization for guiding catheter ablation. J Am Coll Cardiol 39:500–508

Penela D, Fernandez-Armenta J, Aguinaga L et al (2017) Clinical recognition of pure premature ventricular complex-induced cardiomyopathy at presentation. Heart Rhythm 14:1864–1870

Priori SG, Blomstrom-Lundqvist C, Mazzanti A et al (2015) 2015 ESC Guidelines for the management of patients with ventricular arrhythmias and the prevention of sudden cardiac death: The Task Force for the Management of Patients with Ventricular Arrhythmias and the Prevention of Sudden Cardiac Death of the European Society of Cardiology (ESC). Endorsed by: Association for European Paediatric and Congenital Cardiology (AEPC). Eur Heart J 36:2793–2867

Simantirakis EN, Koutalas EP, Vardas PE (2012) Arrhythmia-induced cardiomyopathies: the riddle of the chicken and the egg still unanswered? Europace 14:466–473

Viskin S, Rosso R, Rogowski O, Belhassen B (2005) The „short-coupled" variant of right ventricular outflow ventricular tachycardia: a not-so-benign form of benign ventricular tachycardia? J Cardiovasc Electrophysiol 16:912–916

Yokokawa M, Kim HM, Good E et al (2012) Relation of symptoms and symptom duration to premature ventricular complex-induced cardiomyopathy. Heart Rhythm 9:92–95

17

Felix Bourier and Daniel Steven

17.1 Introduction

Patients affected by ischemic cardiomyopathy after myocardial infarction are at a significantly increased risk for the occurrence of scar-dependent ventricular tachycardias (VT). Although the use of implantable cardioverter-defibrillators (ICD) can terminate VT and thereby reduce the cardiac mortality of this population, ICDs do not lead to a reduction in VT incidence. The life-saving ICD therapies themselves represent a serious deterioration in the quality of life for the affected patients.

Supplementary Information The online version contains supplementary material available at https://doi.org/10.1007/978-3-662-65797-3_17. The videos can be accessed individually by clicking the DOI link in the accompanying figure caption or by scanning this link with the SN More Media App.

F. Bourier (✉)
Klinik für Herz- und Kreislauferkrankungen, Deutsches Herzzentrum München, München, Germany
e-mail: bourier@dhm.mhn.de

D. Steven
Abteilung für Elektrophysiologie, Herzzentrum der Uniklinik Köln, Köln, Germany
e-mail: daniel.steven@uk-koeln.de

▶ A catheter ablation, on the other hand, enables a causal therapy of ventricular tachycardias by modifying the regions of scar-induced myocardial conduction delay in such a way that VT originally caused by the scar can no longer be triggered.

17.2 Etiology of VT, Pathogenesis of the Scar and the Substrate

Undisturbed propagation of excitation in the ventricular myocardium depends on intact cell-to-cell connections. This communication can be disrupted when scars form within the myocardium. This can be mediated by ischemia or by dilation of the left ventricle, which then leads to a remodeling of myocardial cells into connective tissue and fibroblasts. This increase in fibroti tissue can be represented in common mapping procedures as zones of low signal amplitude, which is then referred to as the "substrate" for VT and describes the myocardial texture disturbance.

The predominant mechanism of VT in post-infarction patients is a reentry in the area of a scar (Fig. 17.1). Here, non-conductive parts of the scar represent a barrier through which myocardial fibers or bundles with preserved—but usually slower—electrical conductivity pass. This zone is referred to as a protected isthmus.

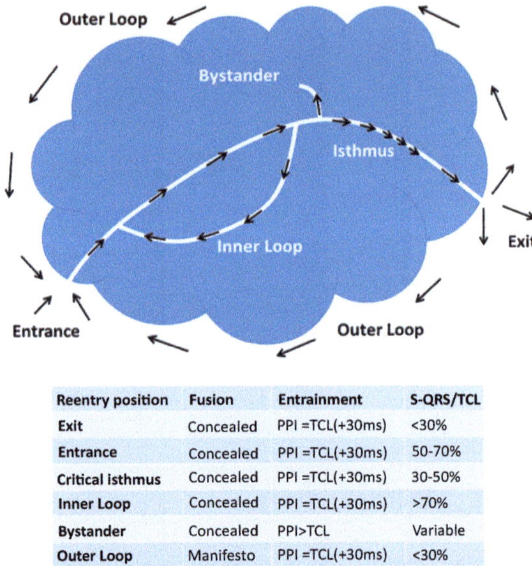

Fig. 17.1 Schematic representation of the mechanism of a scar-associated ventricular reentry tachycardia and observable phenomena during conventional mapping maneuvers

Reentry position	Fusion	Entrainment	S-QRS/TCL
Exit	Concealed	PPI =TCL(+30ms)	<30%
Entrance	Concealed	PPI =TCL(+30ms)	50-70%
Critical isthmus	Concealed	PPI =TCL(+30ms)	30-50%
Inner Loop	Concealed	PPI =TCL(+30ms)	>70%
Bystander	Concealed	PPI>TCL	Variable
Outer Loop	Manifesto	PPI =TCL(+30ms)	<30%

The excitation in the context of VT describes a figure-of-eight movement from the exit—that is, the coupling of the isthmus to the non-scarred myocardium—returning to the entrance (i.e., the entry into the protected isthmus). Due to the inhomogeneity of the scar, muscle fibers within the non-conductive areas, which also lie within the conduction barriers but are not an active part of the reentry, instead being passively excited. These areas are referred to as bystanders.

17.3 Indication

A catheter ablation is indicated with a recommendation lass IA for incessant VT, electrical storm (ES), or recurrent ICD therapies despite medical therapy. Furthermore, there is a class IIa recommendation after the first ICD shock delivery (Priori et al. 2015).

17.4 Ablation Procedure

Due to the increased periprocedural risk in patients with pre-existing cardiac conditions, careful planning and safe execution of the procedure are of particular importance, especially in VT ablation. The following provides an overview of practical implementation.

17.4.1 Procedure Planning

Patients for whom VT ablation is being considered should undergo a thorough cardiovascular evaluation. In addition to the physical examination, routine laboratory tests should exclude a reversible cause (acute ischemia, electrolyte disturbances, hyperthyroidism). A 12-lead documentation of the VT (ECG, long-term ECG) should be pursued. An echocardiography with assessment of the ejection fraction and to exclude left ventricular thrombi is recommended before the procedure. In patients affected by atrial fibrillation, exclusion of left atrial thrombi should also be performed.

This imaging information can help to plan access routes and provide crucial insights into understanding the cardiac and thoracic anatomy.

17.4.2 Procedure Management

One of the challenges of the procedure is the hemodynamic instability after the induction of a VT, making it particularly important to ensure ideal conditions for the procedure during VT ablations. The EP lab should be equipped with all the necessary facilities for an intensive care treatment setting. There should be the possibility for echocardiographic examination, intubation and ventilation, pericardiocentesis, defibrillation, and cardioversion. On the personnel side, the assisting staff should have experience with critically ill patients and be trained in resuscitation situations.

Many investigators today are no longer limited to a retrograde approach with passage of the aortic valve but extend the reach into the left ventricle through an anterograde transseptal approach and stabilize the catheter here with a steerable sheath.

An anterograde approach is associated with better contact pressure on the lateral wall and anteroseptal, while a retrograde approach has higher contact inferobasal and anterior. The anterograde approach is particularly preferable in patients with peripheral arterial disease, aortic valve stenosis, or prosthetic valves.

17.4.3 VT Induction

An essential step is the induction of clinical VT by means of programmed stimulation. For this purpose, the documentation of the VT using a 12-lead ECG is particularly important to match the morphology and cycle length of the clinical VT.

▶ A catheter positioned in the right ventricle is then used to stimulate with 5–7 beats at a fixed coupling interval followed initially by an extrastimulus, which is coupled 10–20 ms shorter per cycle. This stimulation is then performed with two basic cycle lengths and up to four extrastimuli, possibly also from alternative catheter positions.

▶ This initial examination forms the basis for success control. Only if at the end of the ablation procedure at least the clinical VT, but preferably no VT at all, can be induced, can further event-free survival be expected in the medium term.

17.4.4 Mapping and Ablation Strategies

The following describes the mapping techniques established for VT catheter ablations.

Entrainment Mapping

Under sustained VT, entrainment stimulations can be performed. They should be conducted at positions whose electrograms or activation patterns (e.g., mid-diastolic) suggest involvement in the reentry mechanism. Based on the post-pacing interval (PPI) and the 12-lead QRS morphology generated during entrainment stimulation, the position of the stimulation site within the VT reentry mechanism can be identified (Fig. 17.2). The reentry mechanism includes critical components whose conduction properties are crucial for the mechanism and are usually confined to the diastolic conduction part of the reentry (Stevenson et al. 1993). In addition to anatomically fixed barriers, functional barriers also exist during the ongoing reentry. Ablation of these areas is highly likely to result in VT termination. An entrainment stimulation within the protected isthmus activates the myocardium from the same exit, so the resulting 12-lead QRS morphology is identical to the ongoing VT morphology. This is referred to as "concealed fusion." An entrainment stimulation that occurs precisely on critical components (e.g., isthmus) also results in a PPI corresponding to the VT cycle length and a matching local activation sequence during stimulation and ongoing VT (stimulus-QRS interval corresponds to electrogram-QRS interval). Based on these criteria, the reentry components can be identified (tabular overview in Fig. 17.1). Ablation of the critical components, particularly the isthmus, can result in a theraeutic target. Performing an entrainment stimulation requires at least short-term hemodynamic stability and can—analogous to entrainment stimulation in atrial flutter—lead to termination, acceleration, or modification of the tachycardia.

Activation Mapping

An activation mapping of hemodynamically tolerated VT registrates the temporal sequence of myocardial electrical activation, particularly the zones of slow conduction relevant to VT. For this purpose, local electrograms are recorded at various positions in the ventricle during VT, and their activation time is compared with a uniform, common reference (usually a clearly identifiable point of the QRS in the surface ECG). 3D mapping systems enable a color-coded visualization of the activation, allowing the examiner to assess the ventricular activation and zones of slow conduction. A possible isthmus of a scar-related reentry tachycardia is typically recognizable in the activation mapping by a very early, mid-diastolic activation. The local electrogram is typically fractionated and of low amplitude (Figs. 17.2, 17.3 and 17.4).

Activation mapping can be the basis for a successful ablation, but in practice, it should always be combined with the above-described entrainment maneuvers. This is because even passively activated areas within the ischemic scar area can show early, mid-diastolic activation, although they are not an active part of the reentry mechanism (Fig. 17.5).

Even very late activated areas, which are far outside the reentry, could be misinterpreted as mid-diastolic activation. Activation mapping requires hemodynamic stability for the duration of the mapping. Although modern 3D mapping systems allow a certain degree of automation of the mapping through automated annotation and filter algorithms, a valid activation mapping still requires some time. Therefore, in individual cases, it may be useful to limit an activation map under ongoing tachycardia to specific areas where the critical isthmus of the tachycardia is suspected—for example, based on the recorded ECG morphology or a previous substrate or pace mapping.

Pacemapping

Pacemapping is an addition to entrainment and activation mapping, for example, when the clinical VT is only temporarily inducible or hemodynamically unstable. Here, a QRS complex generated by stimulation is morphologically compared with the clinical tachycardia. The degree of orrespondence is usually given in percentage. In ventricular tachycardias of focal origin, a high morphological agreement between pacemapping and clinical VT morphology suggests stimulation at the site of origin. In scar-associated tachycardias, a high agreement indicates stimulation near the VT exit. Pacemapping is subject to certain limitations that should be considered in clinical use. For example, stimulation from sites within the active reentry components, which are anatomically further from the VT exit, can result in completely different QRS morphologies. The coupling of

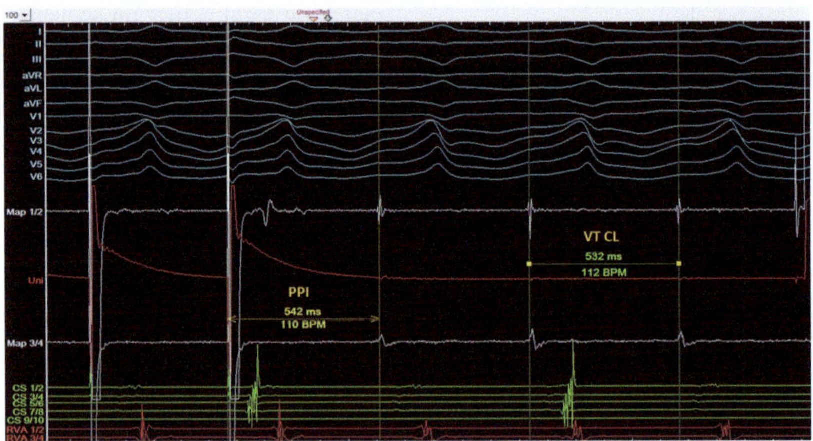

Fig. 17.2 Entrainment stimulation via the ablation catheter (MAP 1/2). The measured post-pacing interval (PPI) is 542 ms, the cycle length of the ongoing VT (VT CL) is 532 ms

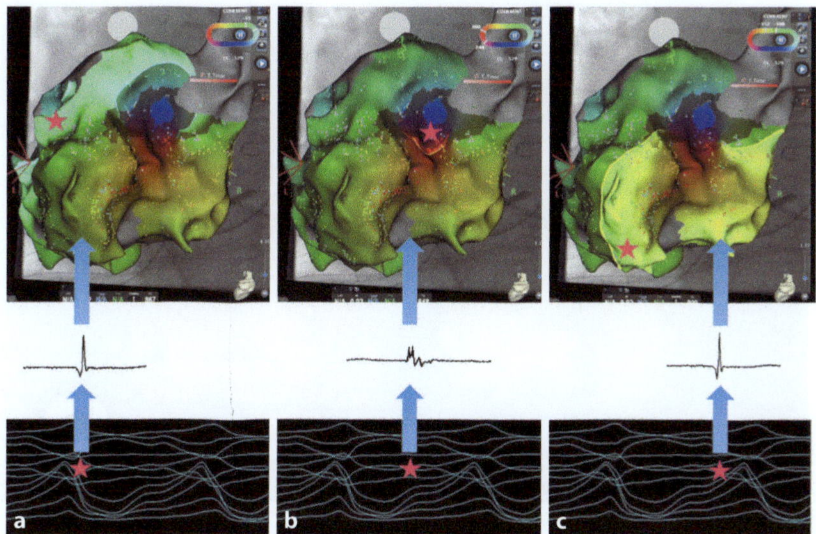

Fig. 17.3 Activation mapping of a VT caused by an inferior left ventricular scar. Posterior view of a high-resolution map created using a multipolar catheter. The activation times shown in the upper part of the image (**a** Late—end of the QRS complex; **b** Mid-diastolic—VT isthmus; **c** Early—beginning of the QRS complex) are correspondingly marked in the 12-lead ECG by *blue arrows*. Representation of the intracardiac signals in the middle part of the image

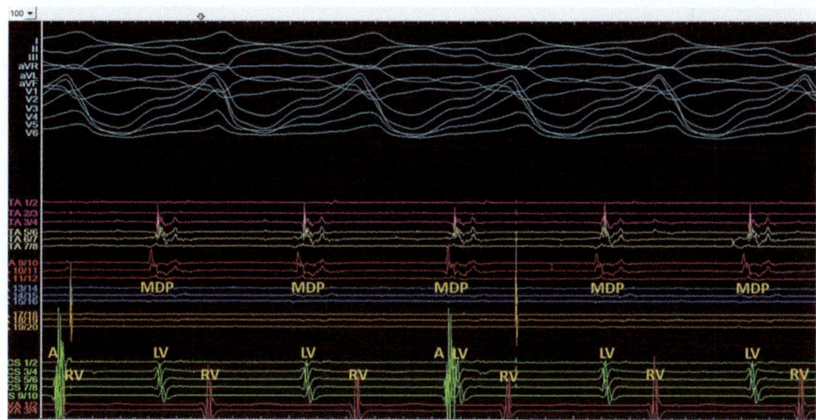

Fig. 17.4 Mid-diastolic potentials (MDP) registered during activation mapping with a multipolar catheter under sustained VT. A: Atrial signal; RV: right ventricular signal; LV: left ventricular signal

the excitation to the healthy myocardium then occurs in the area of the entrance of the clinical tachycardia. The phenomenon of a sudden QRS morphology transition under stimulation of adjacent areas with varying stimulation output can even indicate proximity to the VT isthmus. The spatial resolution of pacemapping is relatively low, so in some cases, a perfect match of the QRS morphology can be produced in areas up to 2–3 cm away from the actual origin. This depends on activation the activated myocardial mass. By choosing a stimulation output as low as possible close to the local pacing threshold (e.g., 2–5 V, 1–2 ms or 2–10 mA, 1–2 ms), capture of larger myocardial areas can be avoided (Fig. 17.6).

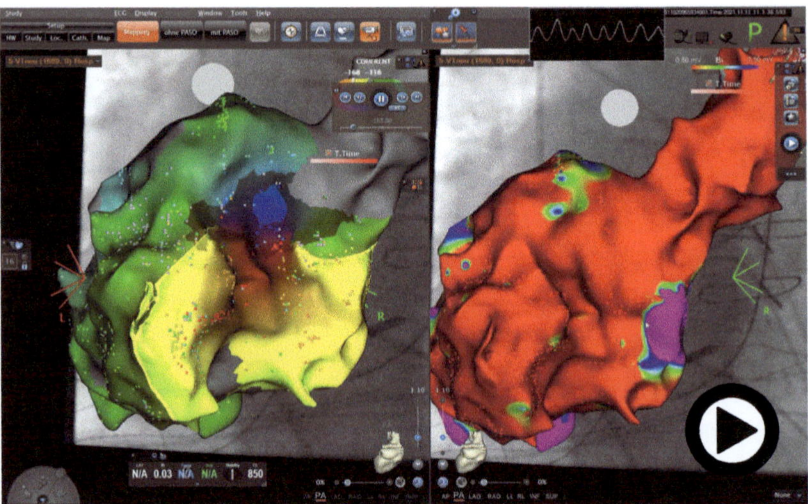

Fig. 17.5 Activation map of a scar-dependent VT with visualization of slow conduction in the area of the critical isthmus and representation of the "Early-meets-late" area with figure-of-eight activation of the outer loop ("Figure of eight pattern") (https://doi.org/10.1007/000-d2z)

Nevertheless, pacemapping is an easy-to-perform maneuver that can provide the operator with simple information about catheter and reentry positions. If the stimulated QRS morphology is, for example, less positive in the inferior leads than the clinical QRS morphology, the next stimulation site should be chosen further superior.

Substrate Mapping

Complementary to the VT mapping strategies mentioned above, substrate mapping is a valid option. this is of particular importance when the aforementioned mapping strategies are not applicable due to hemodynamic instability. In this procedure, arrhythmogenic substrate is identified under sinus rhythm or ventricular stimulation based on abnormal electrograms, which are presumably part of the clinical VT reentry mechanism and thus a promising target for catheter ablation.

The characterization of the arrhythmogenic substrate is carried out based on the analysis of local electrograms and is enabled by an electro-anatomical 3D mapping system (Fig. 17.7).

Mapped areas with a signal amplitude < 1.5 mV are considered electrically abnormal, areas with a signal amplitude < 0.5 mV are considered dense scar. The concepts of substrate-based mapping are based on the fact that areas that are active components of VT reentry (Fig. 17.5) are also recognizable in sinus rhythm or under ventricular stimulation through characteristic electrograms and due to their properties (especially delay of electrical activation, fractionation, late potentials, and Late Abnormal Ventricular Activity (LAVA); Figs. 17.6 and 17.8).

Late potentials occur after the QRS complex, isolated by an isoelectric interval. They indicate slow-conducting, surviving myocardial bundles in a surrounding area of fibrotic scar tissue and thus indicate possible VT isthmuses. Pacing mapping of the late potentials identified in substrate mapping and comparison with the documented clinical VT can be useful, as only about one-third of all late potentials identified in substrate mapping are associated with the active components of VT reentry. The majority of mapped late potentials represent passive components of the reentry, such as bystanders. Late potentials with a long QRS-late potential interval, long electrogram duration, and long stimulus-QRS interval during an additional pacing mapping are considered more specific for active reentry components.

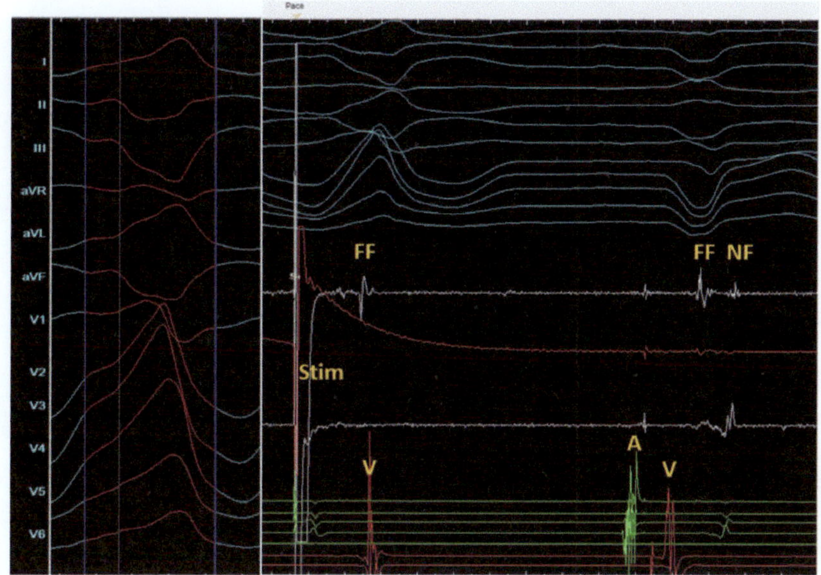

Fig. 17.6 Pacemapping (Stim) with low output. Capture of the late local signal (NF; LAVA) under ventricular stimulation, separated far-field electrogram (FF), long S-QRS interval, and high degree of correspondence with the clinical VT morphology. A = atrial signal; V = ventricular signal

LAVA electrograms are characterized by sharp, high-frequency potentials, which are usually found after the far-field QRS complex. In contrast to late potentials, LAVAs can also remain hidden within or at the end of the QRS complex. LAVA electrograms can be separated and unmasked from the ventricular far-field component by ventricular stimulation or spontaneous ventricular extrasystole. LAVA electrograms indicate areas that are electrically only weakly coupled with the rest of the myocardium and represent a promising ablation target (Jaïs et al. 2012).

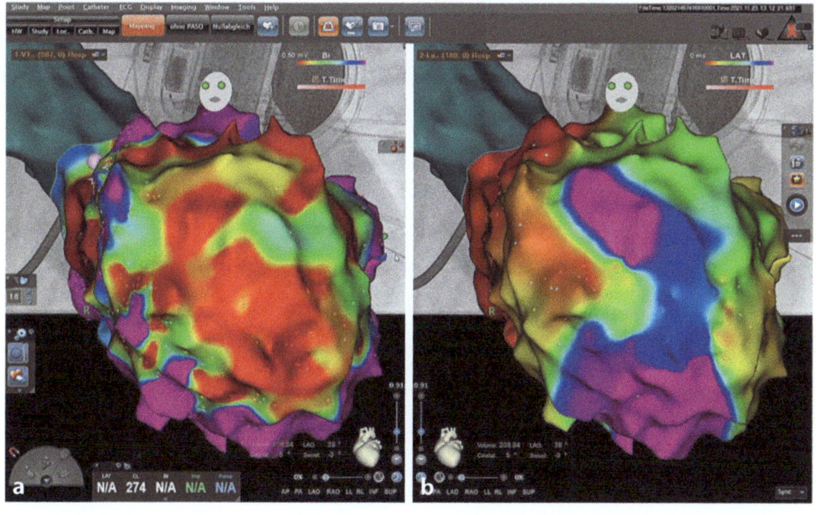

Fig. 17.7 Electroanatomical left ventricular mapping in LAO view during a VT ablation. In the voltage map (**a**), a large apical left ventricular scar is depicted. Numerous late potentials are found in this area (**b**).

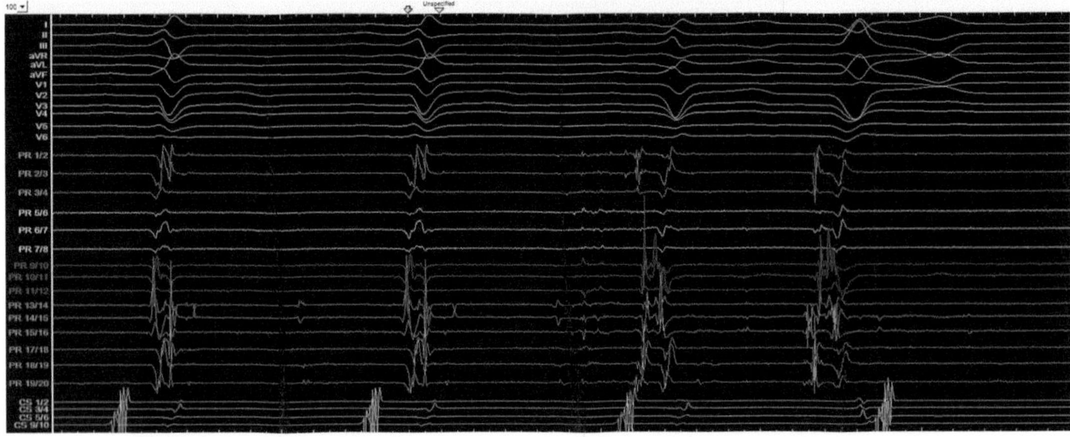

Fig. 17.8 Electrograms derived from a multipolar HD mapping catheter in the left ventricular apical scar area (Fig. 16.6). The LAVA hidden in the far-field QRS complex (PR 19/20) are unmasked during the ventricular extrasystole as early, high-frequency local electrogram components.

High-Density Mapping

Due to the often high complexity of the substrate, the partially low signal amplitude of some late potentials, and the higher amplitude of the far-field compared to the atrium due to the larger myocardial mass, the use of HD mapping procedures has become established for both substrate and activation mapping. For HD mapping procedures, modern multipolar mapping catheters with a high number of electrodes, small electrode size, and small electrode spacing are used to enable better discrimination of individual electrogram components. The multitude of electrograms acquired in parallel with multipolar mapping catheters makes largely automated electrogram detection and annotation (automated mapping) by computer algorithms necessary for efficient clinical use (Viswanathan et al. 2017).

Further Mapping Strategies

A limitation of substrate-based mapping is that areas of delayed conduction, which form the critical isthmus of a reentry VT, are not anatomically fixed in all cases but can also be of function character during ongoing VT and thus may not be identifiable through pure substrate mapping. Even anatomically fixed isthmuses can be masked by global ventricular activation and its directed electrical activation direction (Irie

et al. 2015). Therefore, various strategies for advanced substrate mapping exist, such as the creation of late potential maps (annotation of the latest local potential as an expression of maximum conduction delay) under (fixed-frequency) stimulation from different stimulation sites to achieve different activation directions. The annotation of late potentials under visualization of multiple (e.g., nine) isochrones is called ILAM ("**i**sochronal **l**ate **a**ctivation **m**apping"). Zones where multiple isochrones lie close together indicate areas of local deceleration and can suggest a VT isthmus.

Furthermore, with the so-called DEEP-Mapping ("**de**crement **e**voked **p**otential"), the functional significance of late potentials regarding decremental conduction properties can be investigated. Here, programmed stimulation with different intervals is performed (e.g., S1S1 600 ms; S1S2 450 ms; S2S3 350 ms). The intervals should be chosen so that VT is just barely not induced but close to the VT induction threshold. A late potential map of all three cycle lengths is created. Modern algorithms of 3D navigation systems allow for the completely automated annotation of potentials depending on the stimulated cycle length. Comparing the maps allows conclusions about the decremental conduction properties of the investigated areas and thus insights into a functional substrate.

Combination of Multiple Mapping Strategies

In most VT ablations, a combination of the mentioned mapping strategies is used. The procedural steps presented should be understood as individual components of successful VT ablation. The sequence and individual weighting depend on patient characteristics, procedural situations, and center-specific aspects.

The following is an exemplary workflow:

▶ In the first step, the induction and thus determination of the VT ECG morphology is performed. In the second step, the substrate is mapped in sinus rhythm using a high-resolution mapping catheter and a three-dimensional map. During mapping, areas that are already late-activated or show high fractionation or a good match with the ECG morphology are annotated. In a third step, the identified areas are then mapped during short, re-induced VT phases using entrainment. If the critical isthmus can be identified near or within a scar area, ablation can be performed in this region in the fourth step, for example, until the endpoint of LAVA elimination is reached.

17.4.5 Ablation Procedures and Endpoints

The generator settings chosen for RF ablation are less standardized compared to atrial ablations and largely depend on the subjective experience and assessment of the investigator. Irrigated RF catheters should be used. In clinical practice, RF powers between 30 to 60 W for a duration of 30 seconds to several minutes are chosen. The higher the power and the longer the duration of an RF application, the larger the resulting ablation lesion. From a duration of 30 seconds, a maximum lesion size can be assumed. However, the maximum achievable size of a lesion is predetermined by the chosen RF power. While RF ablations with a power of 30–40 W primarily target endocardial substrate, higher powers of 50–60 W over a longer duration can reach intramural or even epicardial

substrate (Bourier et al. 2020). However, with increasing RF power, the risk of complications (e.g., steam pop, charring) also increases.

Various ablation strategies are available, particularly the ablation of late potentials or LAVA, scar homogenization, the creation of linear lesions through the ventricular scar area, dechanneling, or core isolation (Guandalini et al. 2019; Briceño et al. 2018).

▶ If the critical isthmus of the VT could be successfully localized using the described mapping methods, RF ablation in this area leads to termination. This represents a classic procedural endpoint of ablation. Additionally, there are further endpoints with LAVA elimination and achieving non-excitability in the scar area.

Ultimately, the lack of inducibility of any VT under programmed stimulation at the end of the procedure is the gold standard of success control. The non-inducibility of all clinical VTs should be the minimal goal in any catheter ablation of structural VTs.

17.5 Summary

Patients with ischemic cardiomyopathy are at significant risk for the occurrence of scar-related VT, and catheter ablation enables a causal and effective therapy. Ablation should always be considered in the occurrence of monomorphic VT and is indicated with a recommendation grade IA in incessant VT, electrical storm, or recurrent ICD shocks.

When planning a VT ablation, preprocedural examinations are necessary, and reversible causes should be excluded. The importance of the 12-lead ECG of the clinical VT, which is helpful for the ablation strategy, should be emphasized. A late-enhancement MRI or a CT can be used for substrate characterization, selection of the ablation strategy (endocardial or epicardial), and possibly for image integration. Access to the LV can be antegrade, retrograde, or combined. Only irrigated RF catheters are used for ablation, and high power may be required to reach intramural substrate.

The basis for the formation and sustension of scar-related VT is a reentrant ircuit involving a region of slow conduction. The ablation strategy consists of identifying and eliminating channels of slow-conducting surviving myocardium within the scar. Substrate mapping, ideally high-resolution mapping, is required for the precise characterization of the substrate. Here, "interesting" areas with late potentials and/or LAVA are marked. Complementary use of pace mapping and/or activation mapping is recommended, depending on the inducibility and hemodynamic stability of the VT. In stable VT, activation mapping in combination with entrainment maneuvers is useful. In unstable VT or lack of inducibility, pace mapping can be effective if a 12-lead documentation is available. In all cases, characterization of the underlying substrate is performed, so potential target regions can also be identified for more targeted mapping, and purely substrate-based ablation strategies can be developed.

▶ The goal of ablation is the elimination of VT-critical conduction zones (VT channels, isthmus). Additional procedural endpoints such as the elimination of all late potentials/LAVA or non-excitability in the scar area can help improve the long-term success rate of the ablation. At the end of the procedure, no VT should be inducible by final programmed stimulation.

In all cases, VT ablation is a demanding procedure that should be performed in experienced centers with appropriate equipment and personnel. The application of the standardized and structured approach presented here can help to avoid complications and enhance the success rate.

References

Briceño DF, Romero J, Villablanca PA, Londoño A, Diaz JC, Maraj I, Batul SA, Madan N, Patel J, Jagannath A, Mohanty S, Mohanty P, Gianni C, Rocca DD, Sabri A, Kim SG, Natale A, Di Biase L (2018) Long-term outcomes of different ablation strategies for ventricular tachycardia in patients with structural heart disease: systematic review and meta-analysis. Europace 20(1):104–115. https://doi.org/10.1093/europace/eux109

Bourier F, Ramirez FD, Martin CA, Vlachos K, Frontera A, Takigawa M, Kitamura T, Lam A, Duchateau J, Pambrun T, Cheniti G, Derval N, Denis A, Sacher F, Hocini M, Haissaguerre M, Jais P (2020) Impedance, power, and current in radiofrequency ablation: insights from technical, ex vivo, and clinical studies. J Cardiovasc Electrophysiol 31(11):2836–2845. https://doi.org/10.1111/jce.14709

Guandalini GS, Liang JJ, Marchlinski FE (2019) Ventricular tachycardia ablation: past, present, and future perspectives. JACC Clin Electrophysiol 5(12):1363–1383

Irie T, Yu R, Bradfield JS, Vaseghi M, Buch EF, Ajijola O, Macias C, Fujimura O, Mandapati R, Boyle NG, Shivkumar K, Tung R (2015) Relationship between sinus rhythm late activation zones and critical sites for scar-related ventricular tachycardia: systematic analysis of isochronal late activation mapping. Circ Arrhythm Electrophysiol 8(2):390–399. https://doi.org/10.1161/CIRCEP.114.002637

Jaïs P, Maury P, Khairy P, Sacher F, Nault I, Komatsu Y, Hocini M, Forclaz A, Jadidi AS, Weerasooriya R, Shah A, Derval N, Cochet H, Knecht S, Miyazaki S, Linton N, Rivard L, Wright M, Wilton SB, Scherr D, Pascale P, Roten L, Pederson M, Bordachar P, Laurent F, Kim SJ, Ritter P, Clementy J, Haïssaguerre M (2012) Elimination of local abnormal ventricular activities: a new end point for substrate modification in patients with scar-related ventricular tachycardia. Circulation 125(18):2184–2196. https://doi.org/10.1161/CIRCULATIONAHA.111.043216

Priori SG, Blomström-Lundqvist C, Mazzanti A, Blom N, Borggrefe M, Camm J, Elliott PM, Fitzsimons D, Hatala R, Hindricks G, Kirchhof P, Kjeldsen K, Kuck K-H, Hernandez-Madrid A, Nikolaou N, Norekvål TM, Spaulding C, Van Veldhuisen DJ, ESC Scientific Document Group (2015) 2015 ESC Guidelines for the management of patients with ventricular arrhythmias and the prevention of sudden cardiac death: The Task Force for the Management of Patients with Ventricular Arrhythmias and the Prevention of Sudden Cardiac Death of the European Society of Cardiology (ESC). Eur Heart J 36(41):2793–2867

Stevenson WG, Khan H, Sager P, Saxon LA, Middlekauff HR, Natterson PD, Wiener I (1993) Identification of reentry circuit sites during catheter mapping and radiofrequency ablation of ventricular tachycardia late after myocardial infarction. Circulation 88(4 Pt 1):1647–1670. https://doi.org/10.1161/01.cir.88.4.1647

Viswanathan K, Mantziari L, Butcher C, Hodkinson E, Lim E, Khan H, Panikker S, Haldar S, Jarman JW, Jones DG, Hussain W, Foran JP, Markides V, Wong T (2017) Evaluation of a novel high-resolution mapping system for catheter ablation of ventricular arrhythmias. Heart Rhythm 14(2):176–183. https://doi.org/10.1016/j.hrthm.2016.11.018

VT in Non-Ischemic Cardiomyopathy

Christian Sohns and Vanessa Sciacca

18.1 Introduction

The term non-ischemic cardiomyopathy (NICM) refers to a disease of the ventricular myocardium that is associated with mechanical, electrical, or combined electromechanical dysfunction in the absence of coronary blood flow disturbance. It is a large and heterogeneous group of diseases with different morphological and functional phenotypes that can lead to the development of NICM. An overview of the underlying diseases of NICM is shown in Fig. 18.1.

The prevalence of ventricular tachycardias and ventricular fibrillation is significantly increased in patients with NICM compared to the general population, and their occurrence is associated with an increase in mortality and morbidity. The establishment of antiarrhythmic

medication and the implantation of a cardioverter-defibrillator (ICD) form the basis of therapy for many patients. Furthermore, catheter-based ablation treatment has been established as an additional therapy for ventricular tachycardias for a large number of patients with NICM, especially within the last decade. In some forms of NICM, ablation of ventricular tachycardias has been shown to effectively reduce arrhythmia recurrences, ICD shocks, and the need for antiarrhythmic medication.

▶ Knowledge of the underlying disease of NICM before planning an ablation treatment is of particular importance. Substrate expression and distribution, the necessity of extensive ablation, and long-term prognosis are directly related to the etiology of the disease.

Supplementary Information The online version contains supplementary material available at https://doi.org/10.1007/978-3-662-65797-3_18. The videos can be accessed individually by clicking the DOI link in the accompanying figure caption or by scanning this link with the SN More Media App.

18.2 Tachycardia Mechanisms and Substrate Localization in Non-Ischemic Cardiomyopathy

The occurrence and maintenance of ventricular tachycardias can be attributed to three fundamental mechanisms: triggered activity, increased focal automaticity, and scar-dependent reentry. Knowledge of these arrhythmia mechanisms is of practical relevance for performing ablation procedures. Areas with triggered activity or

C. Sohns (✉) · V. Sciacca
Klinik für Elektrophysiologie/Rhythmologie,
Herz- und Diabeteszentrum NRW, Ruhr-Universität
Bochum, Bad Oeynhausen, Germany
e-mail: csohns@hdz-nrw.de

V. Sciacca
e-mail: vsciacca@hdz-nrw.de

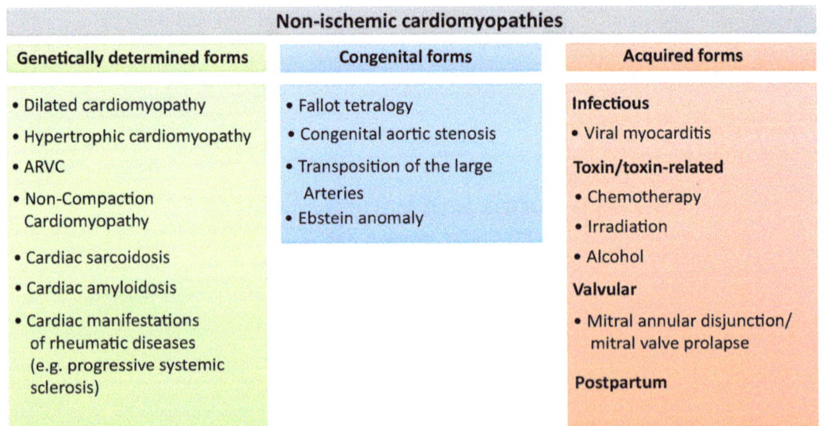

Fig. 18.1 Overview of various entities of non-ischemic cardiomyopathy. Simplistically, a subdivision into genetically determined diseases, inflammatory/infiltrative diseases, congenital diseases, and acquired diseases can be made. For a large number of patients with variously caused non-ischemic cardiomyopathy and recurrent ventricular tachycardias, ablation treatment can represent an effective therapy.

increased automaticity respond particularly well to focal ablations, whereas tachycardias based on scar-dependent reentries often require more complex endocardial or even epicardial substrate modifications.

Despite the etiological diversity of NICM, scar-dependent reentries have been identified as the most common mechanism for ventricular tachycardias (Hsia et al. 2003). In contrast to ischemic cardiomyopathy, where the arrhythmogenic substrate is based on ischemia-induced cardiomyocyte death with the formation of scar areas, inflammatory processes with the formation of fibrosis in all myocardial layers are predominant in NICM. The diffuse fibrosis causes reduced electrical conductivity of the tissue as well as functional and anatomical block, leading to the formation of reentries. The progression of the underlying disease can lead to further expansion of myocardial fibrosis over time.

▶ The distribution of myocardial fibrosis in patients with NICM often leads to an intramural and epicardial expansion of the substrate. Important indications for this can be found in pre-procedural imaging and in the unipolar voltage map, which, in contrast to the bipolar map, represents the voltage of all wall layers.

Specific groups of NICM have been identified with particular distribution patterns of the arrhythmogenic substrate.

In dilated cardiomyopathy (DCM), the most common form of NICM, two main predilection sites for the development of arrhythmogenic substrate can be observed in patients. On the one hand, it is a basal anteroseptal region of the left ventricle in the area of the aorta, the aortomitral continuity, and the basal septum, and on the other hand, it is a basal inferolateral and often epicardially located region of the left ventricle (Haqqani et al. 2011; Oloriz et al. 2014; Glashan et al. 2018). Effective ablation can be complicated by the deep intramural location, proximity to specific conduction tissue, or an epicardial location.

▶ In NICM of the dilated type (DCM), the arrhythmogenic substrate is often located in the area of the basal anteroseptal left ventricle or in the area of the basal inferoseptal left ventricle with epicardial components.

Arrhythmogenic right ventricular cardiomyopathy (ARVC) is a genetically determined form of NICM, characterized by structural remodeling primarily in the right ventricular myocardium. This involves the transformation of cardiomyocytes into adipose tissue cells and, in later stages, into fibrotic tissue (Kirubarakan et al. 2017; Corrado et al. 2015). These structural changes lead to a high incidence of ventricular arrhythmias based on reentry mechanisms in patients with ARVC. Therefore, ablation therapy has become an important treatment strategy for patients with ARVC (Souissi et al. 2018). In this patient cohort, the specific substrate is most commonly located in the right ventricle below the tricuspid valve annulus and in the area of the free right ventricular wall (Liang et al. 2020). A significant proportion of patients with ARVC exhibit a substrate that is primarily accessible through epicardial ablation. Figure 18.2 exemplifies an electroanatomical mapping of a patient with pronounced ARVC and the corresponding substrate.

Hypertrophic cardiomyopathy (HCM) represents another form of NICM, for which a specific substrate distribution is known. In patients with HCM, genetically determined hypertrophy of the myocardium occurs without the influence of secondary causes. Ventricular tachycardias and sudden cardiac death occur in a significant proportion of patients with HCM. In particular, in patients with ventricular obstructions or

ventricular aneurysms, these may manifest as recurrent monomorphic ventricular tachycardias. The substrate of ventricular tachycardias in patients with HCM is predominantly located in the area of the left ventricular apex and the right and left ventricular junction (Igarashi et al. 2018). A significant proportion of patients with HCM and recurrent monomorphic ventricular tachycardias exhibit an intramural or epicardial course of reentries, so an epicardial approach may be required for successful ablation (Santangeli et al. 2010). Figure 18.3 exemplifies an electroanatomical representation using 3D mapping in a patient with HCM.

In the area of ion channel diseases associated with ventricular tachycardias, specific substrate distribution patterns have also been identified for certain patient groups, enabling the establishment of successful ablation strategies. Brugada syndrome is a genetically determined disease in which mutations leading to changes in the structure or function of the fast cardiac sodium channel metabolism have been identified as a common cause of the disease. Brugada syndrome usually does not involve pronounced structural cardiac changes in affected patients. Any structural variants are usually discrete and

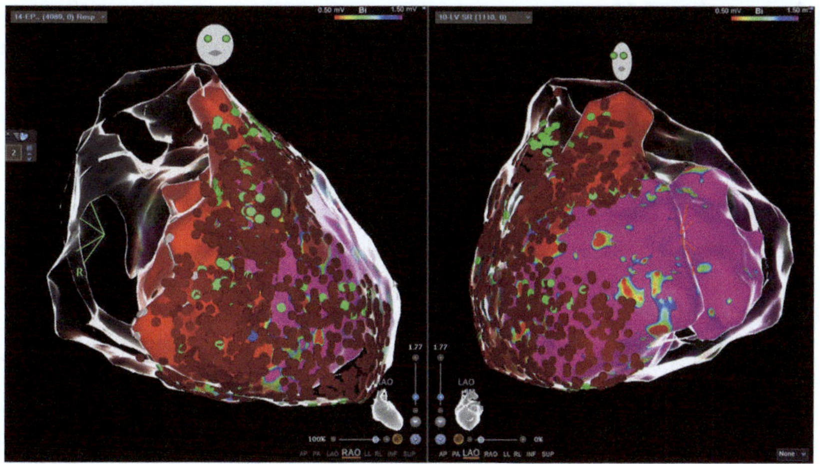

Fig. 18.2 Electroanatomical representation using endo- and epicardial 3D mapping of a patient with arrhythmogenic right ventricular cardiomyopathy. The extent of the substrate (coded in red for areas with voltage < 0.5 mV) in the area below the tricuspid valve annulus and the free wall of the right ventricle with pronounced epicardial involvement is clearly visible

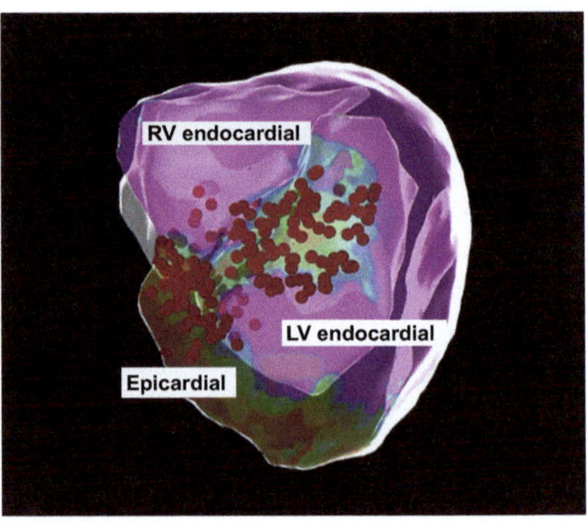

Fig. 18.3 Electroanatomical representation in a caudal view during ablation treatment in a patient with hypertrophic cardiomyopathy. A septally emphasized substrate distribution with predominantly epicardial components was observed. Targeted ablation was performed from the right and left ventricles as well as epicardially as septal substrate modification

localized in the right ventricle, particularly in the area of the right ventricular outflow tract (RVOT) (Chokesuwattanaskul and Nademanee 2021). In smaller case series, the occurrence of arrhythmias and ICD therapies could be reduced or prevented through ablation treatments. These measures usually required epicardial ablation procedures with ablation applications in the RVOT area. Due to the complexity of the procedure and the limited data available so far, this procedure should be considered in individual cases for patients with otherwise therapy-refractory arrhythmias.

18.3 Periprocedural Management

The preprocedural planning before performing a ventricular ablation procedure in NICM essentially correspond to the standardized preparations before ablation procedures in general.

An exact assessment of the patient's history with particular attention to previous cardiac surgeries such as bypass grafts and valve prostheses should be conducted before each procedure. This allows for the pre-procedural assessment of potential difficulties with access routes or anticoagulation management.

Documentation of the arrhythmia to be treated should be available before performing the ablation treatment. Ideally, this is a documentation of clinical tachycardia using a 12-lead ECG. Multiple algorithms have been evaluated in the literature that allow for a non-invasive assessment of the localization of ventricular arrhythmias (Berruezo et al. 2004; Segal et al. 2007). This way, the complexity of the ablation procedure can be assessed pre-procedurally, access routes can be planned proactively, and patients can be specifically informed about the upcoming invasive measures. A common problem is the lack of 12-lead ECG documentation before ablation treatment. Alternatively, the reading of pacemakers and ICD systems can provide documentation of clinical tachycardia in the form of stored electrograms. Therefore, it is recommended to perform a device interrogation before ablation treatment in every patient who has a permanent pacemaker, ICD system, or other monitoring systems such as implantable loop-recorders. Additionally, any pre-existing dysfunctions of a pacemaker or ICD system can be detected before ablation. Before starting the ablation, the antitachycardia functions in patients with ICD systems should also be deactivated to prevent unwanted ICD shocks during the procedure. Intraprocedurally, the patient should be connected to an external defibrillator during every ablation of ventricular tachycardias to enable emergency defibrillation in case of hemodynamic instability under induced tachycardia. After the ablation is performed, a deactivated ICD system should be reactivated immediately, and adjustments to the antitachycardia treatment should be made according to the procedure results.

Other pre-procedural basic measures include the laboratory determination of inflammatory markers, blood count, and coagulation values before performing the ablation. Pre-existing anticoagulant medication therapy must be individually adjusted during the periprocedural period. Usually, oral anticoagulation is paused on the morning of the procedure day. Oral anticoagulation can be resumed on the evening after the ablation treatment if the procedure course is uneventful. If particularities in the periprocedural course prevent the prompt resumption of oral anticoagulation, the indication for bridging therapy with heparin or corresponding analogs must be examined and initiated if necessary. In patients with existing medication with vitamin K antagonists, an INR value of up to 2.5 is accepted before performing the ablation treatment. Standardized bridging therapy with heparin is not recommended for patients with vitamin K antagonists. Medication therapy with platelet aggregation inhibitors usually does not need to be paused. In patients with an indication for oral anticoagulation due to an increased thromboembolic risk from atrial arrhythmias, the indication for performing a transesophageal echocardiography to exclude intra-atrial thrombi before the ablation treatment must be examined. Many patients with NICM also present with highly impaired systolic left ventricular function as part of their underlying disease, with a correspondingly increased risk for ventricular thrombi. In these patients, the indication for performing pre-procedural imaging to exclude ventricular thrombi should also be examined. The method of choice here can be contrast-enhanced transthoracic echocardiography. Alternatively, cardiac magnetic resonance imaging (MRI) can also be performed to exclude ventricular thrombi.

▶ Before the ablation of ventricular tachycardias, the indication for excluding intra-atrial or ventricular thrombi using advanced imaging should be examined and performed if necessary to avoid periprocedural thromboembolic complications.

The performance of pre-procedural imaging before the ablation of ventricular tachycardias in NICM should ideally be routinely done using MRI or computed tomography (CT). Using modern analysis software, it is now possible under experimental conditions to non-invasively predict potential ablation locations pre-procedurally, so that the required access routes, such as an epicardial access route for the planned procedure, can be determined in advance.

▶ Pre-procedural imaging using MRI or CT can identify potential ablation targets in advance and be helpful in procedure planning.

Before performing the ablation treatment, the form of sedation or anesthesia and hemodynamic monitoring should also be determined. In patients with NICM and often highly impaired systolic left ventricular function, an approach with general anesthesia may be indicated. In cases of low morbidity or contraindication to intubation anesthesia, an approach with analgesia and spontaneous breathing can also be considered. Arterial blood pressure measurement during the ablation of ventricular tachycardias in patients with NICM is helpful to identify the need for cardioversion of a ventricular tachycardia due to hemodynamic intolerance. In individual cases, the periprocedural use of left ventricular support systems (e.g., arterial axial pumps) may be necessary to enable ablation treatment in patients with NICM and highly impaired ventricular function.

Post-interventionally, a pericardial effusion should be excluded echocardiographically in every patient before transfer from the catheter lab. In patients with an epicardial access route, it is recommended to leave the pigtail catheter until the following day. After serial aspiration attempts and echocardiographic controls, the pigtail catheter can then be removed if the course is uneventful.

18.4 Catheter Setup

As already described above, a standardized selection of catheters should be available before the ablation of ventricular tachycardias, which can be individually expanded.

The standardized setup should include a right ventricular catheter for mapping and programmed stimulation. Additionally, a coronary sinus catheter and, if necessary, a His-bundle catheter should be available. The coronary sinus catheter can facilitate the transseptal puncture as an anatomical orientation and serve as a valuable catheter in the differential diagnosis of unclear wide complex tachycardias, for example, to differentiate an atrioventricular reentry tachycardia. Furthermore, the region of the mitral valve annulus, which is important in patients with NICM, can be effectively marked using the coronary sinus catheter. A His-bundle catheter can be a valuable diagnostic catheter, especially in patients with NICM who already show an intraventricular conduction disorder in sinus rhythm, in terms of a possibly existing so-called "bundle-branch reentry tachycardia." Specific multi-electrode catheters enable high-resolution electroanatomical representation of the substrate and should be used if possible.

The access routes to the left ventricle include approaches via transseptal puncture and consecutive anterograde passage of the mitral valve as well as approaches via retrograde passage of the aortic valve (Fig. 18.4). Depending on the patient's anatomy and the arrhythmogenic substrate to be treated, a combination of both access routes may also be necessary. An epicardial access may be required in the case of documentation or occurrence of tachycardias originating from the epicardium or if an endocardial treatment target is not detected. The access is enabled by dry pericardial puncture.

In contrast to (diagnostic or therapeutic) pericardial puncture in pericardial effusions or tamponades, the "dry" pericardial space must be targeted here. Therefore, a vertical puncture into the pericardial sac should be avoided; instead, an almost tangential puncture is aimed for. Here, an anterior and an inferior access are distinguished. Typically, a specially curved and sharpened puncture needle (Tuohy needle) is used, whose lumen is directed away from the myocardium. A micropuncture needle can also be used. Usually, small amounts of contrast medium are applied to verify the position of the needle in the pericardial space, followed by the introduction of a Seldinger wire.

▶ Before advancing the epicardial sheath (and possibly prior dilation of the access route

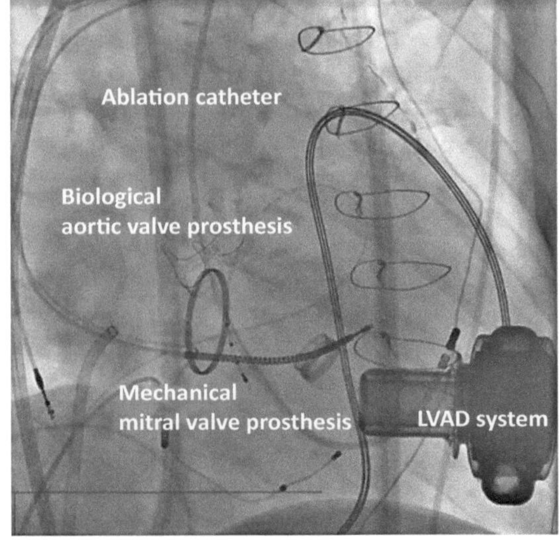

Fig. 18.4 Fluoroscopic image of an ablation treatment of a patient with NICM and severely impaired systolic left ventricular function, who is already provided with a permanent left ventricular assist device (LVAD system). The ablation catheter was introduced retrogradely via the aorta into the left ventricle, as an anterograde access route was not possible due to a mechanical mitral valve prosthesis.

with dilators), the correct position of the wire in the pericardial space must be securely verified. A misplaced wire can often be retracted without serious consequences, while a sheath accidentally advanced intramyocardially or intracavitarily would most likely cause severe bleeding requiring surgical intervention.

Furthermore, it should be noted that the catheter's flushing fluid should be aspirated at regular intervals through the inserted sheath to avoid hemodynamic compromises.

In the case of adhesions, which can occur after previous cardiac surgery or prior pericarditis, the introduction of catheters is usually significantly more difficult or not possible. In individual cases, the introduction of catheters may be successful after catheter-based mechanical adhesiolysis. For the performance of epicardial ablations, a possible proximity of the ablation target to epicardially located structures such as the coronary vessels and the phrenic nerve must be excluded. For this purpose, diagnostic measures such as coronary angiographies and phrenic nerve stimulation maneuvers should be performed. The performance of a coronary angiography may also be necessary for endocardial ablation targets close to the coronary system. For ablation targets in the area of the phrenic nerve, a fluid infusion into the pericardium may increase the distance to the nerve and enable an otherwise unfeasible ablation. Occasionally, PTCA or PTA balloons with a few millimeters in diameter are used for this purpose.

18.5 Mapping, Ablation and Ablation Endpoints

After introducing the diagnostic and therapeutic catheters described above, a mapping of the ventricles should first be performed to visualize and identify the scarred or fibrotic areas and mark corresponding late potentials or LAVAs. In this context, the unipolar voltage map is of greater importance than in ischemic VT. The unipolar voltage map shows the voltage of all wall layers, while the bipolar voltage map predominantly displays the endocardial components. Thus, the finding of extensive low-voltage areas in the unipolar map with less extensive low-voltage areas in the bipolar map suggests an intramural or epicardial substrate.

Under programmed stimulation using specific stimulation cycles, the induction of clinical tachycardia is provoked. If induction of clinical tachycardia is possible, an activation mapping of the tachycardia follows, with identification and, if possible, ablation of the critical isthmus (Fig. 18.5), provided the patient is hemodynamically stable.

If the tachycardia terminates mechanically or has to be terminated by external cardioversion due to hemodynamic instability, pace mapping can be performed. This involves targeted stimulation via catheters followed by morphological comparison of the stimulated ventricular complex and the recorded ventricular complex of the clinical tachycardia. In the case of high correspondence, targeted ablation can then be performed. In patients in whom induction of clinical tachycardia is not successful, ablation is performed according to the electroanatomical representation in the form of homogenization of the substrate area by eliminating all detected abnormal electrical potentials (Jaïs et al. 2012). This approach is also applied additionally in patients with inducible tachycardia. If other than the documented clinical tachycardia can be induced, corresponding ablation of these tachycardias should also be performed. Finally, aggressive programmed stimulation should be performed. The lack of inducibility of any ventricular tachycardias represents the primary endpoint of ablation and is supported by a guideline recommendation (Aliot et al. 2009).

▶ The lack of inducibility of ventricular tachycardias after performing the ablation treatment represents the most important procedural endpoint.

18.6 Summary

The ablation of ventricular tachycardias today represents an important therapy for symptomatic patients with NICM and can contribute to

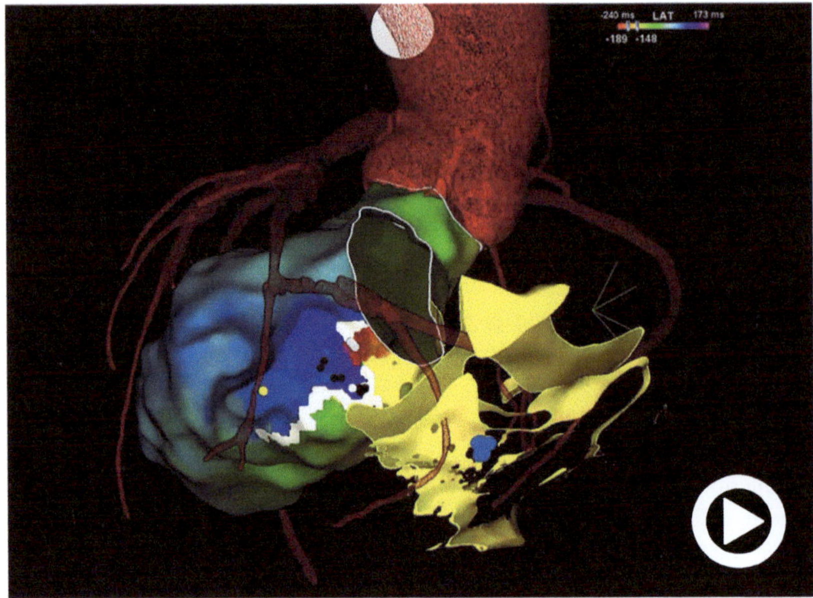

Fig. 18.5 Representation of the electrical activation of a ventricular tachycardia using a three-dimensional electroanatomical mapping system. Note the propagation of the wavefront between the epicardial and endocardial components of the reentry as well as the representation of the critical isthmus endocardially. Overlaid in red is a CT reconstruction of the aortic root and the epicardially running coronary vessels (https://doi.org/10.1007/000-d30)

the reduction of arrhythmia recurrences, antiarrhythmic medication, and ICD shocks. Due to the special substrate distribution in patients with NICM with frequent epicardial extension, ablation treatments must be planned as complex procedures. The use of pre-procedural imaging using MRI or CT should be standardized to non-invasively capture any peculiarities of substrate localization. With the help of temporary left ventricular support systems, ablation treatment can be enabled even for patients with severely impaired left ventricular function.

References

Aliot EM, Stevenson WG, Almendral-Garrote JM, Bogun F, Calkins CH, Delacretaz E, Bella DP, Hindricks G, Jaïs P, Josephson ME, Kautzner J, Kay GN, Kuck KH, Lerman BB, Marchlinski F, Reddy V, Schalij MJ, Schilling R, Soejima K, Wilber D, European Heart Rhythm Association, Registered Branch of the European Society of Cardiology (ESC), Heart Rhythm Society (HRS), American College of Cardiology (ACC), American Heart Association (AHA) (2009) EHRA/HRS Expert Consensus on Catheter Ablation of Ventricular Arrhythmias: developed in a partnership with the European Heart Rhythm Association (EHRA), a Registered Branch of the European Society of Cardiology (ESC), and the Heart Rhythm Society (HRS); in collaboration with the American College of Cardiology (ACC) and the American Heart Association (AHA). Heart Rhythm 6(6):886–933. https://doi.org/10.1016/j.hrthm.2009.04.030

Berruezo A, Mont L, Nava S, Chueca E, Bartholomay E, Brugada J (2004) Electrocardiographic recognition of the epicardial origin of ventricular tachycardias. Circulation 109(15):1842–1847. https://doi.org/10.1161/01.CIR.0000125525.04081.4B

Chokesuwattanaskul R, Nademanee K (2021) Role of catheter ablation for ventricular arrhythmias in Brugada syndrome. Curr Cardiol Rep 23(5):54. https://doi.org/10.1007/s11886-021-01479-2

Corrado D, Wichter T, Link MS, Hauer RN, Marchlinski FE, Anastasakis A, Bauce B, Basso C, Brunckhorst C, Tsatsopoulou A, Tandri H, Paul M, Schmied C, Pelliccia A, Duru F, Protonotarios N, Estes NM 3rd, McKenna WJ, Thiene G, Marcus FI, Calkins H (2015) Treatment of arrhythmogenic right ventricular cardiomyopathy/dysplasia: an international task force consensus statement.

Circulation 132(5):441–453. https://doi.org/10.1161/CIRCULATIONAHA.115.017944. PMC4521905.

Glashan CA, Androulakis AFA, Tao Q, Glashan RN, Wisse LJ, Ebert M, de Ruiter MC, van Meer BJ, Brouwer C, Dekkers OM, Pijnappels DA, de Bakker JMT, de Riva M, Piers SRD, Zeppenfeld K (2018) Whole human heart histology to validate electroanatomical voltage mapping in patients with non-ischaemic cardiomyopathy and ventricular tachycardia. Eur Heart J 39(31):2867–2875. https://doi.org/10.1093/eurheartj/ehy168

Haqqani HM, Tschabrunn CM, Tzou WS, Dixit S, Cooper JM, Riley MP, Lin D, Hutchinson MD, Garcia FC, Bala R, Verdino RJ, Callans DJ, Gerstenfeld EP, Zado ES, Marchlinski FE (2011) Isolated septal substrate for ventricular tachycardia in nonischemic dilated cardiomyopathy: incidence, characterization, and implications. Heart Rhythm 8(8):1169–1176. https://doi.org/10.1016/j.hrthm.2011.03.008

Hsia HH, Marchlinski FE (2002) Characterization of the electroanatomic substrate for monomorphic ventricular tachycardia in patients with nonischemic cardiomyopathy. Pacing Clin Electrophysiol 25(7):1114–1127. https://doi.org/10.1046/j.1460-9592.2002.01114.x

Igarashi M, Nogami A, Kurosaki K, Hanaki Y, Komatsu Y, Fukamizu S, Morishima I, Kaitani K, Nishiuchi S, Talib AK, Machino T, Kuroki K, Yamasaki H, Murakoshi N, Sekiguchi Y, Kuga K, Aonuma K (2018) Radiofrequency catheter ablation of ventricular tachycardia in patients with hypertrophic cardiomyopathy and apical aneurysm. JACC Clin Electrophysiol 4(3):339–350. https://doi.org/10.1016/j.jacep.2017.12.020

Jaïs P, Maury P, Khairy P, Sacher F, Nault I, Komatsu Y, Hocini M, Forclaz A, Jadidi AS, Weerasooryia R, Shah A, Derval N, Cochet H, Knecht S, Miyazaki S, Linton N, Rivard L, Wright M, Wilton SB, Scherr D, Pascale P, Roten L, Pederson M, Bordachar P, Laurent F, Kim SJ, Ritter P, Clementy J, Haïssaguerre M (2012) Elimination of local abnormal ventricular activities: a new end point for substrate modification in patients with scar-related ventricular tachycardia. Circulation 125(18):2184–2196. https://doi.org/10.1161/CIRCULATIONAHA.111.043216

Kirubakaran S, Bisceglia C, Silberbauer J, Oloriz T, Santagostino G, Yamase M, Maccabelli G, Trevisi N, Bella DP (2017) Characterization of the arrhythmogenic substrate in patients with arrhythmogenic right ventricular cardiomyopathy undergoing ventricular tachycardia ablation. Europace 19(6):1049–1062. https://doi.org/10.1093/europace/euw062

Liang E, Wu L, Fan S, Hu F, Zheng L, Liu S, Fan X, Chen G, Ding L, Niu G, Yao Y (2020) Catheter ablation of arrhythmogenic right ventricular cardiomyopathy ventricular tachycardia: 18-year experience in 284 patients. Europace 22(5):806–812. https://doi.org/10.1093/europace/euaa046

Oloriz T, Silberbauer J, Maccabelli G, Mizuno H, Baratto F, Kirubakaran S, Vergara P, Bisceglia C, Santagostino G, Marzi A, Sora N, Roque C, Guarracini F, Tsiachris D, Radinovic A, Cireddu M, Sala S, Gulletta S, Paglino G, Mazzone P, Trevisi N, Bella DP (2014) Catheter ablation of ventricular arrhythmia in nonischemic cardiomyopathy: anteroseptal versus inferolateral scar sub-types. Circ Arrhythm Electrophysiol 7(3):414–423. https://doi.org/10.1161/CIRCEP.114.001568

Santangeli P, Di Biase L, Lakkireddy D, Burkhardt JD, Pillarisetti J, Michowitz Y, Sanchez JE, Horton R, Mohanty P, Gallinghouse GJ, Dello Russo A, Casella M, Pelargonio G, Santarelli P, Verma A, Narasimhan C, Shivkumar K, Natale A (2010) Radiofrequency catheter ablation of ventricular arrhythmias in patients with hypertrophic cardiomyopathy: safety and feasibility. Heart Rhythm 7(8):1036–1042. https://doi.org/10.1016/j.hrthm.2010.05.022

Segal OR, Chow AW, Wong T, Trevisi N, Lowe MD, Davies DW, Bella DP, Packer DL, Peters NS (2007) A novel algorithm for determining endocardial VT exit site from 12-lead surface ECG characteristics in human, infarct-related ventricular tachycardia. J Cardiovasc Electrophysiol 18(2):161–168. https://doi.org/10.1111/j.1540-8167.2007.00721.x

Souissi Z, Boulé S, Hermida JS, Doucy A, Mabo P, Pavin D, Anselme F, Auquier N, Ninni S, Coisne A, Brigadeau F, Deken-Delannoy V, Klug D, Lacroix D (2018) Catheter ablation reduces ventricular tachycardia burden in patients with arrhythmogenic right ventricular cardiomyopathy: insights from a north-western French multicentre registry. Europace 20(2):362–369. https://doi.org/10.1093/europace/euw332

Complication Management

Laura Rottner and Andreas Metzner

19.1 Introduction

The rate of periprocedural complications during a catheter ablation is particularly dependent on the type of procedure and the complexity of the cardiac arrhythmia to be treated. The overall complication rate during an atrial fibrillation ablation is 2.9–5.3%; pericardial tamponade, with an incidence of 0.8–2%, is considered the most common serious complication (Cappato et al. 2010; Chun et al. 2017).

In addition to high quality standards for performing clinics and appropriate infrastructure, such as a cooperation with cardiac/thoracic surgery, experienced interventional electrophysiologists and a sufficient procedure volume of the ablation center are crucial to ensure high safety standards.

Supplementary Information The online version contains supplementary material available at https://doi.org/10.1007/978-3-662-65797-3_19. The videos can be accessed individually by clicking the DOI link in the accompanying figure caption or by scanning this link with the SN More Media App.

L. Rottner (✉) · A. Metzner
Universitäres Herz- und Gefäßzentrum Hamburg-Eppendorf, Hamburg, Germany
e-mail: l.rottner@uke.de

A. Metzner
e-mail: a.metzner@uke.de

19.2 Complications

19.2.1 Intervention-related Vascular Complications

Complications during vascular puncture include mispuncture, hematomas including retroperitoneal hematomas, arteriovenous fistula, and pseudoaneurysm. Vascular complications, with an incidence of 0.2–1.5%, are the most common complication during atrial fibrillation ablations (Cappato et al. 2010). The main risk factors for the occurrence of vascular complications are advanced age, female gender, and a BMI (Body Mass Index) > 30, the necessity of an arterial access, and an existing anticoagulant therapy, especially the combination of oral anticoagulation (OAC) and antiplatelet therapy.

Ultrasound-guided puncture during electrophysiological procedures has been proven to reduce intervention-related vascular complications. Furthermore, the introduction of novel oral anticoagulants (NOACs) has further reduced the rate of periprocedural vascular complications (Sorgente and Cappato 2019).

▶ During vascular puncture, some technical aspects should be considered: 1) A too distal puncture of the femoral vein should be avoided. In this area, smaller arterial branches run together with the vein, increasing the risk of accidental arterial puncture and the risk of bleeding and hematomas. 2) If the artery is accidentally punctured by the examiner, the puncture needle should be removed, and the puncture site should be manually compressed for at least one minute before attempting another puncture. If the sheath has already been accidentally inserted, it is advisable to leave it in place until the end of the procedure.

Patients with vascular complications either present during the procedure or in the immediate postprocedural period with pain or swelling at the puncture site, abdominal or lower abdominal pain, or hypotension. In the case of significant blood loss, there is also a drop in hemoglobin levels. Rapid further diagnostics using duplex sonography at the puncture site is then advisable. The suspicion of a retroperitoneal hemorrhage onstitutes an emergency. Immediate confirmation of the diagnosis using computed tomography (CT) and immediate involvement of vascular surgery are indicated. The treatment of intervention-related vascular complications depends on the severity of the complication and ranges from renewed and prolonged compression to interventional treatment to surgery and should be carried out in consultation with vascular specialists.

19.2.2 Pericardial Tamponade

While the incidence of pericardial tamponade during ablation of right-sided tachycardias is low (0.2–0.3%), pericardial tamponade during atrial fibrillation ablation, with an incidence of 0.8–2%, is the most common, serious, and potentially lethal complication (Cappato et al. 2010). More complex ablations and the necessity for transseptal puncture (TSP) increase the risk of pericardial tamponade (Fink et al. 2020). There appears to be a lower risk of its occurrence when using balloon systems compared to radiofrequency (RF)-based ablation (Chun et al. 2017). During catheter ablation of premature ventricular contractions and ventricular tachycardias, an epicardial access is considered an independent risk factor for the occurrence of pericardial tamponade (Fink et al. 2020).

In principle, pressure recording from the transseptal needle is recommended during the TSP, and in many ablation centers, a TSP that is not only fluoroscopically guided but also echocardiographically guided is performed. Orientation based on two fluoroscopic projections (e.g., "right anterior oblique" [RAO] 30° and "left anterior oblique" [LAO] 40°) can also help to avoid complications, particularly mispunctures resulting in pericardial tamponade, during the TSP. While the height of the transseptal puncture site can be assessed particularly well in the LAO projection, the RAO projection allows for an estimation of how far anterior or posterior within the fossa ovalis the puncture is made. Additionally, the contact with the atrial septum or the fossa ovalis can be assessed through a pulse-synchronous movement of a diagnostic catheter in the coronary sinus (CS) and the transseptal sheath. After the TSP, the introduction of a wire and the advancement of the sheath over this wire into the left atrium is a ommon strategy to first detect a mispuncture early and second ensure safe maneuvering in the left atrium. The assumption that the use of a force-sensing catheter system reduces the incidence of pericardial tamponades has not yet been sufficiently confirmed in clinical studies.

▶ The first clinical sign of a pericardial tamponade is sudden hypotension. In this case, rapid orientation using fluoroscopy in the LAO 40° projection is recommended. In the event of a pericardial tamponade, the distance between the CS catheter and the lateral heart shadow increases, and the contraction of the lateral heart shadow is significantly reduced or completely absent. The diagnosis should then be immediately confirmed echocardiographically (Figs. 19.1 und 19.2).

If the suspected diagnosis is confirmed, a pericardial puncture—about 1–2 cm subxiphoidal—should be performed to access the pericardial space and allow the insertion of a sheath and subsequently a pigtail catheter (Fig. 19.3). A pre-prepared pericardial puncture set with all necessary materials should be readily available in the EP lab (Fig. 19.4).

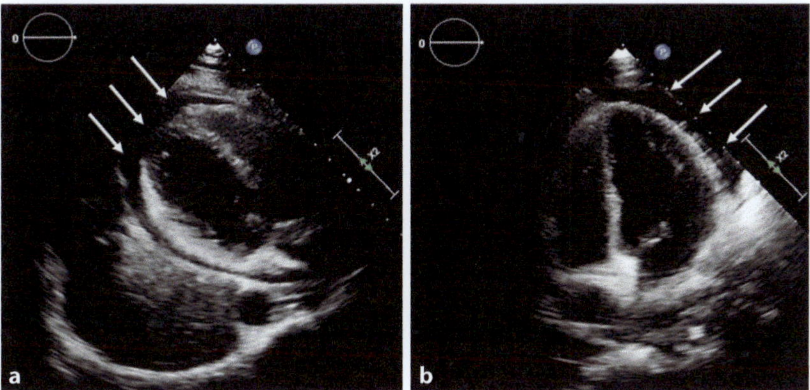

Fig. 19.1 The figure shows a typical echocardiographic image of a significant pericardial effusion from subxiphoidal (**a**) as well as in the four-chamber view (**b**). The *white arrows* mark the effusion margin

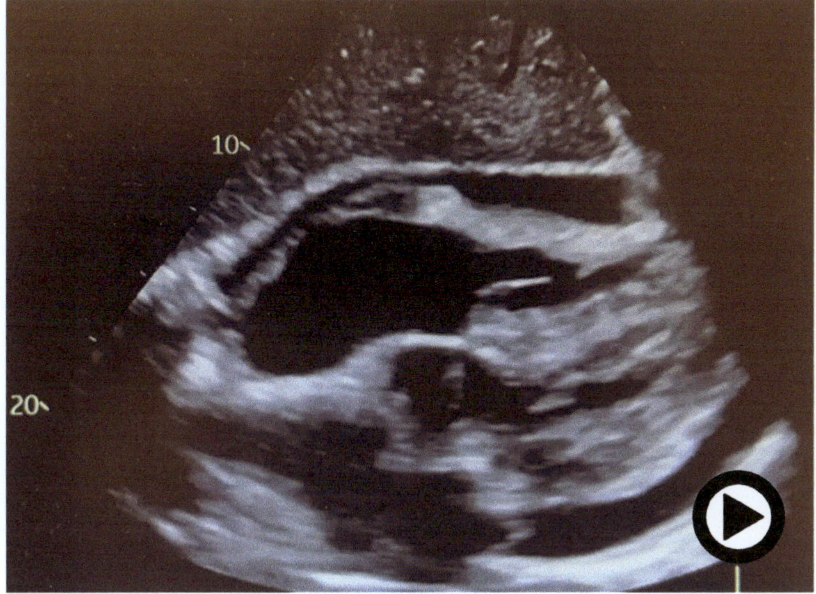

Fig. 19.2 Echocardiographic evidence of a pericardial tamponade with swinging heart phenomenon. Compression of the right heart chambers during diastole (https://doi.org/10.1007/000-d32)

It is recommended to perform the pericardiocentesis fluoroscopically supported in an anteroposterior (AP) or LAO-90° projection. During needle insertion, ventricular extrasystoles in the ECG may indicate penetration of the right ventricular myocardium. A correct puncture can be verified fluoroscopically by the positioning of the wire in the pericardium. The wire should project over the entire heart shadow or all heart chambers (Fig. 19.5).

Additionally, a contrast agent injection can confirm the position of the sheath or pigtail catheter in the pericardial space. After relief, the hemodynamic situation can usually be stabilized immediately. When administering protamine, the risk of hyperreactive coagulation with thrombus formation, especially in the pericardial space itself or in the drain, should be considered, as aspiration is no longer possible. Therefore, the administration of protamine is discussed

Fig. 19.3 Pericardial puncture
in AP orientation, recognizable
by the central position of the
spine. The correct position of the
wire is indicated by its course
along the heart shadow. This can
be confirmed in a second plane.
Then follows the advancement of
the sheath and the drainage via a
pigtail catheter (not shown here)
(https://doi.org/10.1007/000-d31)

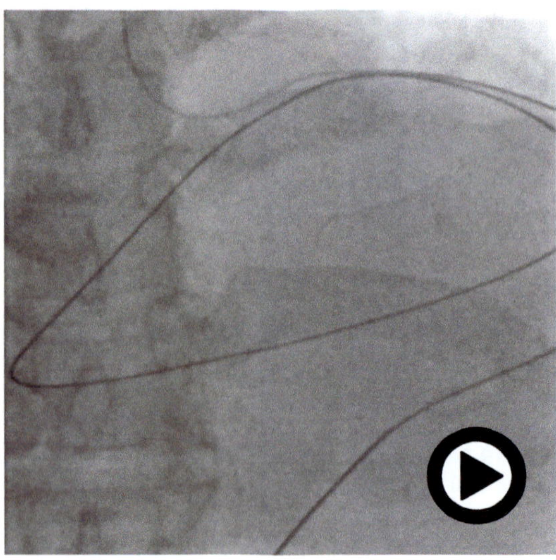

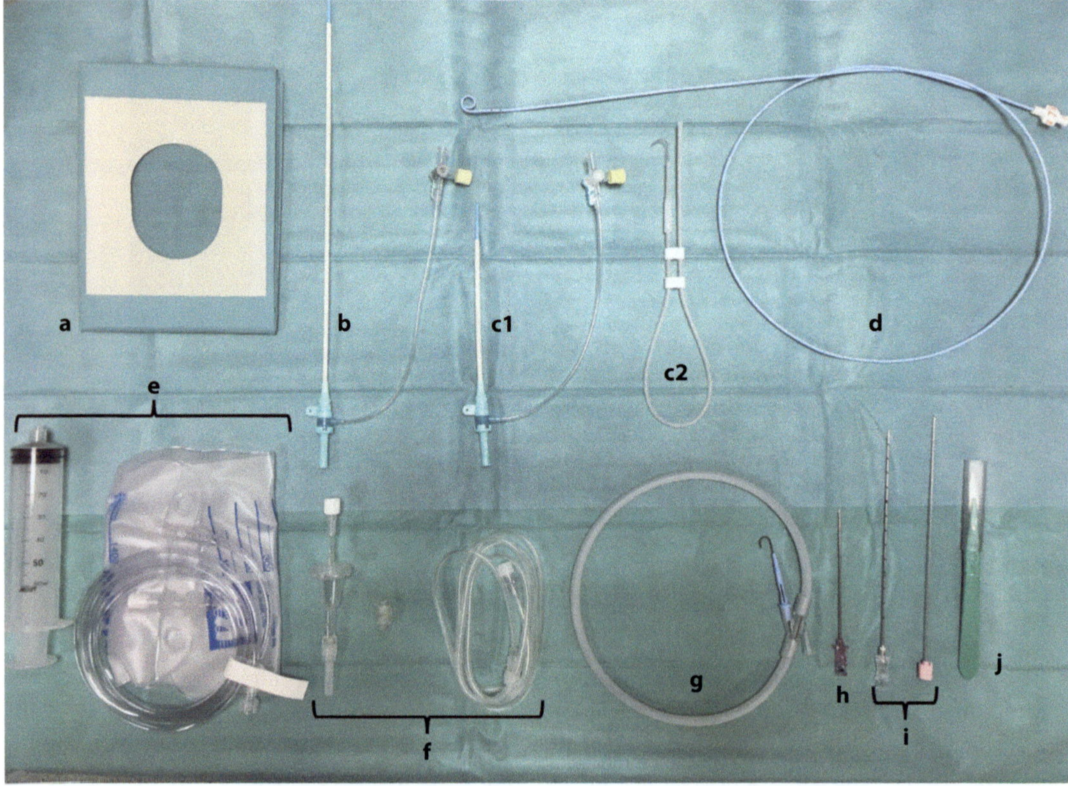

Fig. 19.4 The figure shows a typical pericardiocentesis set with the corresponding materials. **a** Drape, **b** optional long sheath (8 French), **c1** or short sheath (8 French), **c2** and corresponding wire, **d** pigtail catheter (7 French), **e** aspiration syringe with corresponding bag, **f** filter including connection for autotransfusion, **g** long J-wire, **h** conventional puncture needle, **i** Tuohy puncture needle, **j** scalpel

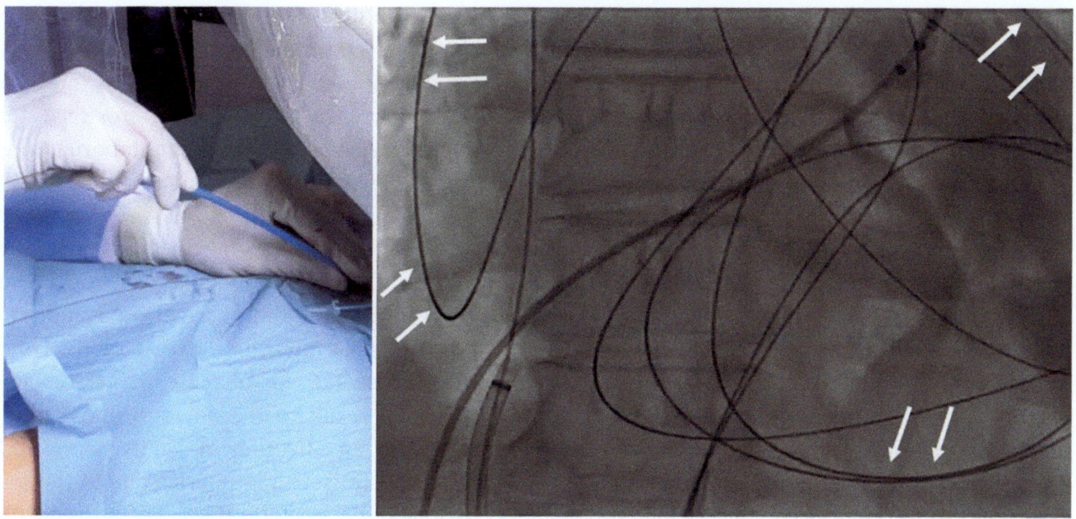

Fig. 19.5 The inserted wire covers all four heart chambers after pericardiocentesis, confirming the correct position of the wire in the pericardial space

only after complete drainage of the pericardium. The administration of specific antidotes in patients on NOAC therapy or the substitution of blood components must also be considered as potential options (Hindricks et al. 2021).

Complication management includes the early involvement of cardiac surgery with interdisciplinary case discussion, especially and at the latest in the absence of hemostasis with persistent pericardial effusion. About 13% of all pericardial tamponades require surgical treatment (Fink et al. 2020).

19.2.3 Aortic Mis-puncture in the Context of Transseptal Puncture

The literature shows a highly variable complication rate for TSP, ranging from less than 1% to nearly 7%. It is particularly dependent on the experience of the operator. Aortic mis-puncture in the context of TSP is a rare but potentially fatal complication. Depending on the location of the mis-puncture (non-coronary aortic sinus, sinotubular junction, or ascending aorta), the consequences range from merely a small pericardial effusion to severe tamponade requiring surgical intervention (Chen et al. 2019).

▶ Strategies for preventing an aortic mis-puncture or for early detection of such include the following: 1) Placement of a His catheter to mark the most caudal aspect of the aortic root (corresponding to the non-coronary cusp of the aortic valve) and, if necessary, the insertion of a wire/(pigtail) catheter retrogradely through the aorta to mark the aortic root; 2) Use of pressure monitoring on the transseptal puncture needle; 3) Contrast agent injection through the transseptal puncture needle to visualize the fossa ovalis or after TSP to stain the left atrium; and 4) Use of transesophageal echocardiography (TOE) or intracardiac echocardiography (ICE) during TSP. An anterior TSP is particularly associated with an increased risk of aortic puncture.

If a transseptal mis-puncture into the aorta is suspected, contrast agent (CA) should be carefully injected through the puncture needle. The puncture with the transseptal puncture needle itself is usually minimally traumatic and rarely results in pericardial tamponade. However, if a dilator or even a sheath has been introduced into the aorta, a long wire should first be inserted through the sheath into the aorta to secure the position and access. The sheath and dilator should initially be left in their existing position. Subsequently, intraprocedural fluoroscopic and echocardiographic imaging of the aortic root is recommended to identify the exact puncture site. For this purpose, a pigtail catheter can be introduced retrogradely through the aorta into the aortic root and CA can be injected. A TOE to evaluate a possible pericardial effusion and/ or shunts between the right atrium and aortic root/ascending aorta should be additionally performed. Involving experienced interventional colleagues as well as cardiac or vascular surgery or interventional angiologists is generally advisable to discuss further means.

19.2.4 Thermal Esophageal Lesions and Atrio-Esophageal Fistula

Radiofrequency and, more rarely, cryoablation in patients with left atrial arrhythmias can cause thermal damage to the esophagus due to its proximity to the left atrium (Fig. 19.6).

The feared, but rare, atrio-esophageal fistula often has a fatal outcome. Its incidence is 0.03 to 0.1% (Cappato et al. 2010; Han et al. 2017). The following constellations can contribute to diagnostic confirmation: the documentation of esophageal ulcers combined with the detection of fistula formation to the atrium, such as

through embolic events and air embolisms or direct visual confirmation of the atrio-esophageal connection at the time of surgical intervention. The presence of esophageal erosions after catheter ablation is considered an important predictor for potential fistula formation and should be regularly monitored by endoscopies (Han et al. 2017). The underlying mechanism of the formation of an atrio-esophageal fistula is not yet fully understood, but thermal injury appears to be the most plausible explanation. Other approaches include an increase in gastric acid content as a result of the ablation, most likely mediated by an affection of vagus nerve endings, as well as ischemic injuries due to thermal occlusions of the end arterioles. The atrio-esophageal fistula seems to occur most frequently in the context of RF-based ablations. Newer ablation techniques such as electroporation appear to have a favorable safety profile in this regard, but long-term data are still lacking. The type of clinical presentation varies but is often a complex scenario consisting of fever, sepsis, and neurological events up to death. The average time from the ablation procedure to presentation is 14–20 days. The diagnostic method of choice is thoracic CT. An endoscopy or TOE is contraindicated in clinical suspicion of fistula formation, as air insufflation massively increases the risk of embolization and mechanical irritation can exacerbate the lesion. Surgical intervention is considered a recognized treatment option. Esophageal stenting is considered an alternative, but there are only case reports on this. Surgical

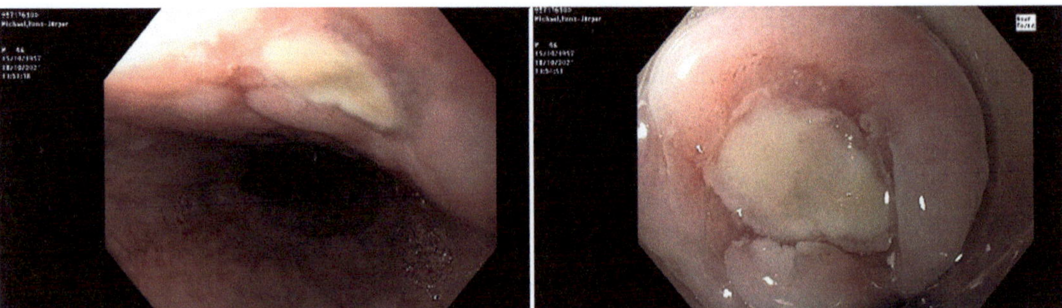

Fig. 19.6 Esophago-gastro-duodenoscopy showing a typical image of a small (5 mm) esophageal lesion three days after RF-based atrial fibrillation ablation

intervention is associated with a mortality rate of up to 34% (Sorgente and Cappato 2019; Han et al. 2017).

▶ To prevent atrio-esophageal fistula, the following points should be observed: 1) Reducing ablation time and energy as well as contact pressure during ablation at the posterior wall of the left atrium, 2) the use of esophageal temperature probes can be helpful through fluoroscopic visualization of the esophagus; particularly in the context of cryo- and laser balloon-based procedures, their use seems effective and safe, although the data for their use in RF-based ablations is inconsistent. 3) The prescription of proton pump inhibitors for four weeks post-procedurally serves to prevent esophageal erosions and ulcers, although there is no reliable data that this therapy is associated with a reduced incidence of fistula formation.

19.2.5 AV Block in the Context of Catheter Ablation

Periprocedural AV blockages in the context of cardiac interventions are not uncommon. In addition to cardiac surgical procedures, transcatheter aortic valve replacement (TAVI), and transcoronary ablation of septal hypertrophy (TASH) in hypertrophic obstructive cardiomyopathy, this occurs most frequently during catheter ablations in anatomical proximity to the AV node region. Atrioventricular nodal reentrant tachycardia (AVNRT) is the most common procedure in this context, with a prevalence of about 0.25%. In cases of recurrent symptomatic episodes, catheter ablation is considered the therapy of choice with a success rate between 95-98% (Hindricks et al. 2021). Complications—particularly AV blockages—are possible during the procedure due to the proximity to the conduction system.

▶ To address significant bradycardia in such cases, the possibility of periprocedural ventricular stimulation—for example, by positioning a catheter in the right ventricle—should be ensured. A prerequisite is stable ventricular capture with adapted output at the beginning of the procedure.

The RF-based ablation or modification of the "slow pathway" is associated with an incidence of acute, complete, and permanent AV blockages of 0.1–2%. Also, in the context of interventional therapy for patients with symptomatic atrioventricular reentrant tachycardias (AVRT), there is a risk of AV blockages, particularly in the case of a paraseptal accessory pathway, but with a prevalence of 0.1%, it is significantly lower (Sorgente and Cappato 2019; Kesek et al. 2019). In the context of catheter ablation of ventricular arrhythmias, the literature reports an incidence of relevant AV blockages of just under 2%, most frequently described for ventricular tachycardias involving the conduction system, such as fascicular tachycardias. The His bundle can also be mechanically compromised during mapping—particularly of the left ventricle—without energy delivery in the area of the conduction system. Patients with pre-existing conduction disorders generally represent a group with increased risk in this context. A mechanically induced AV block usually resolves spontaneously within seconds to a few minutes. Reports from smaller case series show a tendency for AV node recovery in the event of an AV block during ablation after administration of intravenous prednisolone (e.g., bolus injection of 250 mg intravenously, followed by an oral maintenance therapy of 50 mg over five days) and suggest a possible benefit regarding the rate of permanent AV blockages with an indication for definitive pacemaker implantation. Due to a potential recovery tendency of the AV node even after several days, pacemaker implantation should be considered no earlier than 72 hours after an iatrogenic AV block (Parwani et al. 2017).

19.2.6 Air Embolism

Air embolism is a rare but potentially serious complication in the context of endovascular procedures and is associated with increased morbidity and mortality. Air embolism is particularly severe when cerebral vessels or coronary vessels are affected. There are numerous case series that report air embolisms with an acute occlusion—especially of the right—coronary artery, which in extreme scenarios only become noticeable through an acutely occurring cardiac arrest (Ahmad et al. 2016).

The clinical symptoms are nonspecific. Since most electrophysiological procedures take place under analgesia or even general anesthesia, a diagnosis in these cases can often only be made through objective findings. These include hypoxia and hypercapnia, ST-segment changes in the ECG, the occurrence of malignant cardiac arrhythmias, as well as hemodynamic compromise and sinus arrest with asystole or higher-grade AV blockages. If the erebral vessels are affected, intra-procedurally there is often only hypotension, and in the case of pronounced ischemia, a pupil difference can also occur, which in most cases and without regular pupil control—as is not common in most electrophysiological labs peri-procedurally—initially remains undetected. Acute neurological deficits usually only become noticeable after the patient awakens.

Thorough preparation of the equipment necessary for the procedure is crucial, with continuous flushing of the transseptal sheaths being mandatory. Furthermore, particular attention should be paid to thorough aspiration when inserting or changing catheters. The insertion of catheters and catheter changes should, if possible, not occur during deep inspiration (Yokoyama et al. 2022).

▶ If air entry into the vascular system is suspected or has occurred, the sheath flushing should be stopped immediately and extensive aspiration should be performed. Additionally, an immediate withdrawal of the sheaths and catheters into the right atrium is recommended.

Furthermore, treatment with oxygen should be initiated or intensified to improve end-organ oxygenation. High-flow ventilation can also support the reabsorption of nitrogen from the "bubbles" into the blood, thereby reducing the extent of the air embolism. If air embolism into the coronary vessels is suspected and the ST-segment elevations do not spontaneously regress within a few minutes, performing a coronary angiography with possible aspiration of the air using a thrombus aspiration catheter is required. In the case of a cerebral air embolism with neurological deficits, hyperbaric oxygen therapy can be considered. If this is done within the first six hours, a good neurological outcome can be expected (Ahmad et al. 2016).

19.2.7 Thromboembolic Cerebrovascular Events

Catheter ablation is an invasive procedure in which air can enter the circulatory system through the introduction of sheaths and catheters and cause cerebrovascular events as an air embolism, which is considered an important pathophysiological mechanism for periprocedural cerebrovascular complications in the context of catheter ablations (Yokoyama et al. 2022). Other mechanisms include the formation of blood clots on the surface of the catheter systems, charring with clot formation at the tip of RF catheters during energy delivery, and plaque dislodgement, for example, when passing the aortic arch (Sorgente and Cappato 2019).

The incidence of embolisms in the context of atrial fibrillation ablation ranges between 0.1 and 7% (Cappato et al. 2010). Diagnosis can be made quickly in awake patients but can be significantly delayed by sedation. The assessment of neurological status post-procedurally, as well as the exclusion of pericardial effusion, is part of the mandatory follow-up examinations immediately after an electrophysiological intervention. In the event of a cerebrovascular event or for diagnosis and therapy, close collaboration with the department of neurology and (neuro-)radiology is essential and is a mandatory component of the certification process as an atrial fibrillation center by the German Society of Cardiology in Germany.

Avoiding embolic events, in addition to adhering to technical aspects such as catheter flushing and heparin administration according to the respective target ACT ("activated clotting time") during the ablation procedure—at least for all left atrial procedures—is directly related to the anticoagulation regimen before and after ablation. In a meta-analysis of twelve studies, uninterrupted anticoagulation using new NOACs versus vitamin K antagonists (VKAs) in the context of atrial fibrillation ablation was associated with lower rates of transient ischemic attacks and strokes (NOAC 0.08% versus VKA 0.16%) and comparable rates of silent cerebral embolic events. However, severe bleeding was significantly reduced by the use of NOACs (0.9%) compared to VKAs (2%) (Cardoso et al. 2018). Current guidelines recommend resuming anticoagulation in the evening after the procedure (2–6 hours post-procedurally) or the next morning in the case of interrupted anticoagulation. Bridging with unfractionated heparin is no longer recommended due to increased rates of bleeding complications (Hindricks et al. 2021). Since it is still controversial whether atrial fibrillation ablation reliably and long-term reduces the risk of stroke, it is recommended to continue OAC long-term according to the individual CHA_2DS_2VASc score.

19.2.8 Pulmonary Vein Stenosis

Pulmonary vein stenosis is classified as mild (50%), moderate (50–70%), and severe (> 70%), with severe pulmonary vein stenosis being one of the most serious and poorly treatable complications in the context of atrial fibrillation ablations. It mostly affects younger men.

Pulmonary vein stenosis emerged as an unanticipated complication after the introduction of pulmonary vein isolation (PVI) in the early 1990s. The heating of the tissue during RF ablation results in proliferation and fibrotic remodeling, leading to a pulmonary vein neointima, which in the long term causes a reduction in the pulmonary vein lumen and, in the worst case, a complete occlusion. After the first incidents, the approach to PVI quickly shifted from ostial to antral ablation strategy, which dramatically reduced the incidence. Not least because of this, the creation of antral lesions is considered the most important measure to avoid this serious complication (Kuck et al. 2018).

▶ The first symptoms of pulmonary vein stenosis appear significantly delayed after ablation (weeks to months) and range from chest pain, cough, and dyspnea to hemoptysis. The initial diagnosis is often made due to recurrent pneumonia, so any unexpected episode of pneumonia in a patient after atrial fibrillation ablation should raise suspicion of pulmonary vein stenosis. Cryoballoon-based PVI is apparently associated with a lower incidence of pulmonary vein narrowing than ablation using high-frequency current (Kuck et al. 2018).

For diagnosis, a CT scan is recommended. Alternatively, pulmonary vein stenosis can also be diagnosed using TEE and flow acceleration measurement within the pulmonary veins, as well as ventilation-perfusion scintigraphy.

In principle, conservative therapy ("watch and wait"), interventional treatment with pulmonary vein angioplasty and possibly stenting (Fig. 19.7), and surgical treatment are available as therapeutic strategies. Prospective randomized studies on the treatment options are lacking.

The indication for therapy depends on the severity and symptoms. In general, asymptomatic and mildly symptomatic patients only require close follow-up, while symptomatic patients should be referred for pulmonary vein angioplasty. There are only a few case reports or smaller studies on long-term outcomes after interventional therapy. In principle, however, recurrence after angioplasty seems to occur in at least half of the cases. To prevent restenosis, stenting is recommended instead of pure angioplasty, with bare-metal stents apparently being superior to drug-eluting stents (Fink et al. 2018). Regarding the post-interventional anticoagulation regimen, there are no general

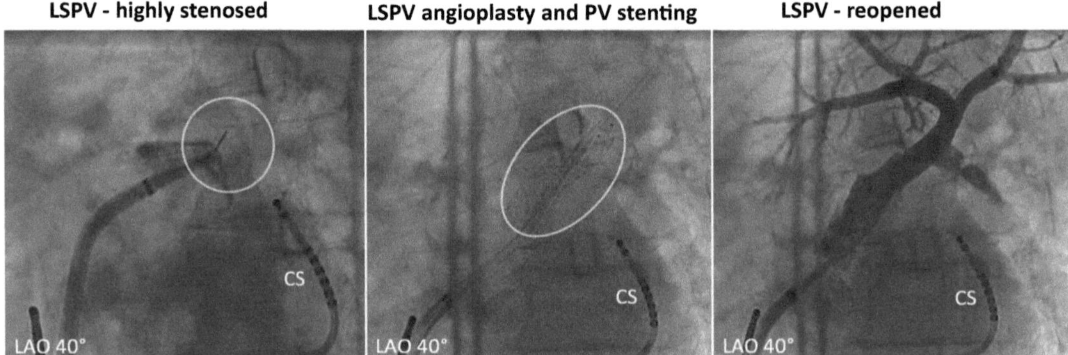

Fig. 19.7 Patient with dyspnea and recurrent pneumonia six months after RF-based PVI. Echocardiographically and in CT, evidence of significant pulmonary vein stenosis of the left upper pulmonary vein. After interdisciplinary discussion, decision for interventional therapy with balloon angioplasty and subsequent PV stenting. Finally, evidence of a good angiographic result. In follow-up, patient free of symptoms. LAO 40° = left-anterior oblique 40°; CS = coronary sinus catheter; LSPV = left upper pulmonary vein

recommendations. Individual decision-making should be based on the stent size and the degree of the treated lesion. Most centers prescribe triple therapy with aspirin, clopidogrel, and NOAC for 3–6 months, followed by long-term aspirin therapy or NOAC depending on the CHA_2DS_2VASc score.

19.3 Summary and Conclusion for Practice

Catheter ablation of cardiac arrhythmias is an established therapeutic option. The incidence of complications is particularly dependent on the type of procedure and the ablation system used; complex ablation treatments are associated with an increased risk. In the context of atrial fibrillation ablation, a pericardial tamponade occurs with an incidence of 0.8–2% and is thus the most common serious complication.

Despite significant technological advancements, serious complications in the context of catheter interventions cannot be completely avoided. In addition to high-quality standards for performing clinics and appropriate infrastructure, experienced operators are crucial to avoid, promptly recognize, and, if necessary, adequately treat periprocedural complications.

References

Ahmad K, Asirvatham S, Kamath S, Peck S, Liu X (2016) Successful interventional management of catastrophic coronary arterial air embolism during atrial fibrillation ablation. Heart Rhythm Case Rep 2(2):153–156

Cappato R, Calkins H, Chen SA, Davies W, Iesaka Y, Kalman J et al (2010) Updated worldwide survey on the methods, efficacy, and safety of catheter ablation for human atrial fibrillation. Circ Arrhythm Electrophysiol 3(1):32–38

Cardoso R, Knijnik L, Bhonsale A, Miller J, Nasi G, Rivera M et al (2018) An updated meta-analysis of novel oral anticoagulants versus vitamin K antagonists for uninterrupted anticoagulation in atrial fibrillation catheter ablation. Heart Rhythm 15(1):107–115

Chen H, Fink T, Zhan X, Chen M, Eckardt L, Long D et al (2019) Inadvertent transseptal puncture into the aortic root: the narrow edge between luck and catastrophe in interventional cardiology. Europace 21(7):1106–1115

Chun KRJ, Perrotta L, Bordignon S, Khalil J, Dugo D, Konstantinou A et al (2017) Complications in catheter ablation of atrial fibrillation in 3,000 consecutive procedures: balloon versus radiofrequency current ablation. JACC Clin Electrophysiol 3(2):154–161

Fink T, Schluter M, Heeger CH, Lemes C, Lin T, Maurer T et al (2018) Pulmonary vein stenosis or occlusion after catheter ablation of atrial fibrillation: long-term comparison of drug-eluting versus large bare metal stents. Europace 20(10):e148–e155

Fink T, Sciacca V, Feickert S, Metzner A, Lin T, Schluter M et al (2020) Outcome of cardiac tamponades in interventional electrophysiology. Europace 22(8):1240–1251

Han HC, Ha FJ, Sanders P, Spencer R, Teh AW, O'Donnell D et al (2017) Atrioesophageal fistula: clinical presentation, procedural characteristics, diagnostic investigations, and treatment outcomes. Circ Arrhythm Electrophysiol 10(11):e005579

Hindricks G, Potpara T, Dagres N, Arbelo E, Bax JJ, Blomstrom-Lundqvist C et al (2021) 2020 ESC Guidelines for the diagnosis and management of atrial fibrillation developed in collaboration with the European Association of Cardio-Thoracic Surgery (EACTS). Eur Heart J 42:373–498

Kesek M, Lindmark D, Rashid A, Jensen SM (2019) Increased risk of late pacemaker implantation after ablation for atrioventricular nodal reentry tachycardia: A 10-year follow-up of a nationwide cohort. Heart Rhythm 16(8):1182–1188

Kuck KH, Fink T, Metzner A (2018) Pulmonary vein stenosis and occlusion following catheter ablation of atrial fibrillation: still worth worrying about? JACC Cardiovasc Interv 11(16):1640–1641

Parwani AS, Schroder AI, Blaschke D, Blaschke F, Huemer M, Attanasio P et al (2017) Third-degree AV block sensitive to prednisolone 72 hours post AVNRT ablation. Clin Case Rep 5(5):671–674

Sorgente A, Cappato R (2019) Complications of catheter ablation: incidence, diagnosis and clinical management. Herzschrittmacherther Elektrophysiol 30(4):363–370

Yokoyama M, Tokuda M, Tokutake K, Sato H, Oseto H, Yokoyama K et al (2022) Effect of air removal with extracorporeal balloon inflation on incidence of asymptomatic cerebral embolism during cryoballoon ablation of atrial fibrillation: a prospective randomized study. Int J Cardiol Heart Vasc 40:101020

Martin Borlich and Philipp Sommer

20.1 Introduction

For many years, the anatomical localization of catheters during the ablation of cardiac arrhythmias was performed exclusively using fluoroscopy. The radiation used is associated with the risk of stochastic and deterministic radiation damage. This applies to both patients and the staff in the EP lab. Users are encouraged to keep radiation exposure during electrophysiological procedures as low as possible (ALARA principle).

The use of modern 3D mapping systems, advances in catheter technology, and the possibilities of additional diagnostic tools such as intracardiac echocardiography (ICE) have significantly reduced or even eliminated the need for fluoroscopic imaging. Given the increase in electrophysiological procedures worldwide, electrophysiologists are more than ever encouraged to be aware of the issue of ionizing radiation and to establish a setup in the catheter lab that includes not only the optimal use of the 3D

mapping system used but also ideal settings of the X-ray system. This chapter provides options for implementing the ALARA principle in electrophysiological procedures as well as options for protection against ionizing radiation.

20.2 General Recommendations

The ALARA principle ("as low as reasonably achievable") is the core statement of radiation protection and demands that radiation exposure (even below limit values) be kept as low as reasonably achievable when dealing with ionizing radiation. The basics rules are rule is the 4A rule: Keep the activity as low as possible, the distance as large as possible, the shielding as strong as possible, and the duration as short as possible.

In addition to the predominantly technical or equipment-based options for reducing radiation exposure described below, appropriate training and "awareness" during education play an outstanding role in avoiding unnecessary radiation exposure for patients and staff.

20.3 Settings on the X-ray Scanner

In principle, permanent changes to the settings for use in pulsed fluoroscopy and video recording ("Cine-loop") can be distinguished from

M. Borlich (✉)
Segeberger Kliniken GmbH, Bad Segeberg,
Germany
e-mail: martin.borlich@segebergerkliniken.de

P. Sommer
Herz- und Diabeteszentrum NRW, Bad Oeynhausen,
Germany
e-mail: psommer@hdz-nrw.de

L. Iden et al. (eds.), *Invasive Electrophysiology for Beginners*, https://doi.org/10.1007/978-3-662-70158-4_20

temporary adjustments required for the respective procedure. For most electrophysiological procedures requiring pulsed fluoroscopy, three pulses per second are sufficient for basic fluoroscopy and 7.5 pulses per second (fps) for video recordings. Collimation to the minimally required visual fluoroscopic field (collimation) and the use of low magnification and low tube voltages also lead to a reduction in radiation exposure (Walters et al. 2012). Fluoroscopy time should be kept as short as possible, and the detector should ideally be positioned close to the patient's body as possible. This improves image quality and reduces skin entrance dose.

The effective reduction of radiation dose through fluoroscopy with low or very low frame rates without relevant impairment of therapeutic efficacy is well documented (Crowhurst et al. 2017; Lee et al. 2017). Manufacturers of X-ray systems also offer low-dose imaging protocols specifically designed for use in electrophysiological procedures. For example, the commonly used Artis-Zee system from Siemens offers such a low-dose protocol, in which only 8 nGy entrance dose of the detector is used for fluoroscopy and 36 nGy for cine-loops. Bourier et al. demonstrated in 2016 that this protocol reduces the X-ray dose by 77% compared to standard protocols, without changes in procedure or RF times and without increasing complication rates.

Fluoroscopic images were taken at 3 fps and a tube voltage of 90 kV, cine-loops at 7.5 fps with a tube voltage of 81 kV (Bourier et al. 2016). In terms of radiation protection, working with these low-dose protocols for electrophysiological procedures should become standard.

20.4 Options for Fluoroscopic Image Integration (CARTOUNIVU™ and MediGuide™)

Another way to minimize the use of fluoroscopy is the combined display of fluoroscopic images or cine-loops with the three-dimensional map (e.g., with CARTOUNIVU). On the other hand, non-fluoroscopic catheter visualization systems such as MediGuide allow catheter navigation in real-time, displayed against the background of stored X-ray sequences. Anatomical localization is facilitated in that repeated use of X-rays for the localization of catheters in relation to anatomical structures is not necessary.

20.4.1 CARTOUNIVU

The CARTOUNIVU™ module (Biosense Webster, Inc., Diamond Bar, CA, USA) seamlessly integrates fluoroscopic images and maps generated by the CARTO® 3 system into a single view (Fig. 20.3). It works with various fluoroscopy systems from different manufacturers. The initial installation of the CARTOUNIVU™ module is specific to the X-ray system used in the respective catheter lab.

An initial registration is performed, during which the position of the registration disk on the "Location pad" is fluoroscopically detected and stored relative to the table position (Fig. 20.1).

This enables the system to calculate the exact position of the localization unit respective to the C-arm of the fluoroscopy system. The now registered relationship between the two systems applies to the acquisition of all other images and cine-loops of each procedure. Every fluoroscopic image or cine-loop captured with the fluoroscopy system is automatically transferred over the network to the CARTOUNIVU™ module and stored precisely in the acquisition projection. When the map is rotated to a projection with a stored fluoroscopic image, the catheter positions are displayed in real-time along with the registered fluoroscopic image. The use of CARTOUNIVU™ leads to a significant reduction in total fluoroscopy time and mean radiation dose without affecting the procedure duration (Cano et al. 2015). This applies to a wide range of treated cardiac arrhythmias (Christoph et al. 2015) (Fig. 20.2).

20.4.2 MediGuide

MediGuide™ (St. Jude Medical Inc., Saint Paul, MN, USA) is a non-fluoroscopic catheter

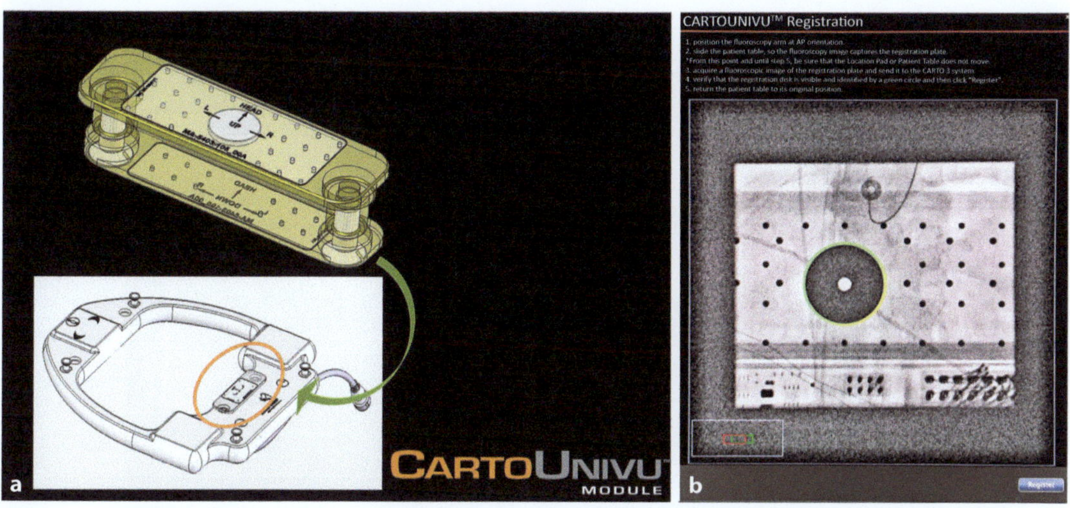

Fig. 20.1 **a** Illustration of the registration disk attached to the Location pad of the CARTO® 3 system (© Johnson & Johnson). **b** Registration window of CARTOUNIVU™ with successful detection of the registration disk

visualization system (NFCV) that enables real-time catheter navigation, which is overlaid with previously recorded X-ray sequences. The system consists of a transmitting unit that generates a three-dimensional electromagnetic field. This unit is connected to the detector of the X-ray system and automatically aligns the fluoroscopy field with the three-dimensional magnetic sensor field. A miniaturized single-coil sensor (< 1 mm^3) is located at the tip of a MediGuide™-enabled catheter and can thus be tracked in real-time in the sensor field without the use of X-ray radiation. A magnetic field reference sensor is attached to the patient and serves as a reference sensor for the calculation of the catheter position and the compensation of motion artifacts caused by breathing and patient activity. MediGuide™ is automatically registered thanks to system integration at the hardware level. Multiple catheters can be displayed by the system simultaneously. For initialization, the recording of two short fluoroscopy loops (usually in RAO and LAO) is required (Sommer et al. 2014, 2018). Subsequently, "sensor-enabled SE" diagnostic and ablation catheters can be visualized in real-time. A three-dimensional mapping system is used in conjunction with the MediGuide™ system for geometry creation (Fig. 20.3).

The most common electrophysiological procedure, pulmonary vein isolation, can be performed using this system with a fluoroscopy time of less than 1 min and a correspondingly low dose-area product (Sommer et al. 2018).

20.5 Intracardiac Echocardiography (ICE)

Intracardiac echocardiography (ICE) enables real-time imaging of anatomical structures during electrophysiological procedures without the use of fluoroscopy. ICE is not widely used in Europe due to high costs and challenging reimbursement situations. There are two types of ICE imaging systems: the mechanical ultrasound catheter radial imaging system (e.g., ULTRA ICE™, Boston Scientific, USA) and the electronic phased-array catheter sector imaging system (e.g., ACUSON AcuNav™, Siemens Medical Solution, USA or ViewFlex™, St. Jude Medical, USA). The former generates a 360° image plane that is perpendicular to the catheter's longitudinal axis. The catheter forms the center of the image. At frequencies of 9 MHz, it provides clear imaging of structures in the near field (up to 5 cm from the transducer) but poor tissue penetration and far-field resolution.

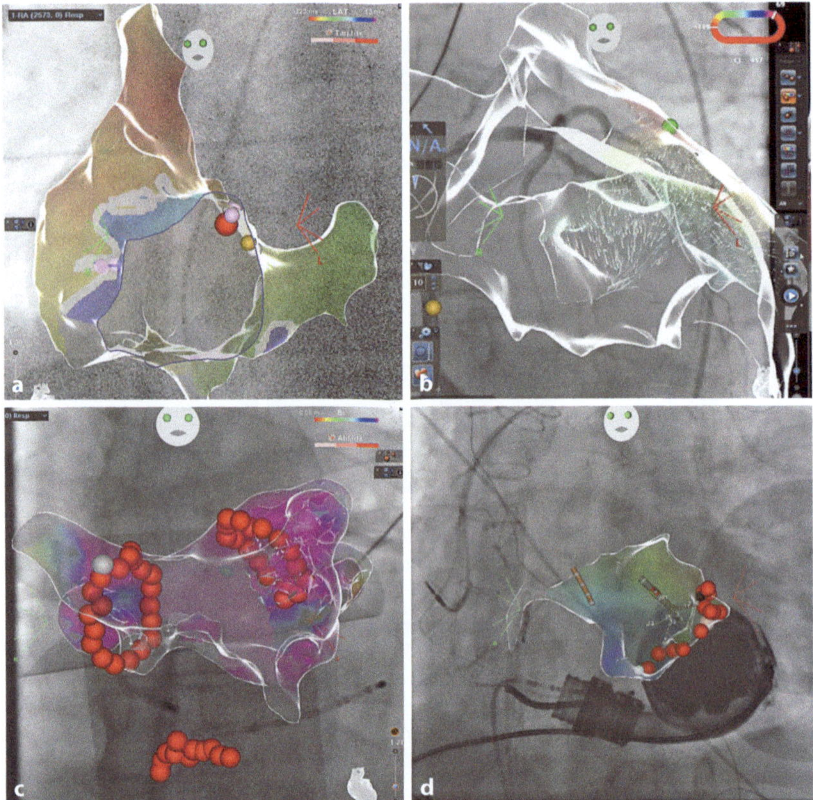

Fig. 20.2 Illustration of the application of the CARTOUNIVU™ module. **a** Ablation of a parahisian accessory pathway in a patient with WPW syndrome; His-marking (yellow) and Visitag at the site of successful ablation. **b** Ablation of a VT with epicardial origin. The angiography of the left coronary arteries was integrated via CARTOUNIVU™ and helped maintain a sufficient safety distance during the ablation. **c** 3D reconstruction and bipolar map of the left atrium and subsequent pulmonary vein isolation and cavotricuspid isthmus block in a patient with paroxysmal atrial fibrillation and typical atrial flutter. **d** LAT map and ablation of a VT in a patient with a left ventricular assist device (LVAD)

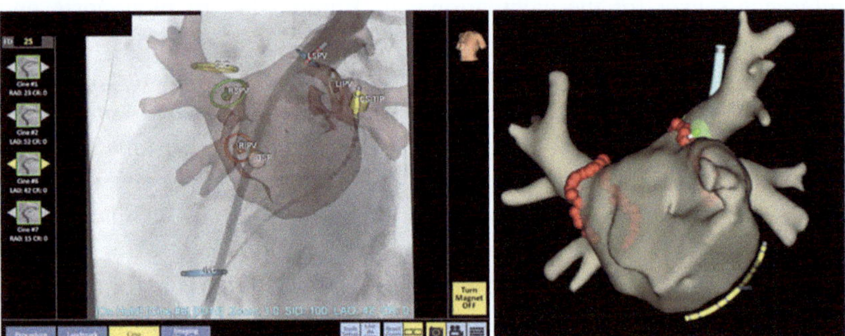

Fig. 20.3 MediGuide™ system and the corresponding three-dimensional reconstruction of the left atrium with EnSite Precision™. The image of a short fluoroscopy loop is displayed on the *left side* in LAO view (42°). The ostia of the four pulmonary veins are marked along with the transseptal puncture site, the tip of the ablation and CS catheter, as well as the inferior and superior vena cava. In the corresponding map on the *right side*, the marked ablation points are shown along with the esophageal probe, the CS, and ablation catheter

In phased-array catheter sector imaging systems, the ultrasound head is attached to the distal end of a steerable catheter. The ultrasound frequencies are variable. Visualization is achieved through a sector transducer that scans along the longitudinal axis, in line with the catheter shaft. This allows for 90° sector imaging, 2D, M-mode, and Doppler imaging with higher tissue penetration (up to 15 cm) and maneuverability of the catheter compared to radial imaging systems. Due to these advantages, phased-array ICE is preferred for most interventional procedures.

ICE is clinically used for transseptal puncture (especially in complex anatomical situations) (see Fig. 20.4), to control catheter position in relation to anatomical structures, to monitor lesion formation, and to quickly diagnose complications such as the development of pericardial effusion.

The ablation of various cardiac arrhythmias with ICE is associated with a significant reduction in fluoroscopy time, fluoroscopy dose, and procedure duration compared to ablation without the use of ICE. These efficiency improvements do not appear to negatively impact the clinical efficacy or safety of the ablation procedure (Goya et al. 2020). Additionally, this method enables fluoroscopy-free catheter ablation of atrial fibrillation and other primarily left atrial arrhythmias (Kautzner et al. 2021). New technologies, such as the NuVision™ catheter (Biosense Webster Inc., USA), allow for real-time intracardiac 3D echocardiography.

Apart from the high costs, this imaging modality has the potential to significantly reduce radiation exposure for patients and examiners and to increase safety in complex procedures, especially in the presence of challenging anatomies.

20.6 Protective Equipment in the EP Lab

A fluoroscopy system will remain an essential component of an electrophysiological lab despite all advancements. In addition to efforts to minimize the use of ionizing radiation, consistent use of fixed and personal protective equipment for radiation protection must continue to be emphasized.

For each X-ray facility used for the application of X-rays on humans, written work instructions must be created for the examinations and treatments frequently performed at that facility. Therefore, reference is made here to the "Work Instructions in the Cardiac Catheterization Laboratory and Hybrid Operating Room," which was created by the German Cardiac Society (DGK) for this purpose in 2015 (Schächinger et al. 2015). Protective measures that comply with the recommendations of the DGK guidelines include fixed permanent protective devices such as lead glass shields or mobile protective walls. Personal protective equipment includes lead aprons, thyroid shields, head coverings, and lead glasses. Additionally, patient-related

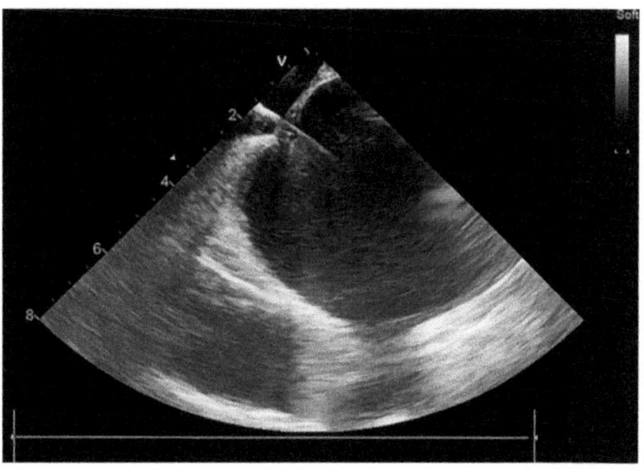

Fig. 20.4 Use of intracardiac echocardiography (ICE) for safe transseptal puncture

coverings such as radiation protection drapes are recommended. The protective equipment used should be regularly subjected to visual and functional inspections.

▶ There are numerous ways today to perform electrophysiological procedures with low radiation exposure for patients and the EP team. Important factors include the regular adjustment of hardware and software settings, attentiveness during the procedure, and the establishment of standardized workflows.

References

Bourier F, Reents T, Ammar-Busch S, Buiatti A, Kottmaier M, Semmler V, Deisenhofer I (2016) Evaluation of a new very low dose imaging protocol: feasibility and impact on X-ray dose levels in electrophysiology procedures. Europace 18(9):1406–1410. https://doi.org/10.1093/europace/euv364

Cano Ó, Alonso P, Osca J, Andrés A, Sancho-Tello MJ, Olagüe J, Martínez-Dolz L (2015) Initial experience with a new image integration module designed for reducing radiation exposure during electrophysiological ablation procedures. J Cardiovasc Electrophysiol 26(6):662–670. https://doi.org/10.1111/jce.12659

Christoph M, Wunderlich C, Moebius S, Forkmann M, Sitzy J, Salmas J, Gaspar T (2015) Fluoroscopy integrated 3D mapping significantly reduces radiation exposure during ablation for a wide spectrum of cardiac arrhythmias. Europace 17(6):928–937. https://doi.org/10.1093/europace/euu334

Crowhurst J, Haqqani H, Wright D, Whitby M, Lee A, Betts J, Denman R (2017) Ultra-low radiation dose during electrophysiology procedures using optimized new generation fluoroscopy technology. Pacing Clin Electrophysiol 40(8):947–954. https://doi.org/10.1111/pace.13141

Goya M, Frame D, Gache L, Ichishima Y, Tayar DO, Goldstein L, Lee SHY (2020) The use of intracardiac echocardiography catheters in endocardial ablation of cardiac arrhythmia: Meta-analysis of efficiency, effectiveness, and safety outcomes. J Cardiovasc Electrophysiol 31(3):664–673. https://doi.org/10.1111/jce.14367

Kautzner J, Haskova J, Lehar F (2021) Intracardiac echocardiography to guide non-fluoroscopic electrophysiology procedures. Card Electrophysiol Clin 13(2):399–408. https://doi.org/10.1016/j.ccep.2021.03.004

Lee JH, Kim J, Kim M, Hwang J, Hwang YM, Kang JW, Kim YH (2017) Extremely low-frame-rate digital fluoroscopy in catheter ablation of atrial fibrillation: A comparison of 2 versus 4 frame rate. Medicine 96(24):e7200. https://doi.org/10.1097/MD.0000000000007200

Schächinger V, Nef V, Achenbach S et al (2015) Arbeitsanweisung in Herzkatheterlabor und Hybridoperationssaal. Kardiologe 9:29–34

Sommer P, Richter S, Hindricks G, Rolf S (2014) Non-fluoroscopic catheter visualization using MediGuide™ technology: experience from the first 600 procedures. J Interv Card Electrophysiol 40(3):209–214. https://doi.org/10.1007/s10840-013-9859-6

Sommer P, Bertagnolli L, Kircher S, Arya A, Bollmann A, Richter S, Hindricks G (2018) Safety profile of near-zero fluoroscopy atrial fibrillation ablation with non-fluoroscopic catheter visualization: experience from 1000 consecutive procedures. Europace. https://doi.org/10.1093/europace/eux378

Walters TE, Kistler PM, Morton JB, Sparks PB, Halloran K, Kalman JM (2012) Impact of collimation on radiation exposure during interventional electrophysiology. Europace 14(11):1670–1673. https://doi.org/10.1093/europace/eus095